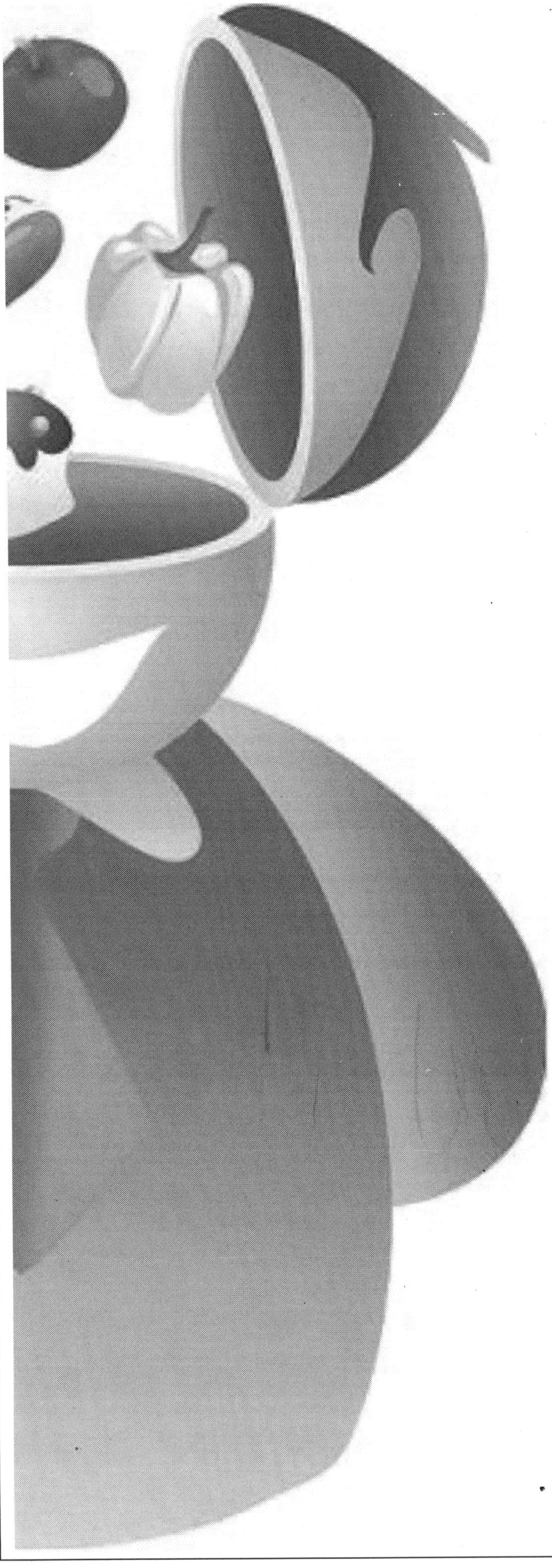

The Mind Diet

Harness the Hidden Power of
Your Mind to Lose Weight Safely
and Keep It Off Permanently

IMPORTANT

Due to the size of this book, printing it in color would be too expensive. Because there are numerous photos and graphics in color, you can receive a free PDF in full color. Simply email me your proof of purchase (irv@mind-diet.com) and I will send you the PDF.

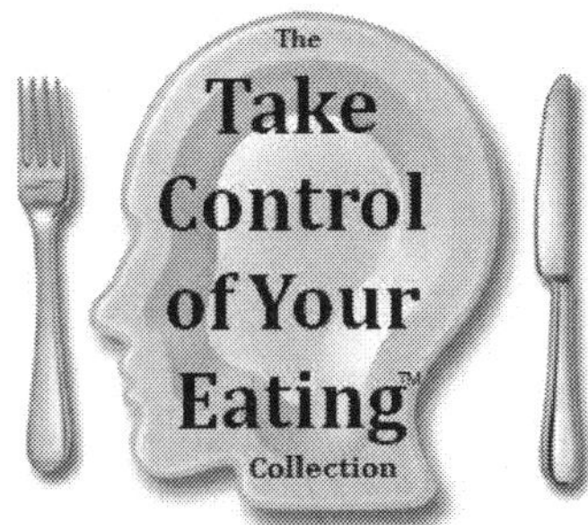

A New, Amazingly Simple Way to
Lose Weight & Eat Healthy
for Adults, Teens, Kids & Parents
by "How-To" Author Irv Brechner

Some of the many ways *The Mind Diet* strategy will help you:

Winner of nine Major Championships on the PGA Tour and a matching nine on the Senior Tour, Player remains in top physical condition at age 77 – with 150 pounds of muscle on his 5'7" frame. He talks about why he's in such good shape:

> *"We must never let ourselves get lazy and stop treating our body as a temple. The reason I am still able to do so much is because have continued my commitment to lifelong well-being."*

Words of inspiration from Gloria Gaynor, whose song "I Will Survive" has inspired people for over three decades. Her words will inspire people to survive obesity and lose weight:

> *"With healthy weight, discipline is the only bridge between desire and accomplishment. It isn't a matter of having discipline, we all do. It's a matter of using it. It's worth it."*

Special sections on "what works" from Dr. Ethan Lazarus of the Clinical Nutrition Center, who has helped treat thousands of people successfully:

- Recipe for successful weight loss: understand what you really need to do.
- Options: once you've reached your Moment of Truth, what to do next.
- Successes: inspiring stories from the archives of his clinic.

Special thanks to a group of people who went through this book with a fine-tooth comb and whose wonderful input enhanced this book: Linda Pretyka, Karen Miller, Stan Miller, Leigh Levy, Susan Head, Valerie McFie, Felicia Servetz, Ellyn Peschitz and Kathryn Howard.

DISCLAIMER

The entire contents of this publication is based on the author's personal experience and publicly available research and contributions from others. The publisher, author and any sellers of this and all other titles by the same author present this information for educational purposes only. This information is NOT intended to provide anything more. The information is NOT presented to replace consultation and guidance from health care and nutritional experts, which should be consulted based on your personal situation. This information is NOT presented as medical advice but as a sharing of information only. You are responsible for your own weight and health care decisions and the author and publisher have no liability or responsibility for any decisions you make after reading this book. This DISCLAIMER applies to all materials, written and verbal, produced by the author and publisher on all venues, including, but not limited to books, ebooks, articles, blog posts, etc., on the author's blog, newsletter and elsewhere, and other third-party publications, websites and newsletters.

ISBN 10: 0-9841043-4-8 ISBN 13: 978-0-9841043-4-5
All Photo Credits: At End of Book | Printed in the U.S.A.

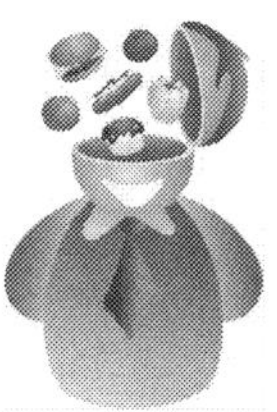

A World of Thanks!

I have five extremely important people to thank.

First is the one who jump-started the process that led to my "a ha" moment – my great friend Paul. His get-right-to-the-point phone call (you'll read about that soon) awakened me from my eating slumber.

Once I reached my "Moment of Truth," my wonderful, phenomenal and supportive wife Nadine, my partner for over 20 years, gave me unwavering support and unbiased input.

I'm grateful to singing legend Gloria Gaynor and championship golfer Gary Player for their inspirational messages and their unique points of view on obesity.

I'm particularly thankful to Dr. Ethan Lazarus, a leading Medical Obesity specialist, for his numerous contributions that greatly enhanced this book.

While I wrote and did my own diet, Nadine did hers. After I finished Guidebook #1, *Truth*, I asked her to read it as a "gut-check" to confirm that I was on the right track. I can always count on her for an unbiased opinion.

Her thoughts after reading *Truth:*

"When I was younger, I had always concentrated on what to eat and that was all I needed to lose weight. As I get older, it's become harder. I realized after reading *Truth* that I needed to do more…I needed to work on my mind as well. So I did. And that helped a lot. What helped even more is following the principles of *The Mind Diet* **together** with Irv:

- We weigh ourselves together every morning.
- We keep each other focused on what to eat and what to skip.
- We're thrilled when each of us loses weight, even small amounts like 2/10th of a pound.

Irv and I follow two different diets. He walks a mile a day. I walk and jog on the treadmill.

But what we do the same, and what works, is make sure that our minds are always focused on the end result of eating healthy – enjoying everything life has to offer."

Here's what people are saying about *The Mind Diet:*

"Irv Brechner's truthful account of how he has successfully lost weight and continues to keep it off is an inspiration to everyone who has tried or wants to lose weight and KEEP IT OFF. His outlook on his own life, both joys and challenges, is a powerful motivating force for us all. As he says, 'I will do everything in my power to get you to really make up your mind, once and for all, to reach your Moment of Truth,' and he does." (Felicia S., Sarasota, FL)

"I found that a number of specific sections in 'The Mind Diet' to be on target. Starting with the book's title, I liked the concept that it represented – something I've believed in for a long time. Irv's writing style is very chatty, which makes it easy to identify with what he says and his personal successful experiences. The 'eating styles' section was fabulous, and the section about 'tomorrow' is a great one to discuss with anyone who is overweight. Finally, I thought the food substitution discussion and examples were excellent." (Susan H., Far Hills, NJ)

"What a no-nonsense, positive-thinking determined strategy. A throw-your-excuses-away plan with a method to succeed. I became very educated on my own eating personality. A great lesson on nutrition labels and how to use them for my good health." (Linda P., Bradenton, FL)

"It was a really easy read with so much usable info, and you made it easy to understand. The format makes it easy to remember key facts – they stuck in my head! "Eat to Live" is my favorite and "14 Chews" is my new mantra. I am inspired to keep a journal of my thoughts, feelings, milestones, compliments. Thank you for the help your book gave me! I see people every day that need it. I saw a woman last week, eating cupcakes in her car at the supermarket. I wanted to say something to her but didn't want to embarrass her. Next time I think I will say something. You never know what might be someone else's "Moment of Truth." (Valerie M, Howell, NJ)

"Irv found that the combination of diet, exercise and self awareness is the key to successful weight loss. The book contains a wealth of information that can be used when making a lifestyle change for improved health and wellness. His candid use of his own battle with weight loss issues should be an inspiration for others facing similar challenges."

Leigh Garfield, Psychotherapist specializing in the treatment of eating disorders, disordered eating and body image issues. She has served on the Board of the New Jersey Chapter of the American Anorexia/Bulimia Association, and is past President of the Eating Disorders Association of New Jersey.

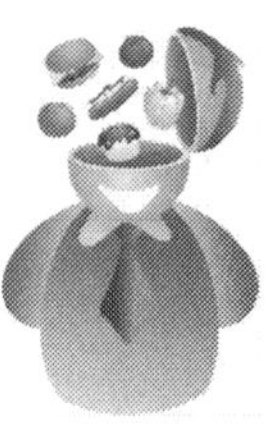

Table of Contents

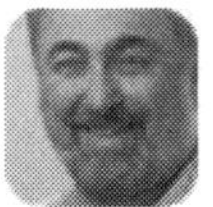

About the Author

Irv Brechner has written 18 books including several best-sellers, and has over 350,000 copies of his titles in print. He writes "how-to self-improvement" books based on his own personal successful experiences, extensive research and in-depth conversations with people and experts. He's been on 100+ TV shows (*The Today Show* four times), 50+ radio programs and has been interviewed by dozens of newspapers. He has written about college, business, health, careers and computers. Brechner has also written 13 business eBooks plus over 100 articles, briefs and white papers. The five titles in the "Take Control of Your Eating" series were written to help kids, teens and adults eat healthy and lose weight, based on his personal weight loss and maintenance journey.

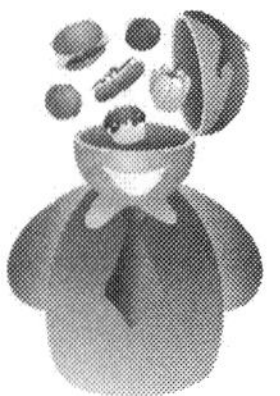

A Most Amazing Discovery about Successful Weight Loss

I've read hundreds of success stories of people who have lost a lot of weight successfully and kept it off for long periods of time. I've read just as many stories for those who did not.

- People from all walks of life.
- People of all ages.
- Men and women, girls and boys.
- From all areas of the U.S. and around the world.
- Representing numerous ethnicities.
- Eating different foods. Following different diets.

No two people were the same.

There was only one common denominator among all of the successes, and that's the discovery that I made and that is the core of *The Mind Diet.* **In every single instance, the successful people had an event in their lives that forced or encouraged them to make a life-changing decision.**

There were three common traits among those who failed:

- Their minds were "not in the right place" for sustained eating changes.
- They did not make a formal commitment to themselves.
- They did not have a well thought-out game plan.

For many, it was the impending birth of a child or the desire to start a family. For others it was being told that if they did nothing, they would very likely get real sick or even die. These events, that I call "Moments of Truth," took many forms. Either they originated with someone else (i.e. a doctor told them they were at great risk) or from within themselves (i.e. they wanted to enjoy their kids).

Before we get started, read inspiring words from singing legend Gloria Gaynor, championship golfer Gary Player, medical obesity expert Dr. Ethan Lazarus, a couple of short stories, and my thoughts on how to get the most value from this book.

And then you'll be ready to learn how to make an extraordinary decision that will change your life for the better!

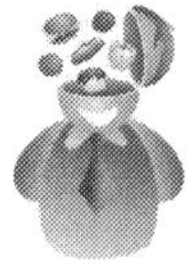

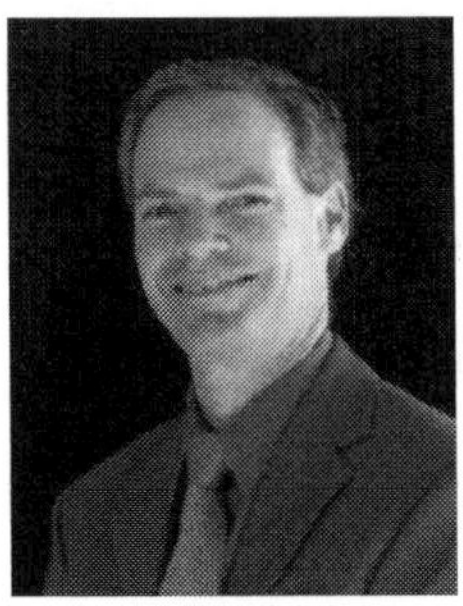

Creating a Successful Weight Loss Plan by Dr. Ethan Lazarus

Dr. Lazarus is an obesity treatment expert. What he and his staff have learned in over 35 years is reflected in his contributions to *The Mind Diet.* He writes here about the need to "get your head in the game" and combine the right mindset with expert guidance for the best possible outcome in terms of weight loss, healthy eating and long-term happiness.

For decades the advice thin people give to heavier people is: "Eat Less. Move More." And for decades, despite increased exercise and more people dieting, we have continued to see America's obesity and overweight rates skyrocket, with 2 out of 3 Americans now obese or overweight by BMI criterion. So, we then as a culture blame people that they aren't motivated enough or are just too lazy to stick with it.

It's time to put this bias and prejudice to rest, and it's time for us to recognize why the instructions to "Eat Less. Move More." inevitably fail. I speak from extensive experience, as I am a Board Certified Family Doctor and a Diplomate of the American Board of Obesity Medicine. I have spent 10 years as the director of Clinical Nutrition Center, in Denver, CO helping countless patients try to achieve a healthy weight and lifestyle.

The Mind Diet is not a book about "Eat Less. Move More." It is a book that looks at our inner thinking. Our psychology. It looks at changing our thinking, changing our environment. Short of changing our genes, all of my successful patients who have lost weight and kept it off long-term have told me the same secrets of their success. "It's not about the weight. It's about the lifestyle." That's what this book is really all about – getting your head in the right frame of mind to address your entire lifestyle.

I hope you enjoy reading The Mind Diet as much as I have. If you take it to heart and really take a look at the reasons why you eat, then perhaps you can start changing how you eat. If you are eating from stress, depression and anxiety, perhaps you need to focus on stress, depression and anxiety! If you are eating because of fatigue, you need to look at why you are so fatigued. And if you are eating because of sky high ghrelin levels from meal skipping, perhaps you need to focus on a strategy to keep ghrelin low throughout the day. Whatever the reasons, this book should provide you with valuable insight on reasons why we eat, and how to get to the point where you're ready to approach healthy eating seriously.

For great tips that build on the success of Dr. Lazarus, check out his blog:
http://www.clinicalnutritioncenter.com/denver-medical-weight-loss-blog

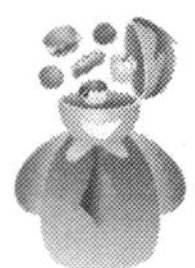

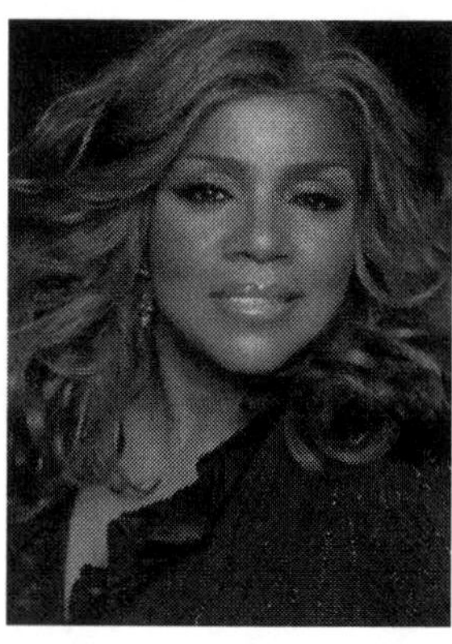

Special Thoughts from Singing Legend Gloria Gaynor

Her iconic song ***I Will Survive*** has been an inspiration to people all over the world for over three decades. As popular as ever, the world renowned singer recently collected inspirational stories from her fans and compiled them into a fascinating book ***We Will Survive***. Whether you're looking to survive a bad relationship, an illness or the loss of a loved one, you'll find inspiration in her book.

In a very real sense, I'm talking about **surviving obesity** in this book. Gloria, who herself has lost a lot of weight and has kept it off, took time out from her hectic schedule to provide these words of encouragement for everyone who needs to take control of their lives, lose weight, eat healthy and get the most enjoyment out of life.

The weight loss industry has created and marketed countless weight loss aids. I have tried more of them than is advisable, yet none of them actually became the catalyst necessary to perpetuate a healthy relationship with food.

Therefore, I have come to realize and accept a few things. The first thing I had to face was that no one should ever be more concerned about my weight loss or gain than I, because no one else was going to benefit or lose more from my being healthy. I love eating good food, and my Mom was a wonderful cook who showed her love by feeding us.

Therefore, it isn't easy to maintain weight loss, but it's a lot easier than trying to recover from the health problems engendered by unhealthy and excessive eating. The alternative is the good feelings that come from compliments about how good you look in your clothes, how young you appear. There's also the peace of mind that comes from knowing you're doing all you can to make sure your body will continue to function properly for as long as you're going to need it.

With healthy weight, discipline is the only bridge between desire and accomplishment. It isn't a matter of having discipline, we all do. It's a matter of using it. It isn't easy, but it's worth it.

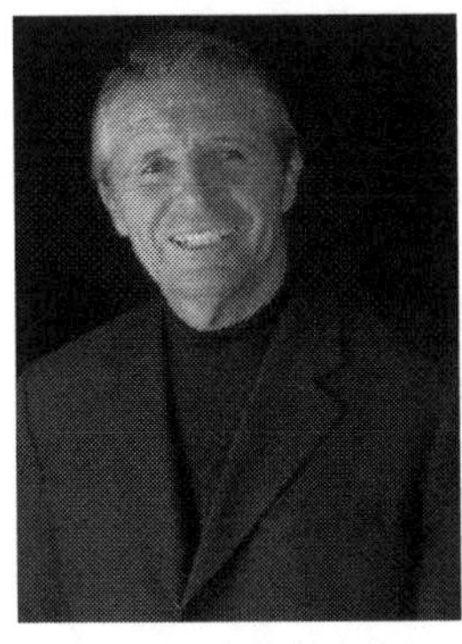

A Perspective on Obesity from Hall of Fame Golfer Gary Player

ESPN The Magazine's 2013 "The Body Issue" features Grand Slam champion Gary Player, who decided to pose for *ESPN The Magazine's* popular issue to in order to draw attention to the global obesity epidemic. Winner of nine Major Championships on the PGA Tour and a matching nine on the Senior Tour, Player remains in top physical condition at age 77 – with 150 pounds of muscle on his 5'7" frame. Despite Player's excellent physique, he often worries about the 14 of his 22 grandchildren who live in the U.S., who are growing up in a society where junk food and sugary drinks are widespread and have resulted in a population with 66% of Americans overweight or obese.

"Mr. Fitness" as many call him, says his commitment to eating healthy and exercising started over six decades ago. Today, when most people nearing 80 are in poor health, he is still works on his ranch, does 1,200 sit ups daily and eats an 80% vegan diet. He's the perfect person to tee off on obesity because he never let it happen to him. Player took a few minutes between sit ups and hard work to give us some keen observations that any person struggling with their weight should read and think long and hard about.

Obesity has been a growing problem in Western cultures for a number of decades now. My unwavering commitment to a healthy lifestyle started at a very young age when my brother Ian went off to war at age 17. Ian made me promise to him that I would always exercise and look after myself. I have now held true to that promise for over six decades. I continue to exercise nearly every day of the week and maintain a healthy, mostly vegan diet. During my career, being in top physical shape was a must. I could have softened up after retiring from competitive pro golf, but rest is rust! That is very important for older generations, especially, to remember. We must never let ourselves get lazy and stop treating our body as a temple. The reason I am still able to do so much is because I have continued my commitment to lifelong wellbeing.

I had achieved a great deal in my professional golfing career, including golf's coveted career Grand Slam. I owe a great deal to my fitness, as well as mental strength. I realized that I would have to exercise and practice harder than everyone else as a young boy. I have always been small in stature, but felt stronger than everyone else. Watching my nutritional intake and fitness is what made me a great golfer, but it can translate to any other facet of life.

When Irv Brechner contacted me and described his radical approach to weight loss, that he wanted to motivate people to use their minds to take control of their health and weight, I knew I had to contribute to that effort because it is something I truly believe. I see people I know making the same mistakes over and over. They just jump from diet to diet to diet, failing miserably. Even though some are getting more exercise, they're still getting fatter because they eat too much. Most people around me eat like it is the last supper. We must feed our body, but with the right foods and not overeat.

What I learned from my personal desire to maintain a healthy lifestyle is that anyone can do the same, by simply making up one's mind. That's really all I did. I made up my mind to stay in great shape and eat well for my entire life. I hope my grandkids and anyone reading this will make the same choices because the rewards are so great. By eating correctly you will have such great energy and feel better well into your life. I am proof of that.

Every human being can either go down the right path or the wrong path. It's totally up to them to take control of their eating habits, weight and health – and keep it up for their entire lives. I hope to be an example. That is the reason why I took the bold step of posing for ESPN's magazine and continue to fulfill one of my greatest passions by helping and inspiring people to lead healthy lives.

An Incredible Inspiring Story

Ten years ago, Marcia weighed some 300 pounds. At around five-feet tall, she carried about 70% too much weight. Today, she is under 150, having lost half her body weight. Even more remarkable is that she's stayed at 150 or under for TEN years. That's unheard of, and her story confirms that dramatic weight loss and not gaining it back is indeed possible.

Long before this book was written, I reached what Irv calls the "moment of truth." I called it my "wake up call," and it came in the form of my doctor reading me the riot act.

He told me if I didn't get serious about my weight and health, I'd never see my children get married, hold grandchildren, or live much longer. Well, that scared the hell out of me. I'd been rationalizing my weight for the longest time, but the doctor's stern warning finally broke through and caused me to take control of my rapidly deteriorating life.

So that's what I did.

After hearing that I could miss out on some of the greatest pleasures life has to offer, I made a firm commitment to myself: that the days of being heavy were over, and I would not fail at getting to a healthy weight, no matter how hard it was.

I thought about how to do this. Knowing my personality well, I knew that counting calories was not for me. I needed something simple that I could easily remember and do at every meal.

I can't remember exactly how I came to it, but I decided what would work for me was simply eating HALF of whatever was on my plate. Whatever I made at home, I'd eat half and save the rest for another meal. Whatever I was served at a restaurant, I'd take half home.

While I also learned to stay away from certain bad foods, the mainstay of my success has been the concept of eating half.

I still eat half of what's on my plate, ten years later. And as a result, I know I will get to dance at my kids' weddings, hold their grandkids, and enjoy a whole lot more. I'm already doing the latter – on a recent visit to New York City, I walked for miles – something I wasn't able to do in my heavy days.

The most important thing I learned from this humbling experience is that it really is all in your mind. Make up your mind and you can achieve anything. Really.

Incredibly Sad Stories

The one thing that became evident the more I researched obesity was the prevalence of inspiring success stories like Marcia's. But for everyone like her, there were hundreds that were the opposite – many so sad that they made me cringe. Weight loss is a positive/negative choice – good things happen when you make a positive choice to lose weight and eat healthy, and bad things happen when you don't. To balance this introductory section, I came across this very sad story that should be enough to get anyone to eat healthy. And to make matters worse, it happened to a three-year-old child.

The BBC NEWS ran a story of a little girl in the UK who was so fat that she died of heart failure at the Royal London Hospital. She weighed about three times what she should have. Close your eyes and imagine the shock of losing a child at this age due to something that is easily preventable.

Specialists at the hospital have also seen four children who were "choked by their fat" – they needed breathing assistance to treat sleep disorders caused by blocked airways. This condition occurs when the airways become blocked by folds of fat.

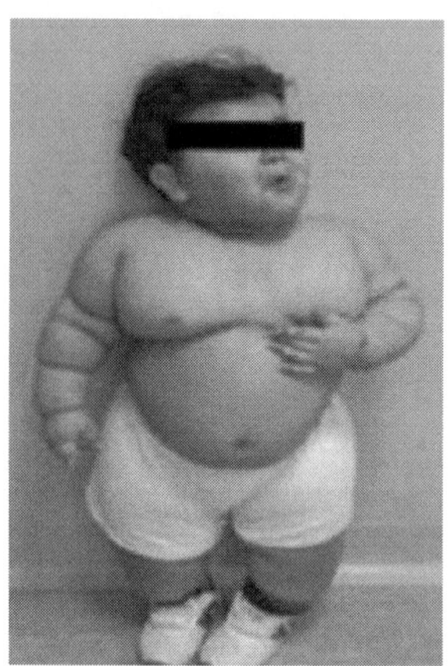

This is the youngest person to ever undergo bariatric surgery. At two years old, this Saudi toddler had a BMI of an astounding 41, leading to sleep apnea and bowing of the legs. Fortunately for him, two years after the 2010 surgery his weight had fallen from 33kg to 24kg and his BMI of 24 was within the normal range.

There are many other sad stories, like the 500 pound man who slept in a recliner and could never get out of it, and had to eventually be cut out of it in order to be transported to the hospital.

Without getting too morbid, the point of this story is part of the overall goal of *The Mind Diet.* The more you are aware of the bad that can happen when you become or stay obese or overweight, the more you will appreciate all the good that can come of making the most important commitment to yourself that you'll ever make – that you will once and for all leave no stone unturned to lose weight safely and keep it off permanently.

Says one of my readers, "This is so true. But it's seldom talked about." The good and the bad are necessary to get you to that point. You'll see exactly what I mean in the first section, *Truth.*

Then: **"Fat & Frustrated"** 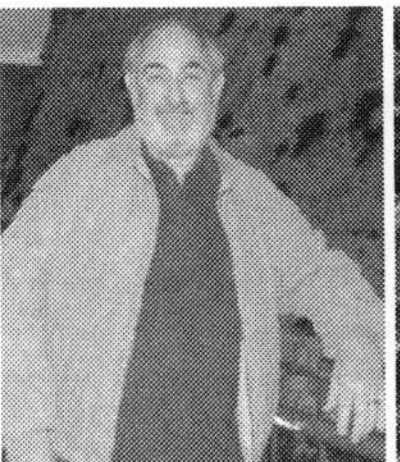 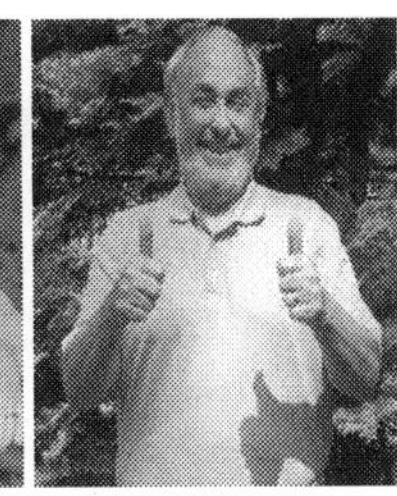 Now: **"Happy & Healthy"**

Introduction

Congratulations for taking a major step towards permanent weight loss by recognizing that you need more than the latest diet program to successfully lose weight and keep it off. I wish I had this book decades ago! For most of my adult life, losing weight was the hardest thing I've ever attempted to do. While I thought about *why* I couldn't lose weight and keep it off hundreds of times, the truth escaped me, year after year. It was puzzling because nothing else in life was so difficult.

Once I finally figured it out, losing weight went from being impossible to actually happening. I'm a different person today than I was when I was "fat and frustrated." Today I'm "happy and healthy."

The one thing I learned from the experience and writing *The Mind Diet Collection of Guidebooks* is that we all have the most important ingredient to lose a lot of weight safely and keep it off permanently: **our minds**. By developing a well thought-out plan with your medical doctor and a nutrition specialist, I have no doubt you'll achieve the same results that I have. With that in mind, let's get right to it!

In case you're wondering about me, I'm a writer by trade and have written 18 books, most of them "how to" based on my personal experience. There are over 350,000 copies in print, and I've appeared on *The Today Show* and numerous TV and radio stations talking about helping people succeed. Losing a lot of weight safely and keeping it off permanently and being able to write about it is a major achievement in my life, one that eluded me for a long time.

While there are dozens of very good motivational posters in Guidebook #10, my all time favorite is **"Nothing tastes as good as being thin feels."** Eating unhealthy foods that taste good result in a few minutes of taste satisfaction. Being thin, on the other hand, is something that feels good every single minute of every day – that's 1,440 minutes every day. When you're at a healthy weight, you feel good, look good and you tend to have a real positive outlook on life. Comparing what life is like when you're heavy vs. thin is a real motivator!

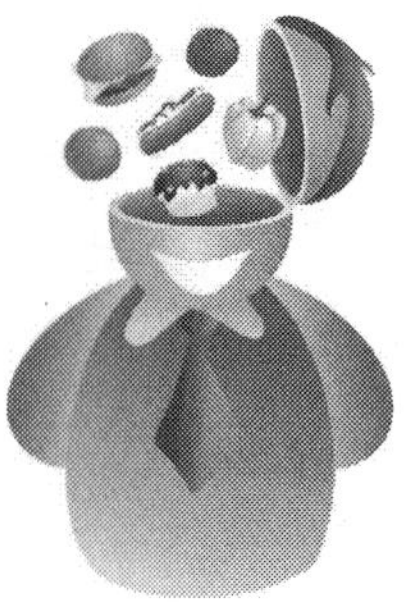

How to Get the Greatest Value from this Book

The Mind Diet Collection was written to give you a plan for success, based on my personal permanent weight loss experience. Follow my plan and you're that much closer to losing a lot of weight safely and keeping it off permanently.

My plan is NOT a diet. It's a roadmap to get you in the right frame of mind.

If you don't follow the plan, it won't work. Do NOT feel like you need to read this book in one sitting like a novel. Take a week or two to read it slowly and think about everything, especially the first three sections.

The critical part of this book are the first 100 pages. That's where you need to focus. Everything else supports the first three sections.

To get started, read the Guidebook #1 – *Truth*, as many times as necessary until you reach your Moment of Truth. If you can't get to that point, re-read it until you do, and don't read other sections until you do. This is critical.

Once you've reached your own personal Moment of Truth, read *Beliefs* and think about each one. In order to implement your weight loss program, you need to believe. I've done all the work to create a list about what to believe in.

Once you've absorbed and embraced the beliefs, move onto *Strategies.* Read each one, especially the section in bold at the end of each strategy. After you finish *Strategies,* make an appointment with a medical doctor and nutrition specialist. The first three sections and your appointments are the core of *The Mind Diet* plan for successful and long-term weight loss.

The other seven sections plus the bonuses are written to support the first three. You should read them prior to your appointments. The core sections with the supportive chapters, combined with input from your doctor and nutrition specialist, will help you formulate an effective plan that will work with any particular foods you have in your diet.

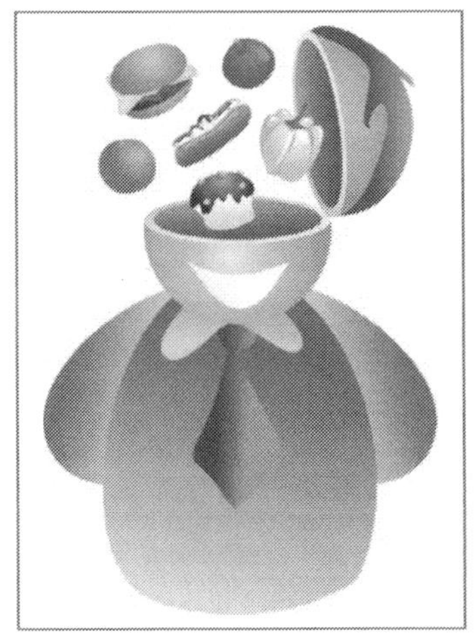

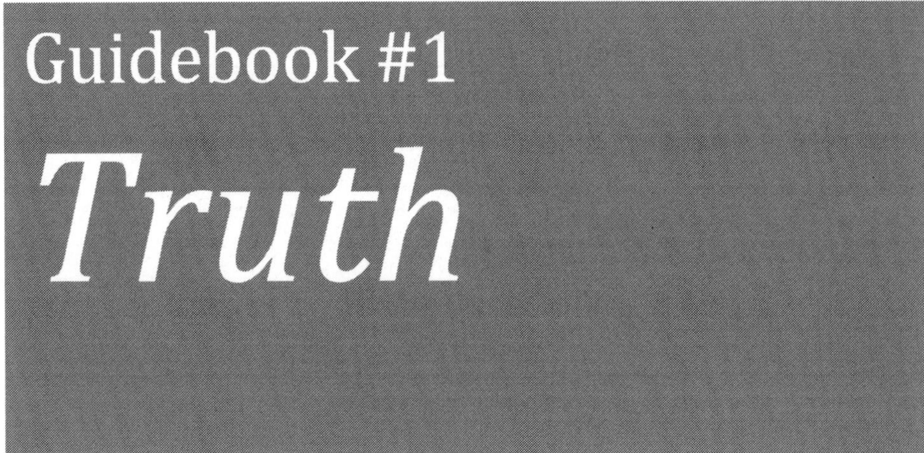

The "Moment of Truth" and What it Means to Your Weight Loss

July 15, 2011. That was the date of my own personal "Moment of Truth." It's etched in my mind, much in the same way the day the U.S. beat the U.S.S.R. in ice hockey in Lake Placid in 1980. It was the date when I decided once and for all, I was going to lose a lot of weight and keep it off. The Moment of Truth as I'll refer to it in these guidebooks is the point when you finally decide that you will do everything humanly possible to lose weight and keep it off. Not "trying" or "taking a shot at it," but making an unbreakable commitment to yourself, your family and your friends that you will succeed. That you will not fail. That you will take weight loss and health seriously.

It was not like all the other countless times that I tried to lose weight and failed. It was not like all those years where I lost hundreds of pounds but also gained every one of them back. In short, I made up my mind like I'd never done before, and the result, is nothing short of amazing.

I looked around me on that summer day, taking stock of my life. I was 58, going on 59, with a very good life. I had (and still have) a wonderful wife and a great marriage, happy family relationships and many great friends.

I was a partner in a marketing and advertising company, working with a great bunch of guys and gals. After working a couple of years out of college, my daughter had been accepted at grad school and was starting soon. She's now working on her doctorate.

But something was nagging at me. I concluded that there was only one thing in my life that was not positive: my weight. Around the same time, my best friend lost a lot of weight, and one day, out of love and concern, he called me up and told me that he was worried about me and said, "I love ya man, **but you look like crap**." He was right. Not only did I **look** like crap, I **felt** like it too.

Between that, thinking about my life, and encouragement from my wife, I reached what I now know to be a very momentous decision: I was going to leave no stone unturned to lose a lot of weight and keep it off forever. Failure was not an option.

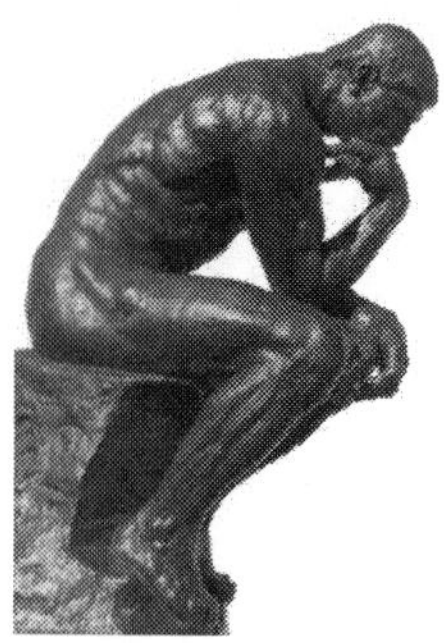

During this period of thinking about my weight and health, I recognized two key facts that were an important part of this soul-searching process:

- If I did nothing about my weight, I could see a long list of ailments and conditions and possible death much too early, and I would miss all the great times with those I love and care about.
- If I did lose the weight and keep it off, I would be able to enjoy life that much more. There would be more travel, grandkids and retirement in the future, more than ever I wanted to be healthy for those special times.

In business, I never said "I'm going to **try** and make a sale today," or "I'll take a shot at writing a good ad." Instead, I said "I'm going to do everything in my power to make that sale or write that great ad."

When people say they're going to "try" to lose weight, "we'll see what happens," "I'll be good today" or "I'll give it a whirl," they are going to fail. They give themselves an "out" and don't really intend to make it happen. If I had a penny for every time people say these things, I'd be the richest man on the planet. I'm reminded of Albert Einstein's famous quote that applies to people who continuously fail at almost anything as I once did at losing weight: **"The definition of insanity is doing the same thing over and over again and expecting a different result."**

American poet and author Maya Angelou summarizes my view on the need to think about your future when it comes to your current weight: "If you don't like something, change it. If you can't change it, change the way you think about it."

This is all about taking **personal responsibility** for your weight and your health. You go to a restaurant and choose from the menu. You shop in a supermarket and choose which items to buy. You decide whether or not to grab a candy bar from the rack. These are all **choices** we make.

What I'm talking about is getting to the point where you say **"I recognize how critically important it is to eat healthy, and I will do everything in my power to make this happen. I will not let anything stand in my way. Period."**

I will help you get to this point in around 30 pages in this first guidebook.

I will do everything in my power to get you to really make up your mind, once and for all, to reach your Moment of Truth. I will:

- Shock you with a long list of dreadful statistics, most of which you've never read before.
- Open your eyes with pages of photographs of medical conditions that result directly or indirectly from being overweight.
- Present you with numerous logical arguments as to why you must finally reach your Moment of Truth, even if you've never done so before.
- Show you how great your life can be if you lose weight and keep it off.
- Show you how awful your life can be if you don't.

It took me a long time to get to this point, but I finally did. Back to 2011...

I realized that everything I did was impulsive. I did not have any plan. Hey, coaches have game plans. Teachers have lesson plans. Business people have business plans.

But I, and 99.999% of dieters, had no plan. That was the proverbial light bulb that went off in my head.

I decided to adapt my business mentality and create a game plan to lose weight, much in the same way I'd write an advertising plan for a client. I developed a simple way of looking at how I had tried and failed to lose weight in the past vs. how I was going to succeed going forward. I created two pie charts:

The Weight Loss Failure Pie

This is how most people approach weight loss. They spend all of their time on tactics (books, videos, diet programs and plans, etc.) and no time thinking about the truth, beliefs and strategies. All three are essential for successful and permanent weight loss. I was one of those people.

The Weight Loss Success Pie

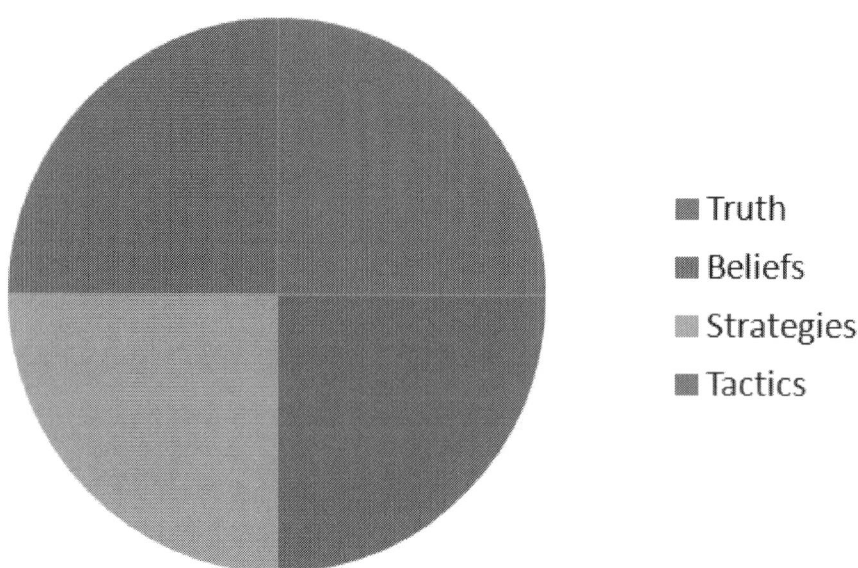

The success pie shows that when you spend about an equal amount of time to seek the truth, decide what to believe in, develop strategies and implement tactics, the results are astounding – and long-lasting.

I found that without "truth," "beliefs" and "strategies," tactics are short-lived and failure is inevitable. With a strong commitment and strategic belief system, success occurs and is long-lasting.

Here's another way to look at how the four components of the Success Pie work with each other in real life:

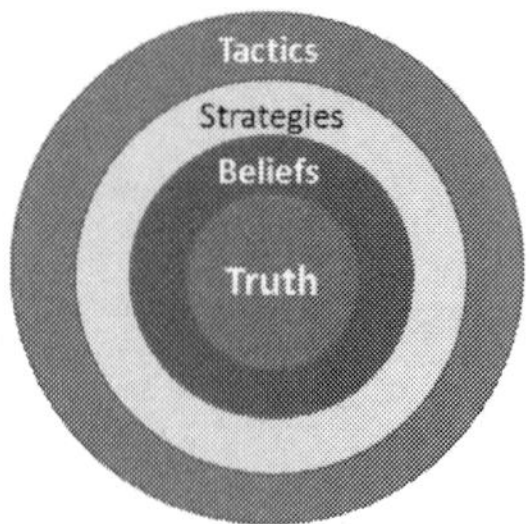

Truth is at the core of your desire to lose weight. You surround Truth with a layer of Beliefs that support Truth. Next is a layer of Strategies that are practical thoughts that bring Truth and Beliefs to life. Last are tactics, the specific foods and drinks you eat and avoid.

Once I reached the Moment of Truth, everything else quickly fell into place. Losing weight went from being one of the most difficult and frustrating things I've ever had to do, to being realistic and attainable.

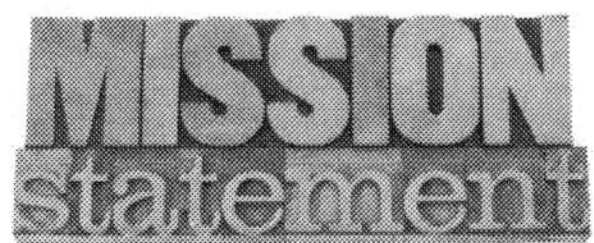

My Mission for You

In this book, I use every which way to help you get to your Moment of Truth – logic, scary statistics, cajoling, humor and more. In other sections of this book, I will give you a boatload of strategies to guide you through all the everyday situations involving food you face.

The Mind Diet is not a diet plan. It is a process that will work with your actual diet plan to train your mind to approach weight loss correctly. As a result, any reasonable program that you've carefully chosen, with input from your doctor and nutrition professional, has a much greater chance of success.

Getting back to the most essential part of my game plan is truth, and what I've referred to as the Moment of Truth. Your Moment of Truth can occur in any number of ways, and in all likelihood, it's a combination of two or more of these events and realizations:

- Your doctor told you that you must lose weight or there's a chance you could become diabetic or come down with some other serious illness.
- Your romantic partner has become less and less attracted to you because of your weight.
- You don't have as much energy as you once did, and it's beginning to affect your performance at work and with your kids and/or grandkids.
- You're more embarrassed than ever because all your friends are thin.
- You've been turned down for a promotion or didn't get a job, and you're sure it's because of your weight.
- You can tell your kid is embarrassed by you.

Chances are that if you're reading this book, you're closer to being ready to make the most important decision in your life.

When you think about it, this whole process is one gigantic trade. I decided to trade food for life. Yes, get rid of bad food and replace it with good things in life. Take a few minutes to let that sink in.

Most of the changes you need to make are small, especially in the area of substitution. Most people won't need to do a complete overhaul of their lives, but rather institute a series of small changes – much easier to do!

There are many ways to reach your Moment of Truth. You could undress and stand in front of a full-length mirror and stare at yourself for a while. Remember that you look worse to other people than you do in a mirror.

Along these lines, one Brit reached his Moment of Truth when Google Street View shocked him into seeing how he looked to others; and a young UK boy reached his Moment of Truth after getting stuck in a slide and also being bullied in school, and subsequently lost 75% of his body weight, and is now a happy and healthy kid.

Google Street View Leads To 100-Pound Weight Loss

Posted 11/15/2010 8:00 am by Ron Hogan

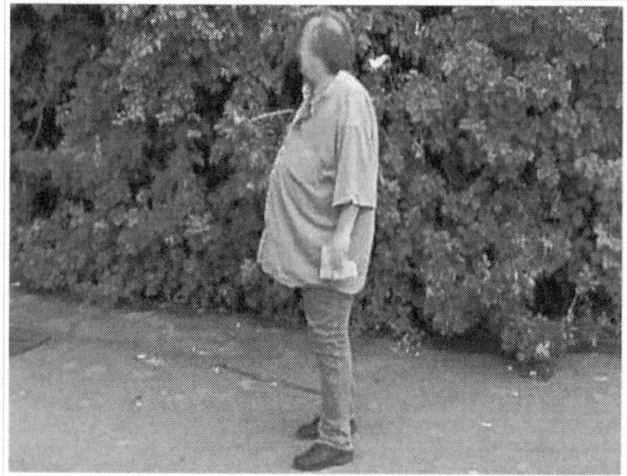

We all need a catalyst to lose weight when we realize we're losing the battle of the bulge. In my case, it was a health scare for my father which made me decide to straighten up and start living a little better. In the case of Bob Mewse, a 56-year-old man from Bristol, England, it was Google Street View. A photograph of himself on Google Street View encouraged Bob Mewse to lose over 100 pounds.

"I was horrified when I saw that photo. I was massive. My belly was sticking out and I looked huge," said Mewse. "I'd been thinking about losing weight for some time but after seeing that picture, I knew that I actually had to do something about it. I was in such bad condition that I was unable to walk and talk at the same time. My blood pressure was sky-high and I was getting back problems due to the excess weight I was carrying around."

So, Mewse went on a diet and exercise program, guided by a personal trainer at Fitness First in his native Bristol. Thanks to a diet rich in vegetables and lean protein, as well as a serious fitness regimen, Mewse has lost about 101 pounds off of his formerly 297-pound frame. Now here comes the hard part: maintaining the weight loss.

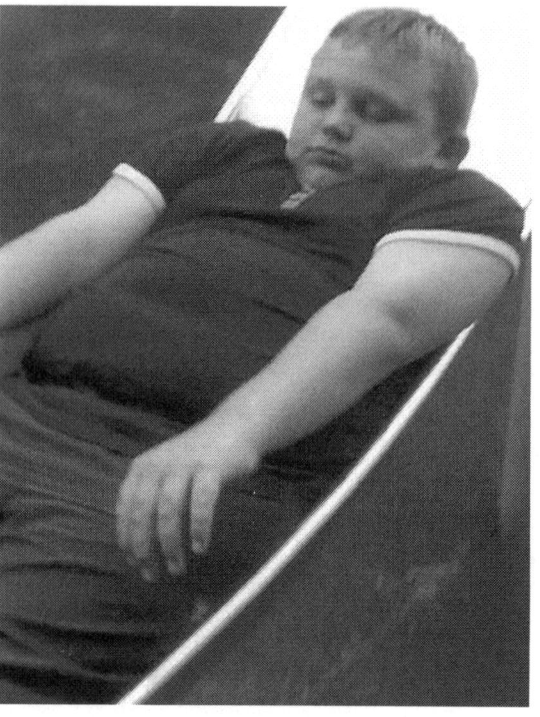

In addition to these stories and my "You look like crap" phone call, here are some "Moments of Truth" from inspiring bloggers:

Roni (www.JustRoni.com) lost 70 pounds: "My defining moment was the birth of my son. I didn't want to let the weight or a bad body image prevent me from missing one second of his childhood. Now, 8 years later, I'm the fun active mom I always wanted to be."

Like Roni, Jennifer (www.ItSuxToBeFat.com) lost 104 pounds: "My motivation to lose weight and keep it off was the desire to start a family. I knew that weighing almost 280 pounds, I would have a hard time getting pregnant. Once and for all, I decided that starting a family was worth my health."

Gabi (www.gabirose.com) went from size XXL to 2: "More than seven years ago I embarked on an incredible journey that transformed my life forever! Back then, this married mother of four weighed over 270 pounds and suffered from depression, chronic back and hip pain with bouts of asthma that nearly took my life. My dress size was XXL and my marriage and self-esteem were at a zero. A near-death experience shook me awake to the reality that if I did not lose weight, my kids would grow up without their mother. Today at a slender size 2 I have learned that 'Training of the Body Begins with the Mind'; my secret to weight loss success and healthy lifestyle maintenance is, first take care of yourself and the rest of life will follow. My 20-year marriage and the continued success of our children are a testament to this principle and a source of joy and inspiration to others."

Read how Callista and Jason Puchmeyer wanted to be good role models for their daughters, so they lost a total of 284 pounds together. Both weighing 300+ pounds, they shed all the weight so that they could have the energy to play with their young daughters. Great read: http://tinyurl.com/nyb797e.

Others reach their Moments of Truth when they have grandchildren (and want to keep up with the toddlers), get a disease like gout, or being prodded, threatened or scolded by their doctor, spouse, sibling, parent or child.

Here are three inspirational stories from the archives of Dr. Lazarus' clinic. They clearly point out the value of a multidisciplinary approach – the "right" way to formulate a plan that you can implement successfully.

John

I met John in 2005. At that time, he was 23 years old and weighed 367 pounds. My evaluation found that he had developed an underactive thyroid. This problem is unusual in men and thus had been undetected. We corrected the thyroid problem and started John on a structured weight management program including partial meal replacement, medications, weekly behavioral visits and medical monitoring.

Over 2 years, John lost a total of 167 pounds and now for the first time in his adult life, weighs under 200 pounds (199!). He was promoted in his job, started hiking in Colorado, and started dating.

When I asked why this had been successful, he replied that the accountability was key. The use of medication was key. He got into a rhythm of having very simple breakfasts, lunches, and snacks, and then varied his dinner. The combination of a simple eating plan, changes in behaviors and lifestyle, and finding an activity he loved (hiking) was the secret to his success.

Sarah

I have known Sarah for 14 years, having played on a sports team with her husband. During that time, I saw her diagnosed with ovarian cancer. In spite of a rigorous treatment program, the cancer recurred. She beat the recurrence, beat ovarian cancer, but during the treatment, gained 100 pounds.

After a careful medical evaluation, we decided to treat with a high-protein, low carbohydrate diet, structured behavior program, and weight loss medication. Even though she had unsuccessfully tried many other weight loss options, this proved to be a better treatment option. Sarah has lost over 70 pounds and now for the first time in her life, joined forces with her husband and is playing on his soccer team.

Cindy

After being diagnosed with diabetes, Cindy lost control of her eating and ballooned to 220 pounds. Her moods were up and down, blood sugars out of control despite a complicated insulin regimen, energy was zero and she had pain in most of her joints.

After a careful medical assessment, we hooked Cindy up with a registered dietitian, used a low-carbohydrate diet to slowly, carefully cut back on her insulin, and used a medical meal replacement to better regulate blood sugars. Over 8 months, Cindy lost 61 pounds and we slowly transitioned back to a diabetes friendly diet.

She now does yoga 20 minutes a day and rides a stationary bike most days, unless it's really nice outside in which case she will walk. She tells me she is "living life rather than watching life pass by because of being overweight." The diabetes is now undetectable and Cindy is no longer on Insulin.

More of Dr. Lazarus' patients' success stories are here: http://tinyurl.com/lug7wux.

Want more inspiration? Read dozens of success stories at www.Health.com: http://tinyurl.com/krkadwe.

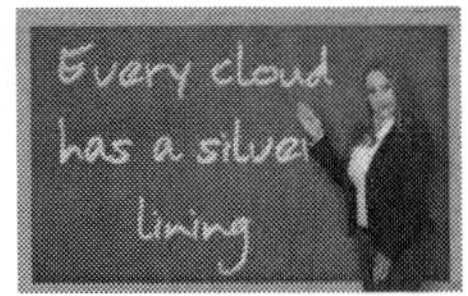

A Silver Lining from James Gandolfini's Death

To his family, friends and fans of *The Sopranos,* and his other acting roles, James Gandolfini was a larger-than-life actor, supremely talented, and taken from life prematurely at age 51. He will be sorely missed by those who appreciated him personally and professionally. Sadly, he is just one of 265,000 Americans age 45 to 64 who suffer a heart attack or fatal coronary heart disease each year, greater than heart attacks in other age groups.

Commenting on his death, American Heart Association president Donna Arnett said, "It is not uncommon to have a sudden cardiac death at his age." The silver lining is that we can learn from this tragedy. If you're carrying around a lot of weight like Gandolfini was, maybe his passing will serve as a way for you to reach your Moment of Truth and take control of your weight, and your life. I sure hope so. About a month after Gandolfini's death, I got word that an acquaintance I knew also died, prematurely. He was a spitting image of the actor in terms of his size, and I'm sure his weight is what did him in as well.

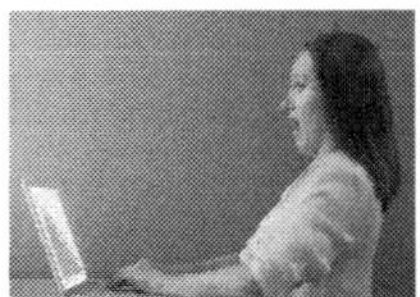

Shocking Statistics

One thing that really helped me during this process was to have a lot of information in one place. We have all heard or read statistics relating to weight loss, but most of us don't remember any of them and they probably didn't have much of an impact on us. Having the most important stats together where you can read all of them in a matter of minutes will help you get closer to your Moment of Truth. This collection of dozens of stats will shock you, and that's the idea. Everyone who is overweight needs to be shocked into understanding just how important weight loss is to their future health.

Most people believe that bad things are **not** going to happen to them. We don't feel we're going to be mugged, burglarized or get cancer. Maybe that's just our sense of optimism; in kids and teens we call it invincibility. But bad things do happen to good people, so being aware of stats is critical to the weight loss process, simply because too much weight affects every aspect of your physical and mental life. **Read all of these stats a couple of times so they really sink in:**

- There are 58 million overweight, 40 million obese and 15.5 million morbidly obese people in the U.S.
- 80% of adults over age 25 are overweight.
- 78% of Americans don't meet basic activity levels.
- 76% increase in Type II diabetes in adults 30-40 since 1990.
- 80% of Type II diabetes is related to obesity.
- 70% of cardiovascular disease related to obesity.
- At least 25% of all children are overweight, up from 4% in 1982.
- 25% of overweight children showing signs of Type II diabetes.
- 60% of overweight children have one risk factor for heart disease.

These stats are from: Get America Fit (www.getamericafit.org)

Children born to obese mothers are 33% more likely to die before age 55 than those of normal weight, and have a 29% higher risk for heart problems, diabetes, angina and strokes (study of 38,000 people by the Universities of Aberdeen and Edinburgh, UK). A study by GlobalData projects the U.S. will have 133 million obese people AND 81 million overweight residents by 2022, leading the world. In every state in the U.S., more than 20% of adults are obese, and in 12 states, the obesity rate is over 30% (CNN, 9/2/13).

In a landmark report "F as in Fat: How Obesity Threatens America's Future" (2013) from the Trust for America's Health (www.healthyamericans.org) and funded by the Robert Wood Johnson Foundation, these really scary stats were presented:

- Children who are obese are more than twice as likely to die before age 55 as kids with a healthy BMI.
- Children who are obese after age 6 are 50% more likely to be obese adults.
- Overweight and obese children and teens face a higher risk for more severe and frequent bullying, rejection by their peers, chosen less as friends and generally not as well-liked.
- The rate of obesity among children age 2-19 has tripled since 1980.
- If nothing is done and Americans remain as fat as they are today:
    - More than 60% will be obese in 13 states.
    - More than 50% will be obese in 39 states.
    - In all 50 states, more than 44% could be obese.
- The medical cost of adult obesity is estimated from $147 to $210 billion **per year**.
- Obese people spend 42% more on health care costs.
- Obesity-related job absenteeism costs $4.9 billion per year.
- As your BMI increases, so does the number of sick days, medical claims and health care costs you incur.
- Obese workers have higher workers' compensation claims.
- More than 25 million Americans have diabetes and another 79 million are pre-diabetic, including 215,000 under age 20 with diabetes and 2 million with pre-diabetes.

- Obese people are 83% more likely to develop kidney disease.
- Weight discrimination has increased by 66% over the last 10 years and is on par with racial discrimination.
- Obese women reported workplace issues related to their weight:
    - 25% experienced discrimination.
    - 54% reported stigma from co-workers.
    - 43% experienced stigma from their supervisors.
- Teachers view overweight students as untidy, more emotional, less likely to succeed on homework and more likely to have family problems; they have lower expectations for overweight kids.
- 63% of children ages 1 to 12 eat out 1 to 3 times per week
- Weight bias is associated with psychological issues including depression, lower levels of self-esteem, dissatisfaction with their bodies and unhealthy eating behaviors.
- More than half of all Americans live with a chronic disease, many of which are related to obesity, poor nutrition and physical inactivity.
- Sedentary adults pay $1,500 more per year in health care costs.
- Sugar consumption is about two times the USDA recommended intake.

More statistics from other sources:

- About 5% of all U.S. youth are "severely obese" according to the American Heart Association (9/9/13). This appears to be the fastest growing sub-category of obesity in youth. Truly alarming.

- Equally alarming, according to a Wall Street Journal article (9/9/13), fatty liver disease, once thought to afflict primarily adult alcoholics appears to be rampant in kids, affecting more than 7 million in the U.S. Some imaging studies of children born from obese mothers show that the infants have more fat on their livers.

- Highlighted in Credit Suisse's "Sugar: Consumption at a crossroads" is a conclusion by the Global Burden of Disease (in 2012) that obesity is a more significant health crisis globally than hunger and/or malnourishment, and as the leading cause of disabilities." In the same report, the United Health Group Modeling group projects that people with pre-diabetes, undiagnosed diabetes, Type I and Type II diabetes will rise to over half the population – 51.9% by 2020. Their researchers could not find one study that suggests that sugar has a protective benefit.

- Back in 2004, 1 in 50 people were morbidly obese (overweight by 100+ pounds). Today it's 1 in 15, according to Rand. Think about it. One out of every 15 people you know is in the worst category of overweight...is it you?

Read all of these scary stats – don't skip any!

- Experts predict the number of cases of diabetes will rise from some 30 million today to 100 million by 2050. That's 15% of the population today rising to over 30% of the population in 2050 (Centers for Disease Control and Prevention, in *Newsweek*, 11/8/10)

- Someone in the U.S. has a heart attack every 29 seconds and dies every single minute. Major contributing factors to heart attack are obesity, high blood pressure and diabetes often caused by obesity and lack of physical exercise (American Heart Association, quoted in *It's Time to Get Heart Healthy* – www.personalliberty.com, 11/11/10)

- Obesity is the #1 reason applicants fail to qualify for military service; an alarming 75% of all young people 17-24 are unable to join the military (*Obesity Threatens National Security* at www.mercola.com)

- The USDA reports that about 63% of the calories Americans eat are from processed foods, 25% from animals and only 12% from plants. Very telling, when you consider that all-important fiber is found only in plants.

- 2/3 of Americans are overweight or obese, and in some ethnic groups, the rate is almost 80% (www.mercola.com)

- Only 6% of us eat the recommended amount of vegetables per day; and for fruits, only 8% (*America's Diet: 3 New Reports,* www.theatlantic.com)

- Americans spend $66 billion per year to lose weight (Marketdata, 2013)

- The consensus among U.S. authorities is that the average male should consume around 2,700 calories per day, as reported by Credit Suisse. Actual consumption is about 1,000 calories MORE in almost every U.S. market.

- We are faced with 200 decisions about food every day, and we make many of them without thinking about the ramifications (*Lose Weight Without Really Trying,* AARP.org magazine, 12/10)

- The risk for colon or bladder cancer in adulthood is 40% higher in adults who were overweight as children (Study by Tel Aviv University in *The Jerusalem Post*).

- If you drink regular soda, other juices and drinks that are sweetened with sugar, you're ingesting at least 3,000 calories per week; it takes 3,500 calories to make a pound of fat (Dr. Travis Stork, host of "The Doctors" on *The Today Show,* 12/10)

Read all of these scary stats – don't skip any!

- About 25% of women misperceive their body weight (they think they are at the correct weight) and as a result, are unlikely to attempt to lose weight. 82% of African American women and 75% of Mexican American women are overweight or obese (University of Texas Medical Branch study, in *Healthy Lifestyles*)

- Children aged 9-12 who have a high BMI (Body Mass Index) from being overweight have risk factors for cardiovascular disease that show up when they are 15-16 years old (Avon Longitudinal Study of Parents and Children in www.OnMedica.com)

- American kids age 2-19 consume about 7.2 trillion calories from sugar in sweetened beverages per year! *(The Obesity Society, 2012 Annual Meeting)*

- An American Medical Association study estimated that an obese 20-year old white male, 5'10" in height and who weighs 288 pounds would lose 13 years of his life due to obesity.

- Consumer responses, when asked about their diets: 52.6% said their diets were "somewhat healthy;" 31.5% - "very healthy" and 5.6% "extremely healthy." But 43% drank at least one regular sugar-sweetened soda or other drink daily, and only 25% limit the amount of sweets and fats they get each day. Americans rarely count calories, and only 13% weigh themselves daily. Their perceptions of healthy eating were clearly contradicted by these responses (*Consumer Reports* telephone poll in www.WebMD.com (1/4/11)

- Along the same lines, 30% of people who are overweight believed they were of normal size, and 70% of those classified as obese felt they were simply overweight. Even worse: 39% of those considered to be morbidly obese thought they were merely overweight. This from a *MedicineNet.com* article titled "Americans Blind to the Obesity Epidemic."

- People who eat eight or more servings of fruit and vegetables combined per day are 22% less likely to die from heart disease than those who eat three or less (*Heart Disease Death Rate Drops With Each Added Fruit and Veggie Serving,* ABC News Medical Unit).

- Obesity is not just an American problem. There are about 1.4 billion overweight people in the world and ½ billion are obese. Some small countries you never heard of have obesity rates in the stratosphere: Nauru (71.1%), Cook Islands (64.1%), Tonga (59.6%), Samoa (55.5%) and Palau (50.7%). Yikes! (HealthCare Colleges).

- Your risk for restless leg syndrome is 45% higher if you are obese (Study in *Neurology*, in Meridian Health, 3/11)

- More than 30% of infants and toddlers who don't get enough sleep (less than 10 hours per night) end up overweight or obese later in childhood (Study in *Archives of Pediatrics & Adolescent Medicine,* in *Woman's Day*, 4/11)

- An obese person is 600% more likely to die after experiencing a critical injury than a thin person (*Archives of Surgery*, in *Men's Health* (3/05)

- A thin woman will make about $4,000 more in salary than a woman who is average size or larger (*Journal of Applied Psychology*, in *Reader's Digest*, 5/11)

- An average child in the U.S. will watch almost 10,000 TV commercials for food and beverages per year (*Journal of Nutrition Education,* in *National Geographic,* 8/04)

- Given the choice, 41% of Americans would eat their favorite less-healthy fast-food item and not choose a healthier option (*Gallup Poll,* in *Men's Health*, 3/04)

- Americans get 11% of their DAILY calories from fast food. Not weekly nor monthly. But daily. That's very scary.

- Obesity kills more people than smoking. According to stats from 2010, nearly 680,000 people die from their dietary habits vs. 465,000 from smoking. (*Institute of Health Metrics and Evaluation at the University of Washington*)

- Doctors in the U.S., Europe and Asia were surveyed, and 90% believed the sharp growth in type II diabetes and the current obesity epidemic are strongly linked to excess sugar consumption. (Credit Suisse report "Sugar, Consumption at a crossroads).

Finally, here's the most incredible "bad news" stat…one that supports everything in *The Mind Diet* series of guidebooks. Read this over and over until it really sinks in:

95% & 65%

A staggering 95% of people who lost weight with a crash diet plan gained it all back. An astronomical 65% of those people gained back more weight than they had lost! (www.TheNewsForYou.com, 11/16/10)

Think of all the wasted time, money and frustration that tens of millions endure every year. Besides going on diets that never work, being overweight or obese exacts a toll on your body.

To further underscore how critical obesity is, on June 18, 2013, the American Medical Association decided to recognize obesity as a disease for the very first time. This is a major development that shines a brighter spotlight on the obesity epidemic.

And Americans are paying attention. 83% of us think obesity is the most important health issue in our country, topping cancer and other diseases (Repass & Partners survey, 2013).

Dr. Walter Willett, Chairman of the Nutrition Department at the Harvard School of Public Health sums it up quite simply: "If Americans could eliminate sugary beverages, potatoes, white bread, pasta, white rice and sugary snacks, we would wipe out almost all the problems we have with weight and diabetes and other metabolic diseases."

If all these stats don't make you sick to your stomach, then you need to keep re-reading them until they do. Weight reduction and maintenance is likely **the** most important aspect of your life that you need to deal with. I'm sure you've heard the expression "to die for" as in "those shoes are to die for" or "that 48 ounce steak is to die for." Well, when it comes to food, you don't want that cliché to happen to you.

Speaking of "to die for," MSNBC *Morning Joe* co-host Mika Brzezinski told her best friend, "You are fat! I love you too much to let your weight kill you." In her book *Obsessed* she talks about how America has become so overweight. The result of a nation of fat people is the subject of this next section.

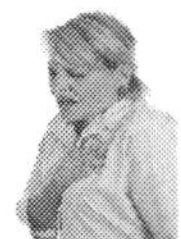 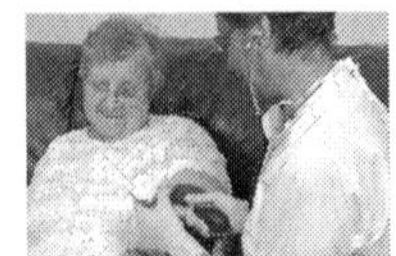 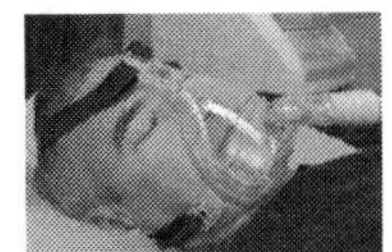 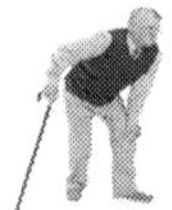 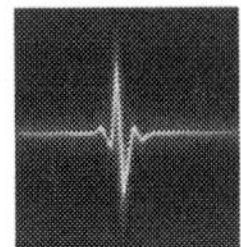

Obesity and Medical Conditions

Losing weight has been proven to reduce or avoid various medical conditions. A study (*Archives of Internal Medicine)* showed that people with severe Sleep Apnea who lose the recommended amount of weight were three times more likely to recover than those who didn't. No surprise, because Sleep Apnea is most common in overweight and obese people. This "two-way street" phenomenon is most important to embrace:

- Remain fat and you may get various diseases and conditions.
- Lose weight and you reduce or eliminate some diseases and conditions.

One reason people gain weight back after dieting is that once they reached their weight goal, they think that's the end of the weight loss program: "I reached my goal, I'm done."

The simple fact is that you have to have two goals. The first is to reach your goal weight AND the second goal is to remain at that level **forever**. According to the American Dietetic Association, good goal setting increases the likelihood that you'll reach your diet objective by a whopping 84%. Writing in www.active.com, Charles Stuart Platkin suggests these tips:

- **Be specific**, like "I will lose 10% of my body weight within one year."
- **Determine how**, like "I will lose 2/10th of a pound a day for 8 months."

Once you hit your goal, it's time for another visit to your nutrition specialist to create a game plan to help you maintain your weight…forever. You must commit to both goals as part of reaching your Moment of Truth. Being fat can lead to a plethora of medical conditions, some serious and life-threatening, including:

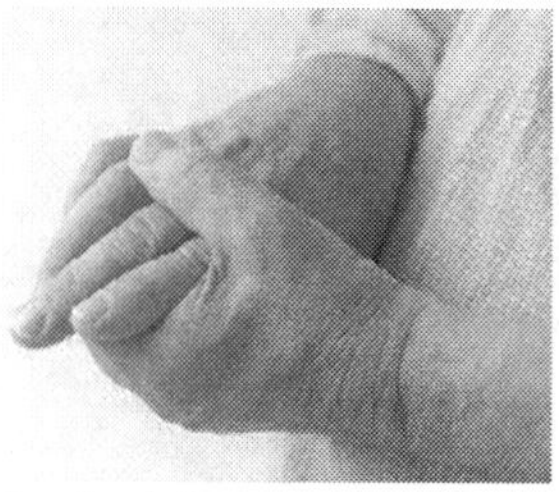

Arthritis

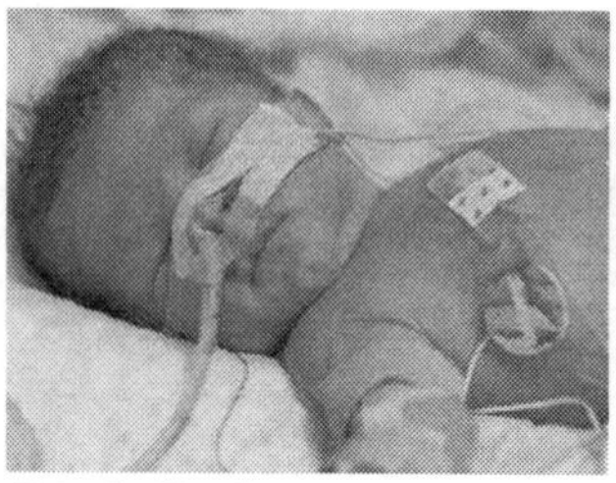

Birth Defects

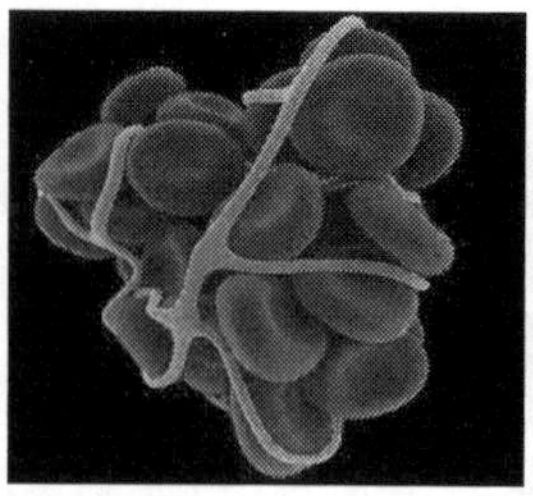

Blood Cots

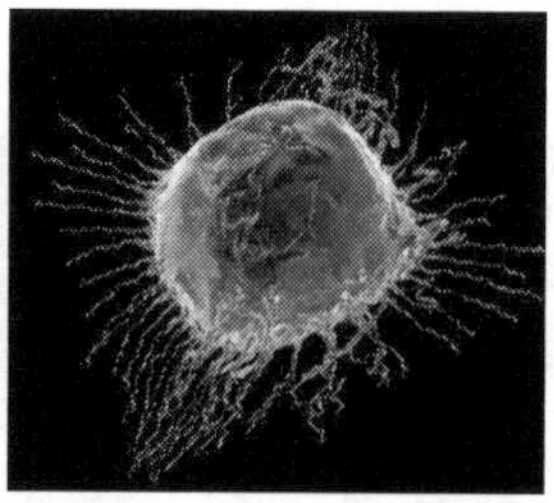

Cancers (numerous)

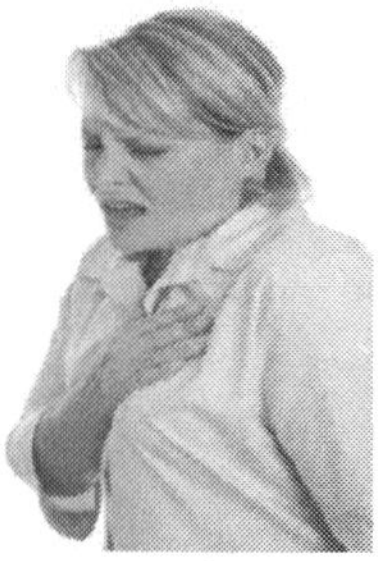

Heart Condition

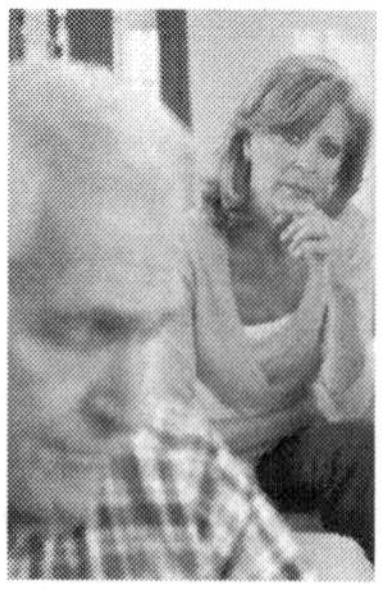

Dementia

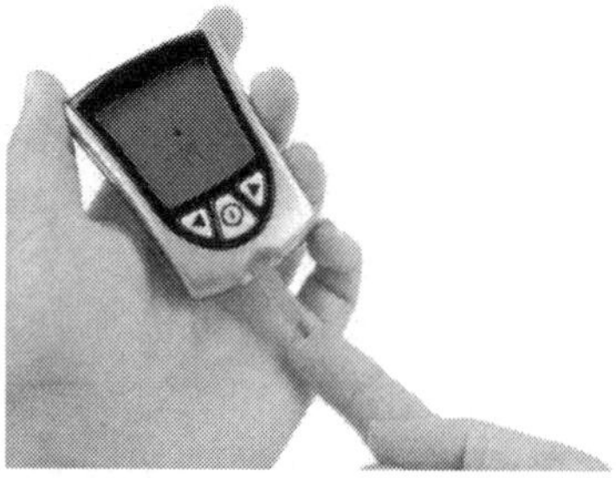

Diabetes

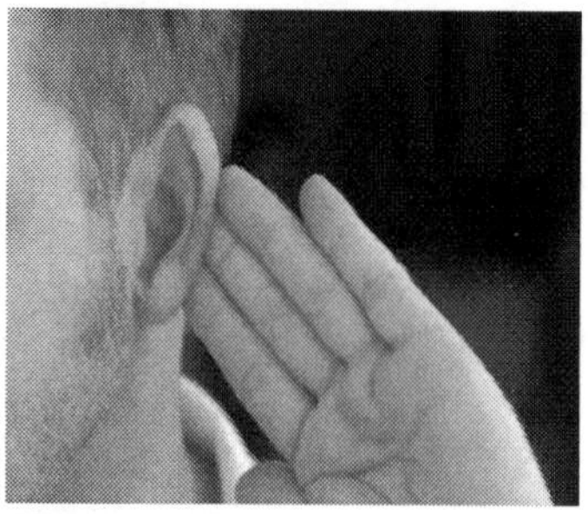

Hearing Loss

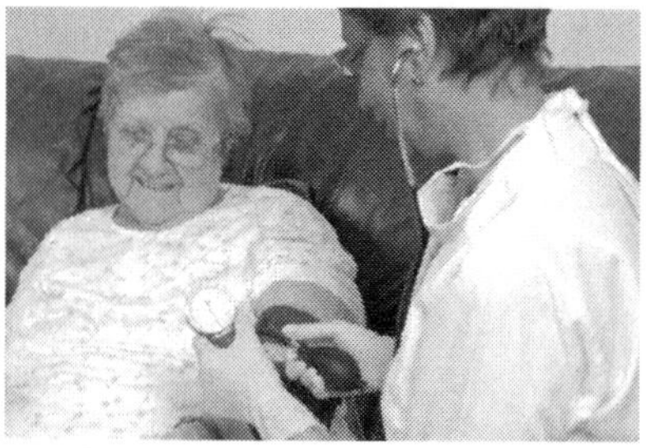

High Blood Pressure

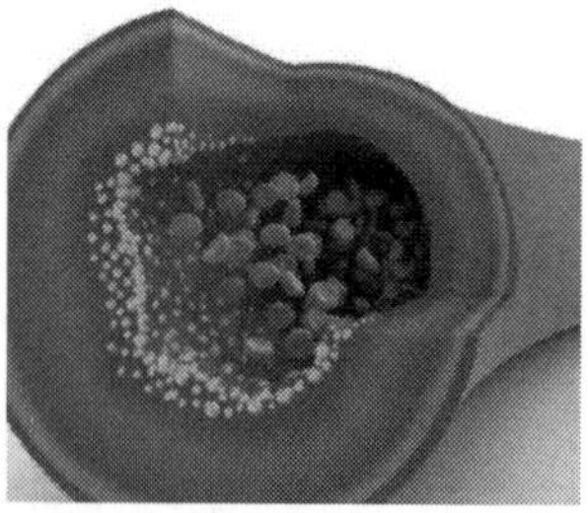

High Cholesterol

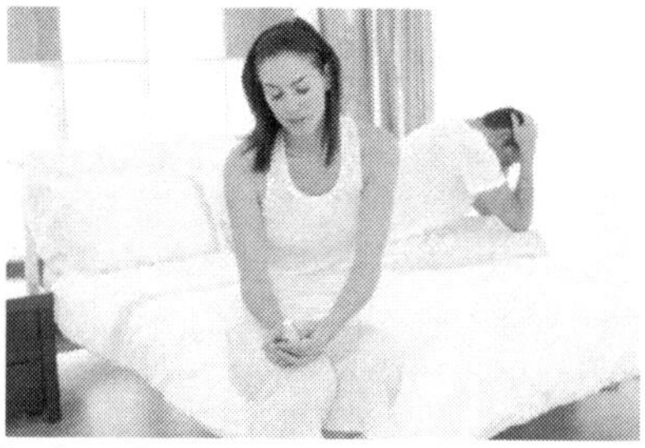

Infertility

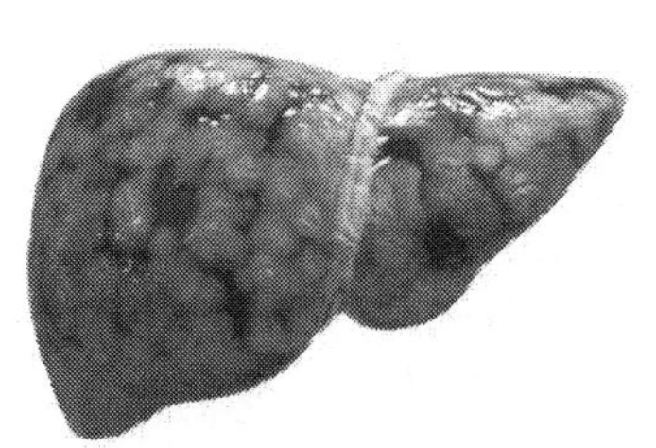
Liver Disease

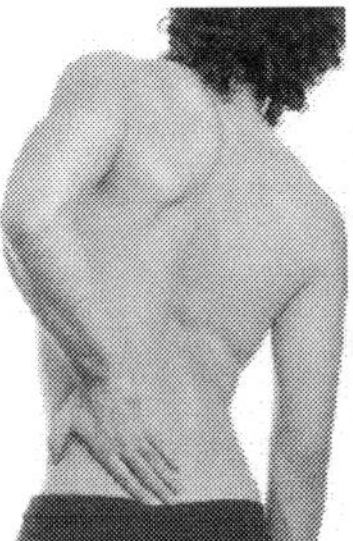
Back Pain

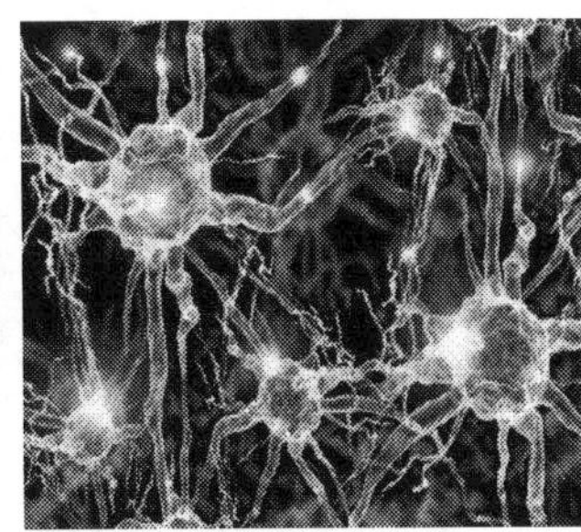
Nerve Damage

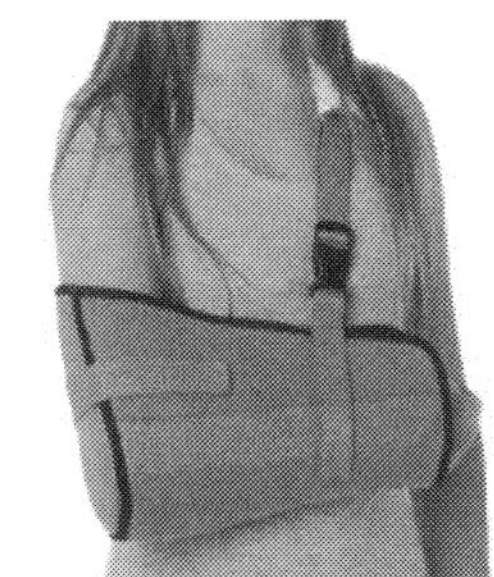
Bone Problems

Skin Problems

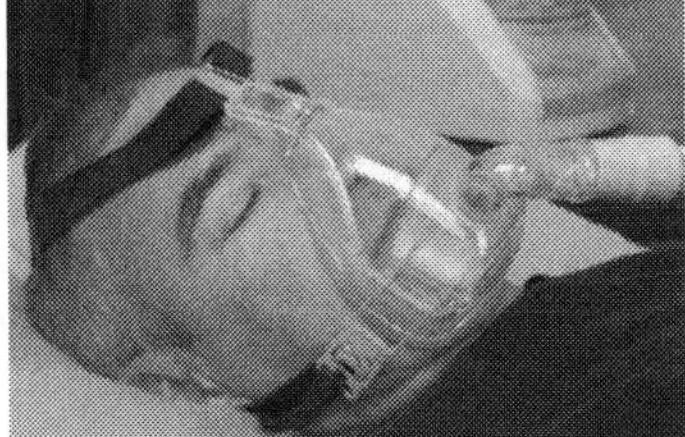
Sleep Apnea

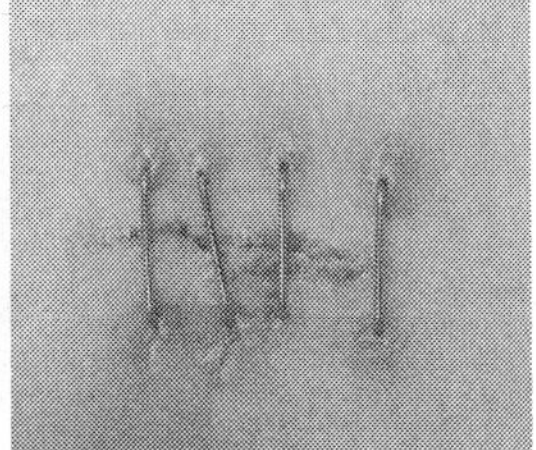
Gallbladder Surgery

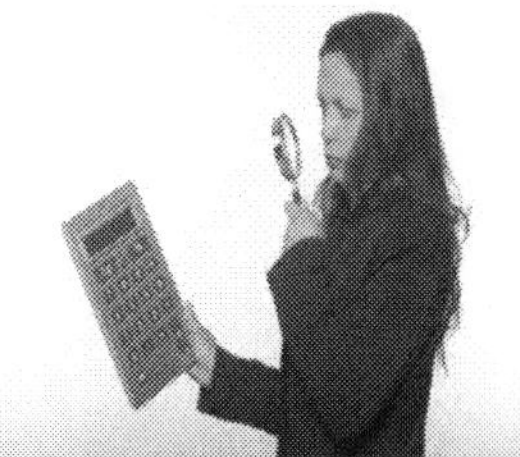
Vision Problems

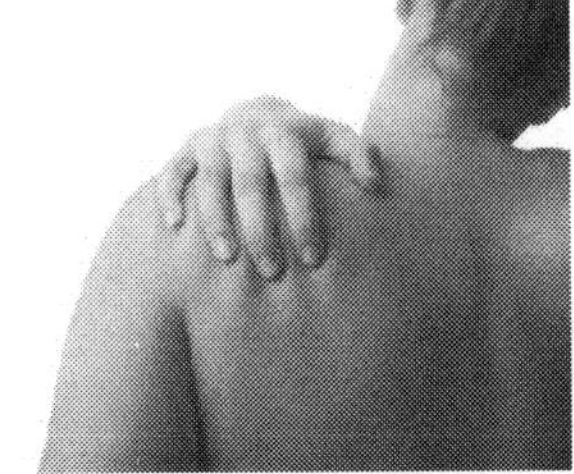
Pain

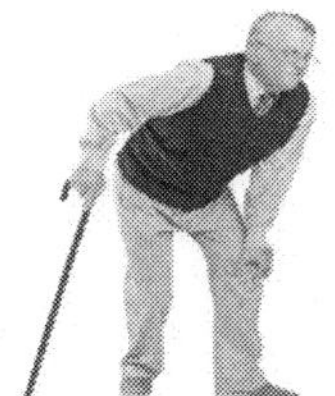
Osteoarthritis

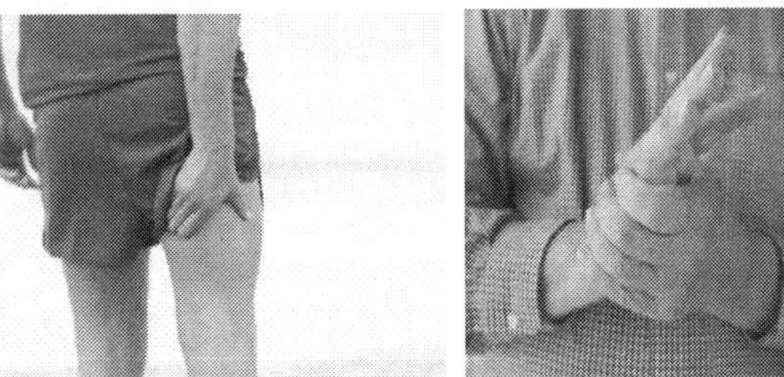
Muscle Problems

Tingling in Hands

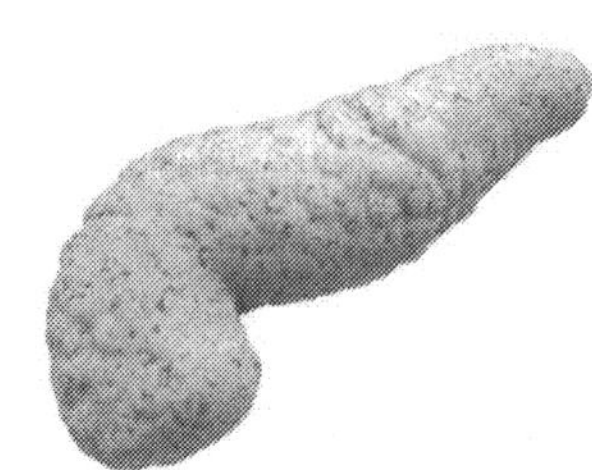
Pancreas Disease

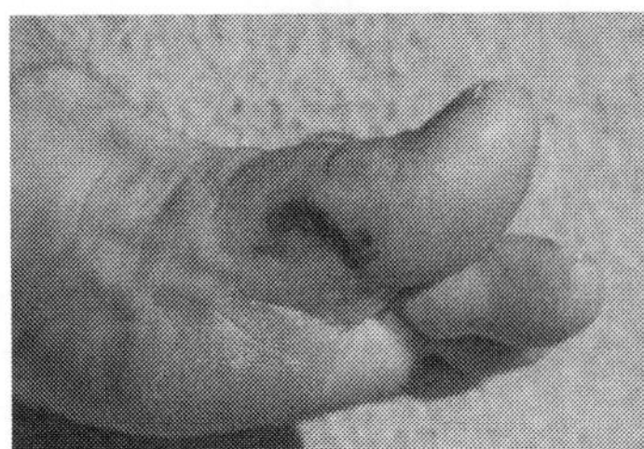
Wound Infections

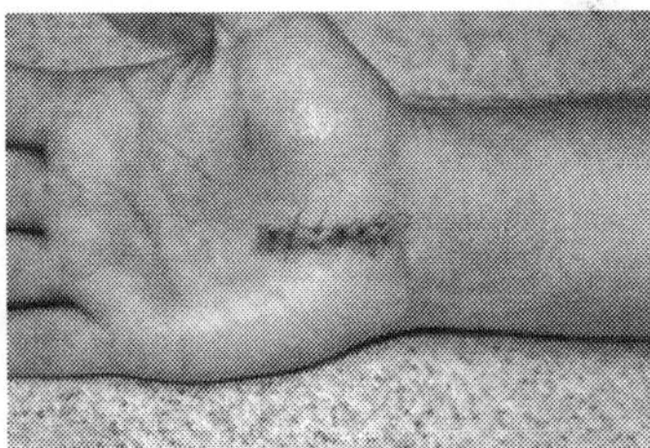
Carpal Tunnel

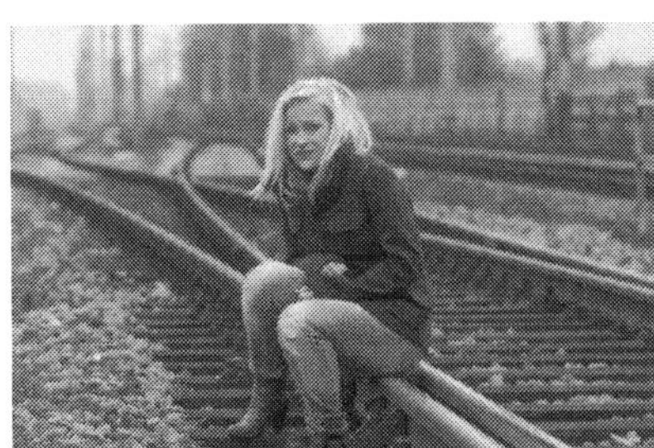
Depression

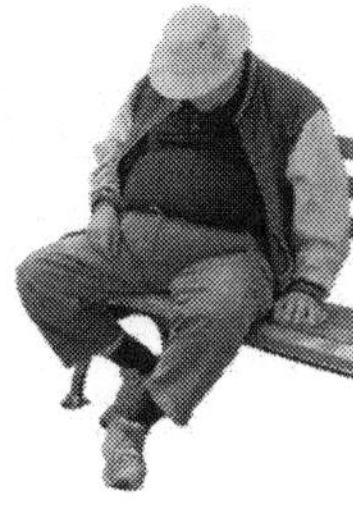
Sleepiness

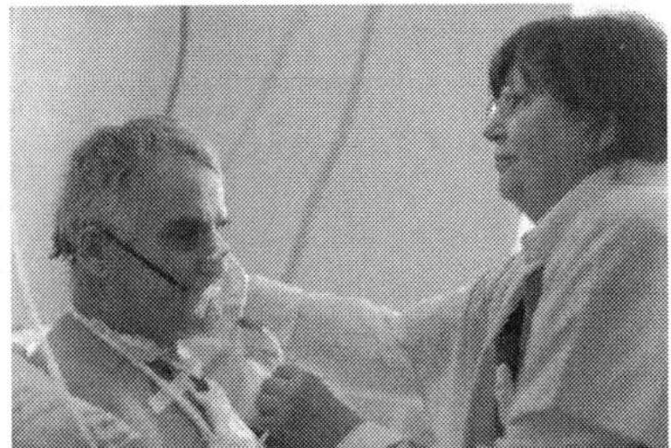
Respiratory Problems

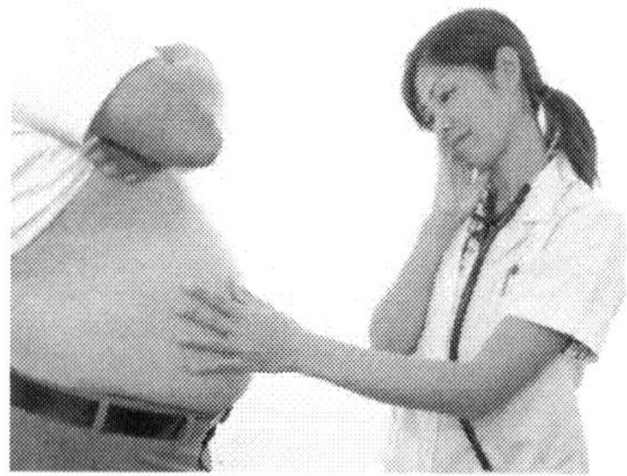
Metabolic Syndrome

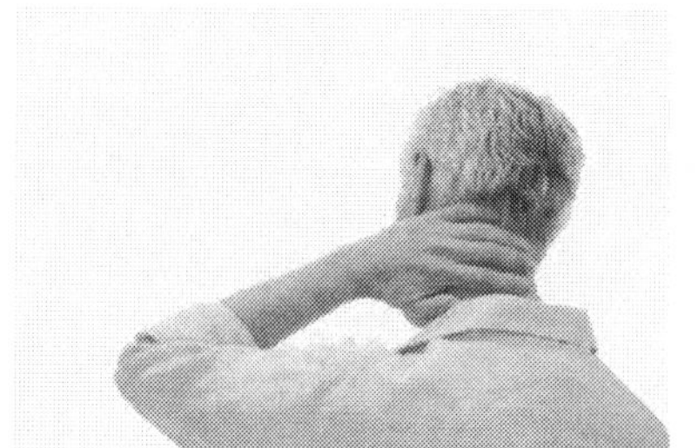
Neck Pain

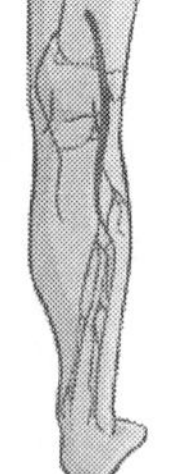
Vein Problems

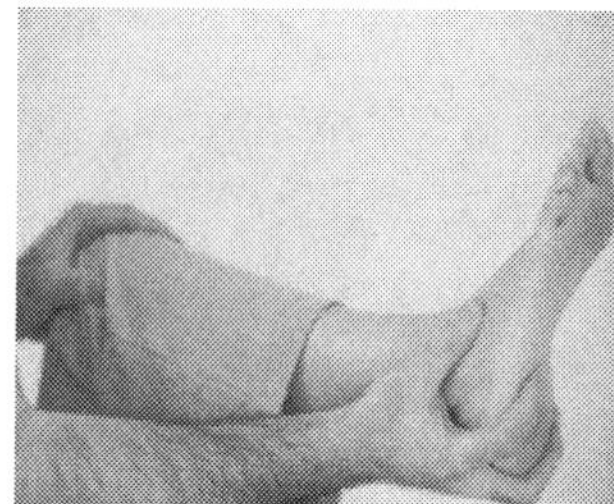
Heel Spurs

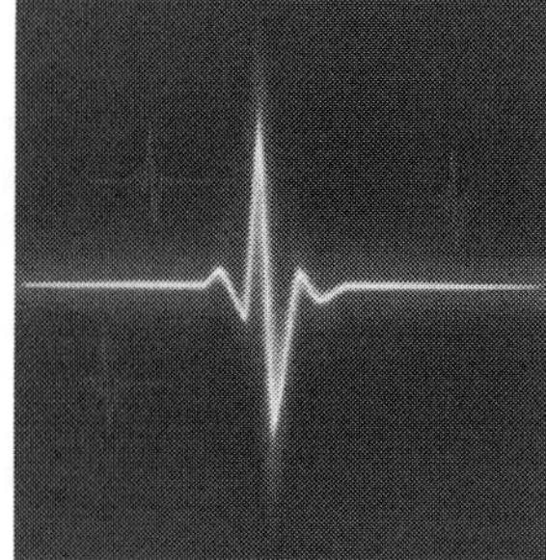
Atrial Fibrillation

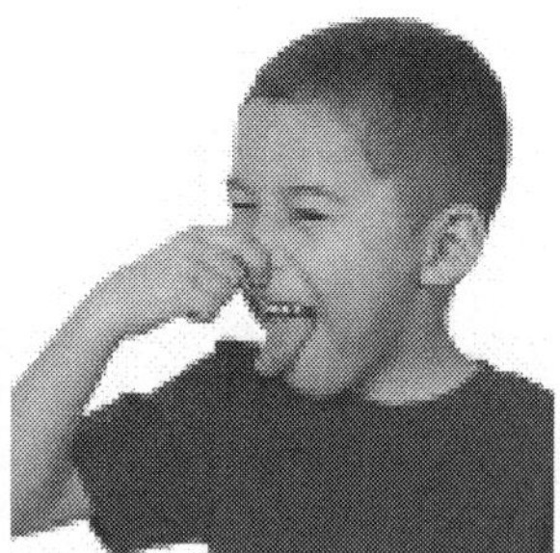
Chronic Odor

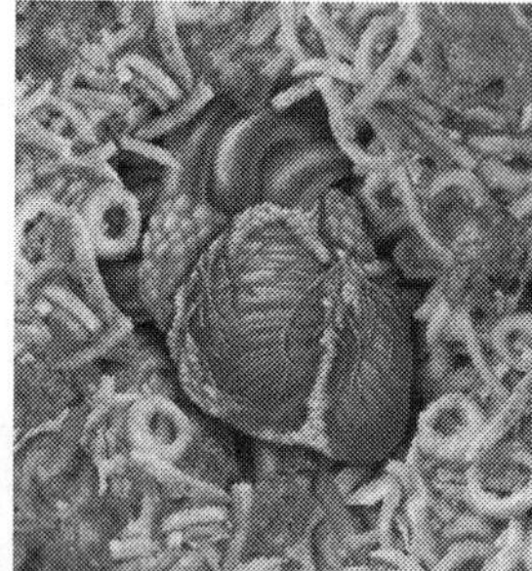
Heart Disease

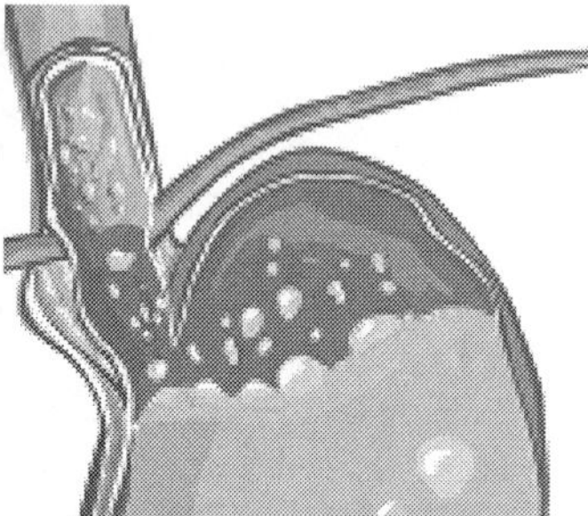
Gastric Reflux

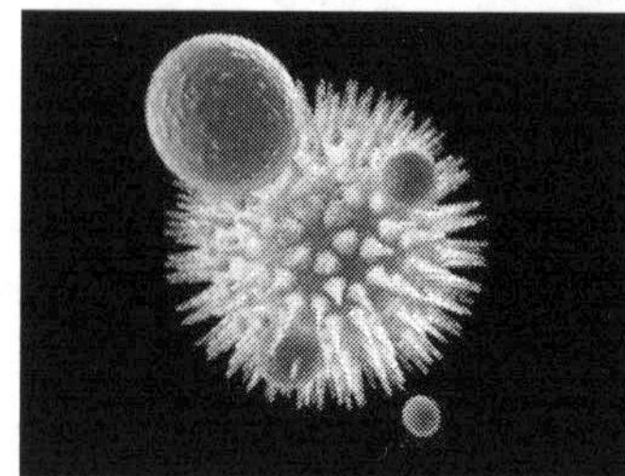
Immune System Problems

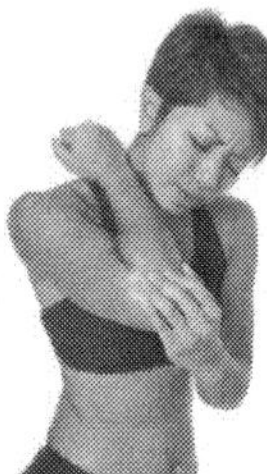
Joint Problems

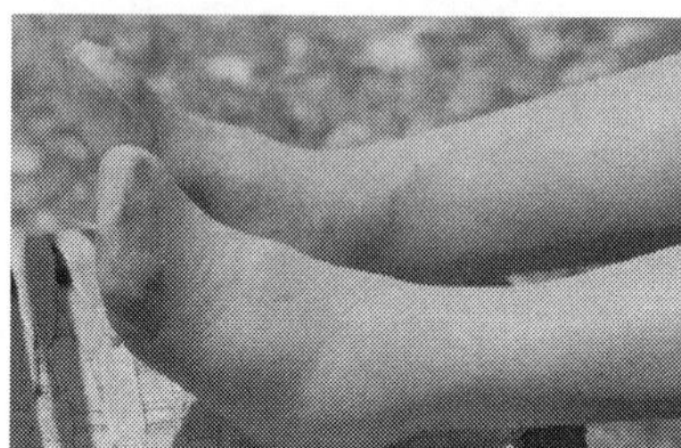
Swelling

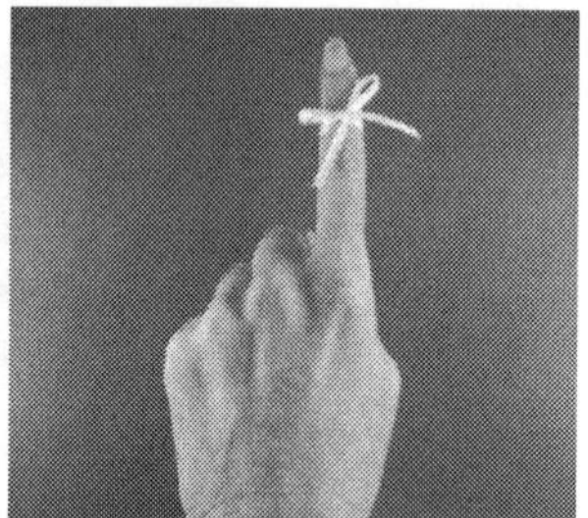
Memory Loss

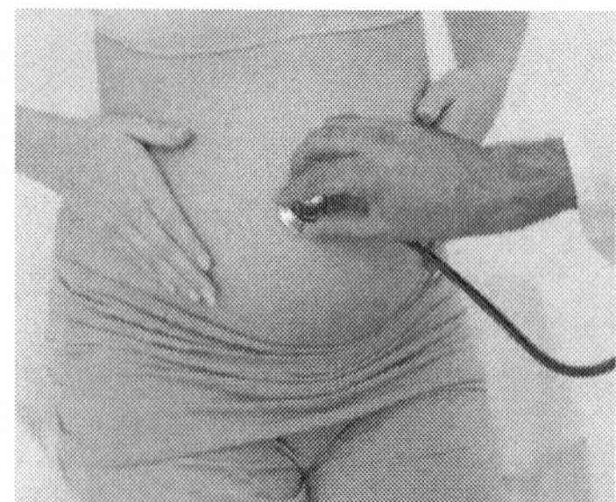
Pregnancy Problems

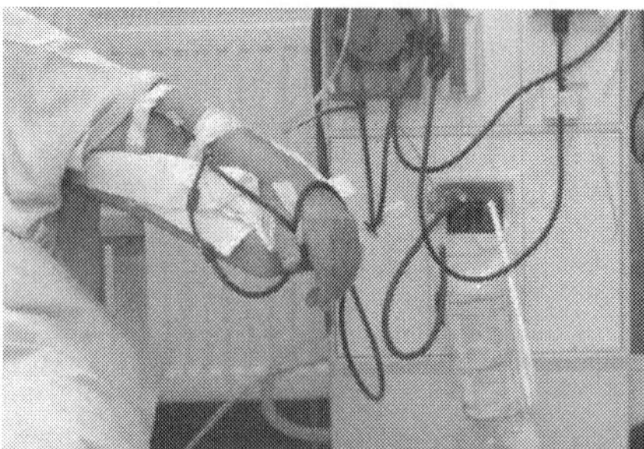
Kidney Problems/Dialysis

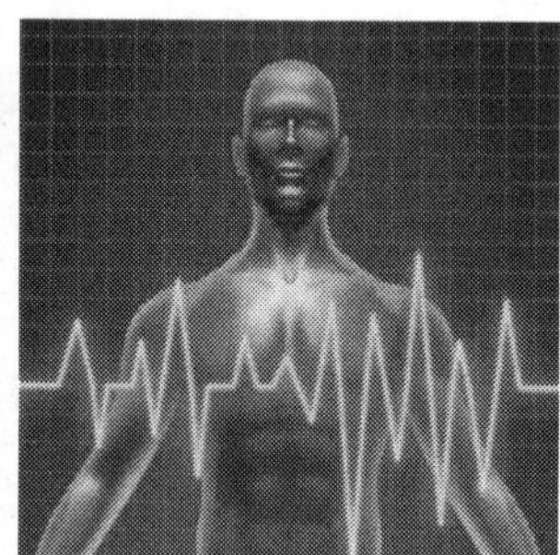
Stroke

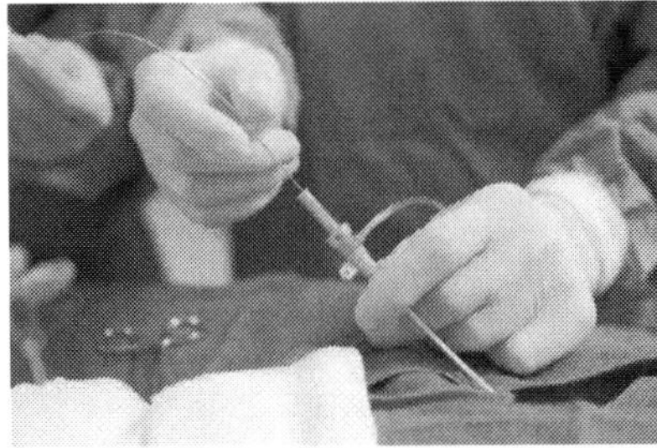
Surgical Complications

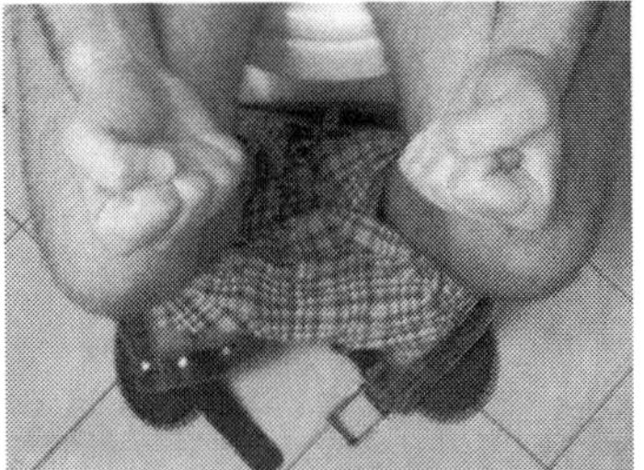
Urinary/Bowel Problems

Plus gout, elephantiasis, Alzheimer's and others. Two of the most common and feared conditions in the U.S. are Type 2 diabetes and Alzheimer's. Researchers believe that having insulin resistance or Type 2 diabetes raises your risk of developing the brain plaques and tangles that are believed to destroy brain tissue, leading to Alzheimer's. The news just gets worse and worse when you're obese. In fact, read "Is Alzheimer's Type 3 Diabetes?" by Mark Bittman on the NY Times blog and you'll be stunned: http://tinyurl.com/92xbane. Want another scary thought? Researchers at Wake Forest and other institutions have determined that rich foods hit the same pleasure centers in our brains that heroin and cocaine activate, and that drug addicts and obese people have similar neurobiological circuitry. What does all this mean? A steady diet of junk food could get you so addicted to food that you may never be able to lose weight! Talking about your brain, a study in *The Journal of Neuroscience* found that viewing images of delicious food lit up the brain's reward center in women, causing them to overeat.

Even if the obesity trend shows no sign of letting up, when you get to the Moment of Truth, embrace it and develop your beliefs and embrace my strategies to deal with food intake on a daily basis, it is my belief that you will not become one of these statistics.

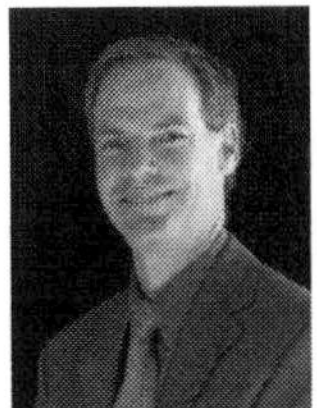

Guest Essay – Dr. Ethan Lazarus

The Truth about Weight Loss That You Don't Know

Every diet program I've seen combines eating less and moving more in some way or another. While they all sound different, they all have these two factors in common. Restricting calories. Getting more exercise. That's been the mantra for decades. I call it "Eat Less, Move More" or ELMM for short.

And that's precisely why 99.999999% of people who try ELMM fail, over and over again. Sometimes I laugh and sometimes I cringe when I see people starving themselves because they binged, or killing themselves at gyms, trying to shed some pounds. Not only is ELMM the reason people fail, it's also the reason why the entire weight loss industry succeeds.

Think about it. The weight loss industry succeeds (i.e. makes a ton of money) because people fail at losing weight, and they keep coming back to buy more products and use more services in the eternal hope that someday they will succeed. Americans spend some $60 billion a year in this regard, and plenty of countries around the world are in the same boat.

The irony in all this is that ELMM flies in the face of what we know about the human body. Your body revolts when you eat less. It revolts when you have ridiculously strenuous workouts. After all, it's not wise to attempt to fool mother nature, which is exactly what everyone is doing, and virtually none of us realize it!

If there's one thing I've learned in working with countless overweight and obese people in my clinic it's that other factors are far more important than how much you eat and how much exercise you get. In fact, here's my list of the top factors that impact one's ability to lose weight:

- Genetics – based on centuries of the development of humankind
- Environment – everything that's around you that impacts your body
- What you eat – the specific foods and drinks you consume
- When you eat – the time of day you eat
- The reasons you eat – most of which are not good reasons
- Your mental state – do you really want to lose weight?
- Constant food temptations – it's everywhere
- The amount of food you eat – surprise, this is way down on the list
- The amount of exercise you get – another surprise

Even though you can't change your genetics, there ARE plenty of things you can do to successfully lose weight and keep it off. Thousands of my patients have done just that, and the phrase that best describes why they were successful is:

Eat Right. Live Right.

ERLR for short. It replaces Eat Less. Move More.

If there's one thing you get from this essay, it's the critical importance of ERLR.

Eating less and moving more are simply tactics.

Eating right and living right are states of mind.

I hope you see the difference.

Our bodies are extremely complex. In order to lose weight successfully, we're balancing how our mind works with various neurotransmitters (chemicals that facilitate communications between nerves) – norepinephrine, serotonin and dopamine. Layer in the lousy nutritional composition of many foods and beverages, and mix in the bad habits and bad advice we've been getting over decades (like the USDA food pyramid which for decades recommended high carb, low fat diets – a great recipe to gain weight), and you begin to see that losing weight is not the slam dunk that many marketers of diet products and services claim it is.

I could go on and on with heavily scientific explanations of all this, but *The Mind Diet* is more about ERLR than anything else, and that's exactly where you need to start.

Let's go back in history, shall we? Remember that our lifetimes represent a miniscule sliver of time in relation to the entire history of the world. Cave men and women were all thin, as were most of their successors throughout the ages. Until recently, people basically ate just enough to survive, unless they were wealthy. In fact, sugar was scarce for the longest time, available only to those who had money.

So why were cave dwellers and pretty much all other societies thin, and why are we all heavy?

It's a pretty simple explanation. Our predecessors didn't have an abundance of food as we do. They didn't have sugar in everything they ate. They didn't have stores to buy supersized meals. They didn't have ads screaming "eat me" all day long. And they didn't have complex personal issues that resulted in emotional eating problems. Nor did they have cruise ships and restaurants with endless buffets.

They basically had simple lives and the food they ate was simply to survive.

Fast forward to the present. It's only been the last 100 years or so that our waistlines have exploded. 100 years is not enough time for our genes to adapt to such a dramatic environmental change.

We live in an environment where food is ever-present, and most of the time we consume food and drink for the wrong reasons.

This first section of *The Mind Diet – Truth*, where Irv has placed this essay, is perhaps the most important chapter in the entire book. The real truth is that almost everything you've been told about weight loss is false, outdated, and not based on reality.

So start thinking about "Eat Right. Live Right." That's the new mantra that actually works.

Dr. Lazarus is one of only 191 (as of 8/13) individuals to have completed the first certification process of the newly formed American Board of Obesity Medicine. Physicians certified in Obesity Medicine are able to positively impact patients of all ages by incorporating weight management into traditional models of medical practice. In addition to completing coursework on obesity medicine at the Harvard School of Medicine, The Obesity Society, and the American Society of Bariatric Physicians, Dr. Lazarus helps teach a certification course in obesity medicine and is frequently invited to teach doctors about the medical management of obesity. He is a delegate to the American Medical Association on behalf of the ASBP. He is the director of the Clinical Nutrition Center in Denver (CO), where he has worked with countless patients since 2004 on the medical management of obesity.

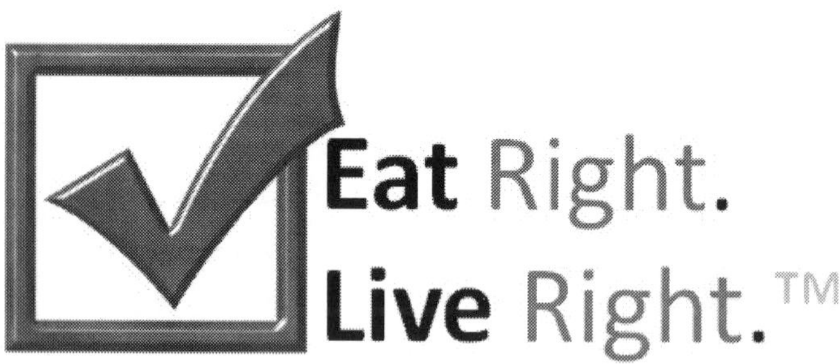

The "Eat Right. Live Right" mantra covered in the previous essay consists of these components:

Eat Right.

- Eating the correct amount of food and drinks.
- Eating food and drinks that are healthy.
- Avoiding food and drinks that are unhealthy.
- Not eating for the wrong reasons.
- Not skipping breakfast and lunch.
- Eating smaller dinners (in most cases).
- Choosing healthy snacks.
- Making good choices when you eat out.
- Drinking water and seltzer, not soda.

Live Right.

- Walking every single day.
- Spending plenty of time outdoors.
- Solving problems not by eating.
- Doing everything to be a happy person.
- Getting plenty of sleep.
- Losing weight slowly, not quickly.

- Discussing food with your family.
- Taking control over what you eat and drink

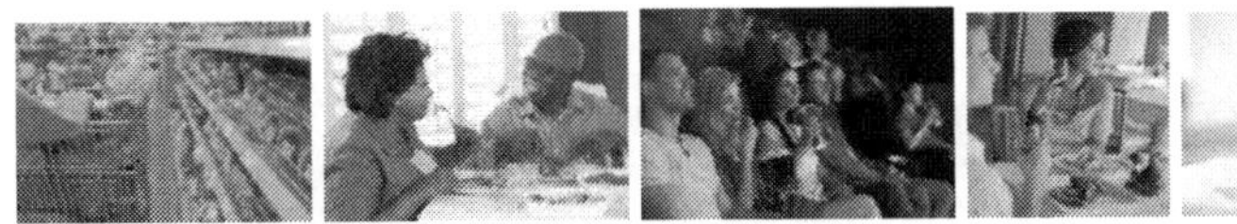

Food and Daily Life

Most people don't think about it, but food is extremely prevalent in our lives, from the moment we wake up until we go to sleep. We are faced with 200+ "eating opportunities" all day long:

- Breakfast
- Coffee/donut/bagel on the way to work
- Coffee breaks throughout the day
- Snacks and candies on co-workers' desks
- Lunch
- Birthday celebrations in the break room
- Dinner
- Couch potato snacking

Plus, the size of meals is completely upside down. We've been conditioned to eat a little breakfast or even skip it, and have big dinners. It needs to be the other way around – the less food you eat after work, the better off you will be. You'll learn more about timing in the next guidebook.

One of the most important tactics is that you (and I know this is going to sound strange) develop a passion for your weight loss program. In the same way you put time and effort to buy a car or house, root for your favorite sports team, enjoy your partner/family/friends, you must put the same effort into weight loss. I've also come to actually despise unhealthy junk food to the point where I'll never eat it again. Even the smell of fried foods has become a real turnoff! The combination of consistent losses, feeling lighter, compliments on how you look and other benefits will keep this passion strong!

Losing weight needs to be elevated from something you avoid like the plague to something you embrace and get passionate about. Being able to lose small amounts of weight every day becomes a special moment for you. Rather than waiting for a once-a-week weigh in, I've found it's better to weigh yourself every day, and be thrilled with 2/10th of a pound loss every day. That was my goal – and the reason is simple: 2/10th of a pound a day equals a one pound loss every 5 days and about 6 pounds lost per month! It's a lot easier to think about losing 2/10th per day than 40, 50, 60 or more pounds.

From a health point of view, Emily Banes, a clinical dietician at the Houston Northwest Medical Center says in www.EverdayHealth.com, "We usually recommend about a half a pound to two pounds a week, which is a lot less than what these fad diets promise." Losing 2/10th a day is right in line with this excellent medical advice.

A study reported in *Woman's World* showed that people who weigh themselves daily lost more weight over two years because they felt more accountable to their weight loss program. I can tell you from my experience that weighing in daily keeps weight loss at the forefront of your mind and seeing almost daily losses, even just 1/10th or 2/10th of a pound, is gratifying and reinforces the overall plan to lose weight slowly and steadily.

After I reached my Moment of Truth, and thought about weight loss throughout the day when situations arose, I also realized that every single thing that is impacted by weight can be viewed in two ways.

As an example, let's talk about how clothes fit us when we're overweight. Here's how to think about this topic:

- **Losing** weight means you'll be able to wear clothes that make you look better and look good on you and you'll feel good about yourself as a result.
- **Not losing** weight means you'll be stuck with less fashionable clothes and clothes specifically designed for overweight people, and they probably won't look very good on you, and you'll likely feel bad about yourself.

How about work?

- **Losing** weight often means you'll perform better on the job, be positively viewed by employers and co-workers, and will make it easier to land better jobs.
- **Not losing** weight means your work performance may suffer, you might be an "outcast" among your co-workers, and it will be harder to land betters jobs.

Even though hiring based on weight is illegal, you can bet it happens all the time. Bottom-line focused employers lament the enormous cost they have to absorb because overweight employees get sick more often and don't have the high energy needed to succeed.

When you think about it, your weight directly impacts:

- How you look
- How you feel
- How you act
- How you sleep
- How you breathe
- How you perform
- How your skin looks

- How others react to you

And on and on and on. Excess weight is a fact of life. Stop fighting it and reach your Moment of Truth. In "7 Tips for Successful Weight Loss" (www.medicinenet.com), there are several that mirror my philosophy:

- The desire to lose weight must come from you, not from anyone else.
- Surround yourself with people who support your efforts and don't undermine you.
- Set small goals and focus on these, rather than the big picture.

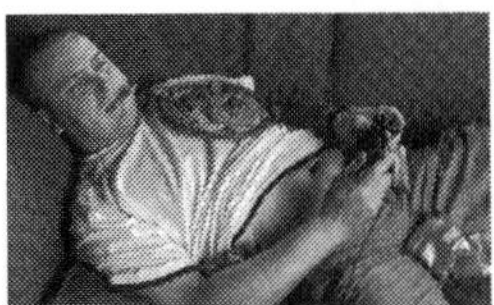

Eating Styles

Let's change course and take a humorous look at the way people eat.

I've identified 13 types of what I call "eating styles," and with one exception, they all are destructive and prevent weight loss. Many people I've watched combine two or more of these styles. Some are so absurd they are humorous; others are sickening.

I'm sure you're familiar with most or all of them. Some of the writing in this book pokes fun at the way people eat. The purpose is not to make you feel bad, but to show you the absurdity of some of the habits you may have developed, in the hope that thinking about them will lead to positive change.

Shovelers. These are people who shovel food into their mouths as if they were excavating their plate and being paid for it. I'm amazed at how much food they can pile on one fork or spoon and how fast they get that food from the plate into their mouths.

Speed Demons. Maybe they are all trying to get into the *Guinness Book of Records*, but these folks place the speed of finishing their meal above all else. Sure, it's OK to eat fast if you're in the Nathan's hot dog contest, but to quickly finish off a meal of steak, potato and vegetables without any "taste enjoyment" makes no sense.

Chunkers. These people have not learned how to use their knife and fork to cut big pieces of food into little ones. They eat the largest imaginable pieces, and practically have to swallow them like snakes because the pieces are so large. They end up eating a big steak in 5 or 6 chunks!

Big Eyes. You're at a party, and you see one of those people who take way more food than anyone else. And not just one item, but lots of everything. They can't possibly like every single item they take, but they take it anyway.

Plate Scrapers. If there's one bit of food left on the plate, you can be sure that person is not a plate scraper. Plate scrapers make sure that nothing is left, even food that didn't really taste that good. If you have a plate of 20 French fries and you leave over 5 of them instead of scraping your plate clean, you've left behind 25% of the fat and calories!

Food Bullies. People in this group will push other people out of the way, cut in front of the line and plant themselves at a buffet table so they can get to the food first. On a cruise recently, I watched as a guy ran down the buffet line, brushing into and bumping into people on his way to the dessert area as they stood between him and the table. For whatever reason – and I can't think of **any** reason that would justify this behavior – he had to be there before anyone else.

Swallowers. People that are Shovelers and Speed Demons also tend to be Swallowers. These people don't chew their food; they just swallow it. They must get some sort of pleasure out of food as it goes down their throats, but I just can't see it.

Messy Ones. Because people in this group eat fast and eat big pieces of food or take big bites, they tend to wind up with food on their faces. It reminds me of a little boy eating a cheeseburger and getting ketchup on his face because it seeped out of the side of the hamburger roll while he was taking a bite. Cute on a kid but not on an adult.

The Supersizers. These people are fast-food chains' favorite customers. They always say "yes" when asked if they'd like to supersize their meals by getting a larger size of fries or onion rings, or whatever the supersize promotion happens to be. They go from ordering a regular size fries with X number of fries to one that is a good value but adds perhaps 10-15 more fries. The amount of fat and calories can be increased by 30% to 50%. A related group might be called "Second Helpers." They always take seconds, even if they're no longer hungry…and they often take seconds before they've finished their first serving!

Food Focused. The first time I saw this I said, "This must be an exception." But then I saw it again and again. Food-focused people sit at a table and the full force of their attention is on the plates in front of them. There could be 10 people at the table, all talking and eating and having a good time, but the food-focused person doesn't participate and only cares about what's on the plate.

Quick Reloaders. Here's an interesting group of people. While they are scarfing down one forkful, they are immediately reloading the next one. In fact, the "on deck" forkful of food is lifted into position so they can jam it into their mouths the split-second the first batch has been swallowed.

Buffet Busters. I believe these people are on a mission – to bankrupt any restaurant that is silly enough to put out a buffet. Whether they're paying $19.95 or $39.95, or if the buffet is included (i.e. on a cruise or all-inclusive vacation), they are ready to grab just about anything and everything for their plate. In many cases (30% in a recent quick sampling) they took two plates full of stuff, as if to say "Take that, buffet manager. You're not going to make any money on me!"

The last eating style is one that I have become. It's the one you need to become. Getting to your Moment of Truth will help you become a "food lover."

Food Lovers. A food lover takes the time to really taste and enjoy the food. Savors every bite. Combines the act of eating with conversation. Eats very slowly. Lets food rest on the palate and the taste buds take over. Deliberately thinks about what to take from a buffet. In short, becoming a food lover is what this book is all about. Once you make up your mind, it's not all that difficult. Like playing golf or chess, it's all in the mind. Go ahead, make a real honest decision to become a Food Lover.

I've also observed from talking with people that there are two types of hunger:

- **Physical Hunger**. This is where you actually feel hungry, with so-called "hunger pangs." The key is that your body is truly telling you that you should eat.
- **Emotional Hunger**. This is where you are really not physically hungry, but you want to eat due to some other positive or negative stimulus. Emotional hunger is what gets us all in trouble, because you're eating for the wrong reasons. And sometimes the clock says it's time to eat, and you do, even if you're not hungry!

When you feel you're hungry and want to eat, it's time to be totally honest with yourself. Ask yourself one simple question: am I eating because I'm truly physically hungry, or is there some other reason. If your answer is the latter, don't eat and spend the time figuring out what's causing your desire to eat even though you're not hungry.

Think about that!

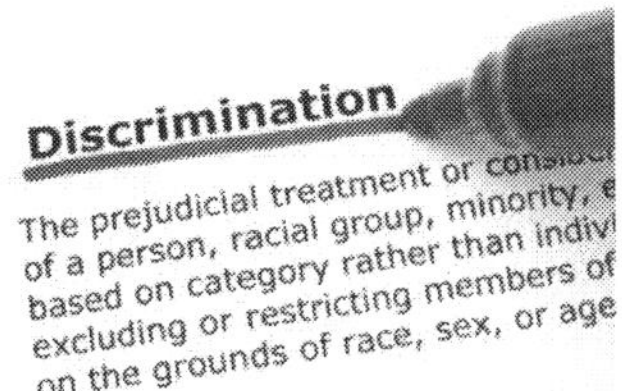

Discrimination

Most people know that overweight and obese people can be discriminated against. Any form of discrimination is immoral and has no place in society, but in fact, it exists and wont' go away. Author Morris M., writing in www.ListVerse.com, points out "Ten Frightening Ways We Discriminate Against Fat People." Quite an eye-opener. Here's the list:

- Medical Bias: Surveys showed that some doctors and medical students have a strong subconscious bias against overweight people.
- Legal Bias: A Yale study revealed that male jurors were more likely to convict a fat woman than a skinny one for the same crime.
- Workplace Bias: Numerous studies show that hiring managers and senior executives really hate fat people.
- Welfare Bias: In 2013, the UK government cut welfare for heavy people who don't go to the gym.
- Homeless Bias: Homeless people are not thin, malnourished people who don't know where their next meal is coming from. Quite the opposite – 66% in a Boston study were overweight or obese.
- Children Bias: Obese kids are less likely to get financial assistance from their parents, and parents often buy into the cultural myth that fat people are lazy.
- Boy Scouts Bias: In 2013, the scouts banned boys with a BMI over 32 from joining in their Jamboree, held every four years.
- Bullying: obese kids are 65% more likely to be bullied at school, and are more likely to remain overweight.
- Patient Bias: patients are less likely to trust an overweight doctor and ignore their advice than if it came from a skinny doctor.
- Global Bias: a 2011 worldwide study showed than obesity has become associated with laziness and a lack of self-control.

This is obviously extremely disturbing and can impact every area of your life. These mental abuses, when combined with physical diseases, are a strong "1-2 punch" to get your weight under control!

Think About This...

In an interesting philosophical article by Katherine Bishop and Margo G. Wootan of the Center for Science in the Public Interest, the authors say, "If obesity was a communicable disease that was transferred from one person to another like avian flu, cholera, or smallpox, there would be an enormous public outcry and major mobilization of the government to protect the American people."

The panic that permeates the population when communicable diseases take hold is vastly different than the apathy that many people have towards obesity. Yet I'll make a brief case that in some very important respects, obesity really is communicable.

Though you can't "catch" obesity from someone else, you can certainly **mimic** behaviors of fat people. Examples:

- A young child mimics the eating habits of his obese parents. The result is exactly the same as if obesity were communicable.
- You hang out with friends who pig out regularly, and by doing so, you gain weight.
- Your family always celebrates milestones with big dinners, buffets and other food-oriented events.

In a practical example, I saw a mother, son and daughter in a restaurant recently. The mom was obese and the son, about 10 years old, was definitely overweight and maybe obese, and the teenage daughter was thin. Their desserts – ice cream sundaes – told the story. Mom and son finished 100%. The daughter left 75% over. Clearly the boy mimicked his mom's eating habits, while the daughter has taken control of her health and eating habits.

Think about that. Obesity is philosophically communicable!

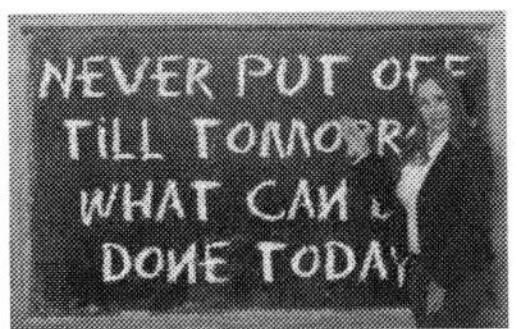

Tomorrow

Now let's talk about "tomorrow." The problem with putting off starting your diet for any length of time is that it becomes harder and harder to get started, and you wind up gaining more and more weight as you get closer to the theoretical tomorrow.

Getting to the Moment of Truth means eliminating tomorrow. When you think about it, tomorrow becomes the day you reach your Moment of Truth. Once you really make up your mind, tomorrow never enters your psyche!

Think of it this way: food will become so unimportant to you and life will get so much better when you declare your Moment of Truth. All of the failed "tomorrows" will be a distant memory, and you'll wish you had gotten to this point a long time ago.

But you're here now, and that's all that counts.

Finally, another benefit, sometimes major, is how much money you save by losing weight and keeping it off permanently:

- You'll never have to spend another dime on products like diet books and weight loss videos.
- You'll never have to join a gym (unless you want to). I've found that simply walking every day is all the exercise I need.
- You'll never need an operation to eliminate fat.
- You may be able to stop taking blood pressure, cholesterol and other medications that cost big bucks.
- You'll eat out less often and save major dollars, year in and year out.
- When you do eat out, you'll eat less food and drink less alcohol, another source of savings.

Add it all up and it means there's a real financial benefit for losing weight and keeping it off!

Want 100 great reasons to lose weight? There's a guidebook in this collection that illustrates them all!

Another way to view weight loss is to examine what goes through your mind when you're eating after a negative event:

> *I know this pint of double chocolate ice cream is bad for me, but I am annoyed at my boyfriend and I'm going to eat it anyway.*
>
> Sound familiar? Here's what you should be saying:
>
> *I'll never eat this pint of double chocolate ice cream because I know it's bad for me, and I will figure out a way to deal with what my boyfriend said.*

Eating the ice cream is avoiding the issue. Ignoring the ice cream and dealing with the issue is the only way to go if you ever hope to lose the weight and keep it off.

While most of this guidebook is focused on you, we can't forget our kids. If you have children, one extremely important reason to gain control of your weight and health are your kids. You know the old cliché: the acorn doesn't fall far from the tree.

Well, the sad truth is that parents who don't eat healthy have kids who don't either. The result: in 2004 the American Heart Association reported than 10% of kids aged 2 to 5 were overweight. Yes, you read that right: kids 2 to 5 are fatter than ever before. Further, 9.3 million kids age 6 to 19 were overweight or obese. Those are staggering numbers. The last thing you want is to raise fat kids. As you learned from the statistics presented earlier, things keep getting worse.

One last point before I ask you what may be one of the most important questions in your life. Most of us, myself included, have made "New Year's Resolutions" to lose weight. I used to make them in November, giving me 4-6 weeks to eat whatever I wanted. If you've really reached your Moment of Truth, you'll make a "today resolution" – and you won't put off this momentus decision, not for a day. www.MedHelp.org has a good piece on resolutions at: http://tinyurl.com/laskblp.

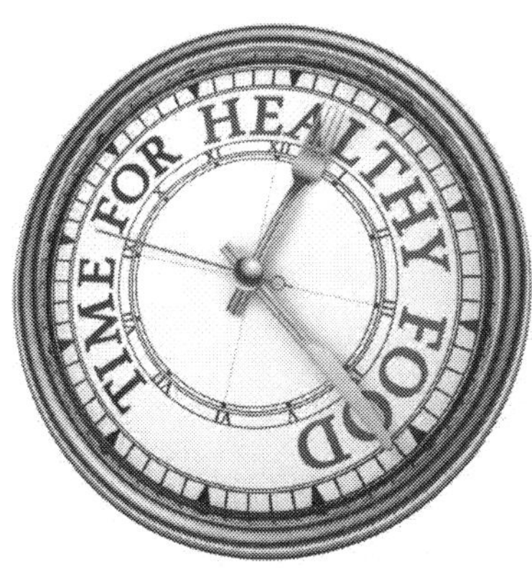

So now I have one simple (but long, on purpose) question. It's simple to ask, yet requires a completely honest answer on your part. Here goes:

Are you absolutely, positively, without reservation 1000% ready to declare your Moment of Truth to yourself and to people who care about you, and get on with successful weight loss, without fail, and are you willing to do everything in your power to be successful at losing weight and keeping it off for the rest of your life?

Are you prepared to open up your refrigerator and throw out all of the junk food and crap that you know is bad for you? Are you prepared to give away clothes that become too big on you when you lose weight?

If your answer is "no" or "not sure," I strongly suggest you re-read *Truth* and think very carefully about each point I made. And re-reading this first section until your answer is a resounding "yes."

If your answer is an uncompromising and definitive "yes," then congratulations. Reaching and declaring your Moment of Truth is a major first step. Next, read "*Beliefs*." This section will discuss how important specific beliefs are to the process and how they impact the strategies you will read about in the third guidebook. It builds upon what you have accomplished by reaching and declaring your Moment of Truth.

I'm tempted to say "good luck," but this is not a game of craps. You don't need luck. You've already begun tapping into the most powerful weapon you have to lose and keep weight off: your mind!

A long time ago, Chinese Philosopher Lao Tzu wrote "A journey of 1,000 miles begins with a single step." I say to you, "A journey of a lifetime of optimal weight and health begins with a single commitment...to yourself."

While on vacation several years ago, my wife's cousin was talking about balancing careers and kids. She said something that stuck with me: "My career is for my mind. My kids are for my soul."

As I wrote these guidebooks, I couldn't help but adapt her quote to losing weight: "Weight loss is for **both** my mind and my soul."

My good friend Kenny likes to use the acronym BLOL when he talks about something of great importance in one's life. He'll say, "It's the BLOL," meaning it's the bottom line of life.

BLOL, or perhaps BLOYL, certainly applies here. Successful weight loss really is the bottom line of ***your*** life.

Think about that. I can definitely tell you that not only your mind and your soul, but every part of your body feels incredibly better when you've lost your weight and kept it off!

The two big lessons from this first guidebook are to reach your

and make up your mind to

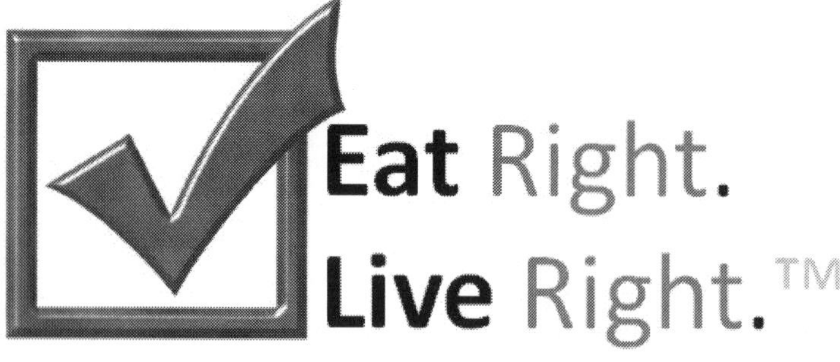

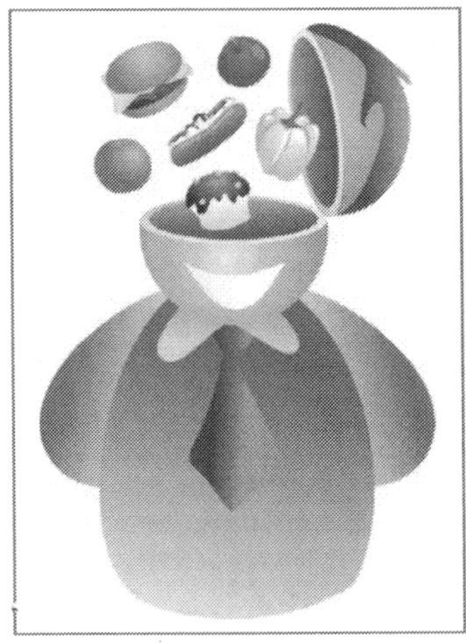

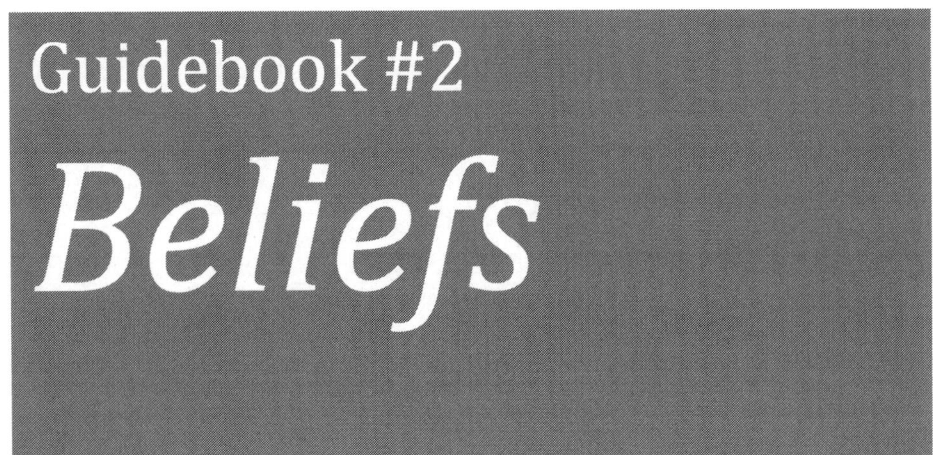

Why do you need a weight loss belief system? And what exactly is it?

Now that you've reached your Moment of Truth, it's time to add a belief system to bring your commitment to life. If you have skipped the first section or have not reached your own personal Moment of Truth, you need to go back to *The Mind Diet: Truth* and read/re-read it. This section builds upon your "moment" and until you have reached it, the rest of this collection of information will not be effective for you.

Reaching your Moment of Truth is a major first step. The balance of the sections in *The Mind Diet Guidebooks* build upon your decision to **absolutely, positively, without reservation, get on with successful weight loss, without fail. To do everything in your power to be successful at losing weight safely and keeping it off for the rest of your life. No more excuses. No more postponement. Just do it now.**

Think of this section of 26 "weight loss beliefs" as building blocks to carry out the goal you set in reaching your Moment of Truth. We all have beliefs in other areas of our lives, such as the value of education, work ethic, treating people fairly and kindly, religious beliefs, etc. When you've made an important decision, you need beliefs that you can hang your hat on – so that your direction is clear.

You will see, through this section and others, that people who lose weight and keep it off share common beliefs and actions. The National Weight Control Registry at the Brown Medical School keeps track of thousands of people who have lost at least 30 pounds and have kept if off for at least a year. Three stats about people in their registry are key for you to remember and believe in:

- 78% eat breakfast every day
- 75% weigh themselves at least once a week
- 90% exercise, on average, about one hour per day

Here are the 26 beliefs I developed. Make sure to read these over and over and over until they become second nature. That's how important they are!

#1 Believe in the Power of Your Mind
#2 Believe in Understanding Why Diets Fail
#3 Believe in the Power of Words
#4 Believe in Discovering Why You Eat
#5 Believe in Knowing Your Numbers
#6 Believe in the Power of Substitution
#7 Believe in Going Slow and Going Small
#8 Believe in the Importance of Knowledge
#9 Believe in Honesty and Sharing
#10 Believe in Learning All About Processed Foods
#11 Believe that Added Sugar is Deadly
#12 Believe in the Value of Exercise
#13 Believe in Understanding Carbs, Insulin, Glycemic Index/Load and Leptin
#14 Believe in the Value of Water
#15 Believe that Cheating Never Works
#16 Believe in Visualizing Your Way to Success
#17 Believe that Myths and Misinformation Can Derail You
#18 Believe that You Must Understand Fat
#19 Believe that Regular and Diet Soda are Very Bad for You
#20 Believe in the Power of Timing
#21 Believe in Frequent Milestones
#22 Believe in Learning About Genetically Modified Foods
#23 Believe in Teaching Your Children Well
#24 Believe in Sleep's Important Role in Weight Loss
#25 Believe that Empty Calories are Horrible for You
#26 Believe that You Need to Forget Most of What You Know About Weight Loss

I finished writing this book in early September, 2013.

Everything I believe in and have written about throughout *The Mind Diet* was recently confirmed by research from Harvard, summarized in this excellent article at one of my favorite health information sites, www.Mercola.com. Read the article and watch the video, and then keep reading this book! Go here: http://tinyurl.com/lowfzes.

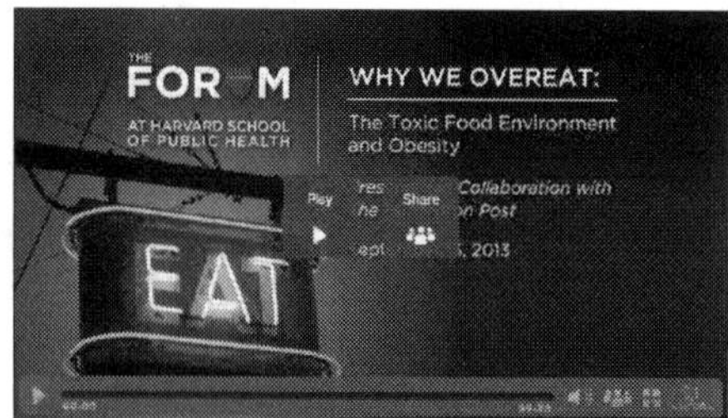

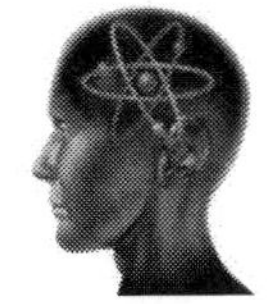

Belief #1

Believe in the Power of Your Mind

If there is one thing I've learned, it is that the power of my mind is an amazing thing.

Once I made up my mind, developed and embraced these beliefs, losing weight became profoundly easier. No longer was I tempted by junk food and my new outlook enabled me to say "no" in almost any tempting situation.

I found myself saying over and over to myself that our minds are so incredibly powerful, leading me to conclude that when you truly have reached your Moment of Truth by absolutely making up your mind, then your mind will reward you by making this journey much easier.

It makes sense. When you think about what you've achieved in life, such as a great marriage, excelling in a sport or having a successful career, you made up your mind to do everything humanly possible to reach that success.

Over time, you developed beliefs about how you were going to reach your goals. In terms of a great marriage or relationship, you probably said to yourself that you were going to be honest (your belief #1), communicate with your partner (#2), develop fun activities that you both enjoy (#3) and so forth.

It's also imperative to focus on the long-term goal. That is an important key to weight loss success. Tip #3 from "6 Weight Loss & Diet Tips" at www.wellsphere.com is a cornerstone of *The Mind Diet:* Create a mindset for change with no time limits. Read the article for detail plus five other very good tips.

Rely on your mind once you've truly made it up, embrace the other 25 beliefs in this section, and then just go reach your goal!

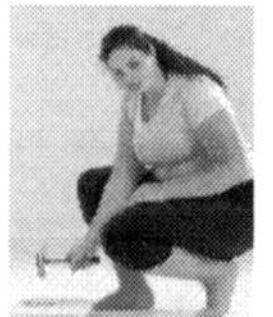

Belief #2

Believe in Understanding Why Diets Fail

It is my conclusion, based on my own experience, extensive research, and talking with a lot of people, that the #1 reason why people fail at *any* kind of diet is that they fail to make an honest and definitive commitment to themselves. There are numerous other reasons (all excuses), but most of them can be traced back to the failure to commit. They are:

- Using food as a reward or a treat after stressful events or when good things happen (I used to do this).
- Believing you can find a quick and easy solution to weight loss, even though intellectually you know it doesn't exist (I did this).
- Thinking you can lose weight by doing it on your own, without any help or advice from health professionals (ditto).
- Expecting major changes without changing your lifestyle (Yeah, that was me).
- Refusing to take personal responsibility for your life – not just weight loss but any aspect that impacts your ability to lose weight and get fit (Sounds familiar).
- Going on diets that do NOT talk about a long-term change in your behavior (did that for a long time).
- Not having a plan, goal and well thought-out strategies (I wish I had done this a long time ago).
- Blaming others when your diet doesn't work, whether out loud or to yourself (well, I didn't do this).
- Not taking the time to learn how foods impact you – negatively or positively, and therefore you can't make informed eating decisions (that was me for sure).
- Eating at "all you can eat" buffets because you want to get your money's worth (could never say "no" to a buffet).
- Skipping breakfast. A University of Minnesota study showed that obesity, high blood pressure, type 2 diabetes and metabolic syndrome was 50% **lower** among those who eat breakfast daily! As reported in *Bottom Line Health,* another study of over

27,000 men over age 45 who reported they regularly skip breakfast, concluded that those who skip this important meal are 27% more likely to suffer heart attacks or die from coronary disease than those who did not skip breakfast.

- Thinking that excess weight is in your genes and that there's nothing you can do about it (yeah, mom and dad were both fat).
- Rationalizing any situation to justify eating what you shouldn't (I was great at that).
- Thinking and believing that pills, powders, drinks and supplements are actually more powerful than they really are (for a while I did).
- Thinking of exercise as work (negative), instead of a positive and enjoyable way to improve your health and your life (that was me).
- Drinking a lot, not thinking that alcohol has calories (fortunately, I don't drink much).
- Watching too much TV, play too many video games or other sedentary things (yep).
- Giving up way too soon and resign yourself to remaining fat (yep again).
- Keeping candies and other sugar-laden foods in the house in case people come over, but you eat it yourself (all the time).
- Thinking that short-term diet sprints instead of long-term slow weight loss is the answer (I was the poster boy for this).
- Looking at a small piece of candy and saying "it's so small…how bad could it be?" and you wind up eating a dozen of them (one of my top rationalizations).
- Thinking "popcorn is so light in weight, how bad can it be?" and you end up eating a lot of it (with extra butter too).
- Taking the advice of others, sometimes even strangers, who don't know what they are talking about, but because what they say "sounds good" you don't research their suggestions (I never questioned their advice, wish I had).
- Not seeking guidance from a doctor and nutrition specialist, the only ones who know your personal situation (now I know better).
- Believing clichés that have been around forever but happen to be untrue, such as "it's OK to eat everything in moderation" or "mom always told me to clean my plate" (yeah, I had a few of these).

- Losing track of your snacks, not realizing how much you've eaten in-between meals (always).

- Loading up on foods marked "low fat" without considering if they are high in sugar (never thought about this). For example, when you remove all the fat out of milk, you're left with too high a concentration of natural sugars. While that may not sound bad, it's not optimal.

- Not drinking enough water (now I do!).

- Skipping meals or fasting for a day or longer (always skipped breakfast).

- Not getting enough sleep (and it wasn't good sleep as well).

- Setting unrealistic goals (yeah, like 20 pounds in one month).

- Taking the drive through at fast food places instead of picking up healthy food at a store (it was easier).

- Taking medications that can cause weight gain, including antidepressants, corticosteroids, antipsychotic and others (thankfully not me).

- Having a thyroid problem or other medical condition (not me either).

- Dieting while quitting smoking (I never smoked).

- Using a diet that is an "artificial" plan that doesn't match your lifestyle (that's for sure).

- Using a "one size fits all" diet that is not customized to your individual situation (guilty again).

- Being impatient wanting to lose weight fast (absolutely).

In addition to these beliefs that result in weight gain, there is another group of factors that impact weight loss. Several researchers (among them Yoni Freedhoff, founder of Ottawa, Canada's Bariatric Medical Clinic) have found that three other factors are better predictors of obesity than the amount of fat in a given diet and the amount of vigorous exercise you do:

- Sleep: the less you get, the greater your chance of being overweight.
- Emotional Eating: the more you eat because of unresolved emotional issues, the heavier you will be.

- Low Calcium Intake: when you're below the daily minimum or the level your doctor indicates, the greater the chance for weight gain.

A reader commented about the last one, "I never heard that before!" That's true of a lot of nuggets in *The Mind Diet* because weight loss is very complicated.

Very few people (myself included until I stumbled upon these studies) think about sleep with respect to weight loss/gain. Here's why:

- Just one night of shortened sleep can raise the level of ghrelin, a hormone that signals your brain to start eating.
- Just two nights of shortened sleep causes a drop in leptin, the hormone that tells your brain when your stomach is full. You'll learn more about leptin later on.

Below is an infographic from The Hartman Group (www.hartman-group.com) that puts these reasons in vivid detail. I've shown the top 10 factors:

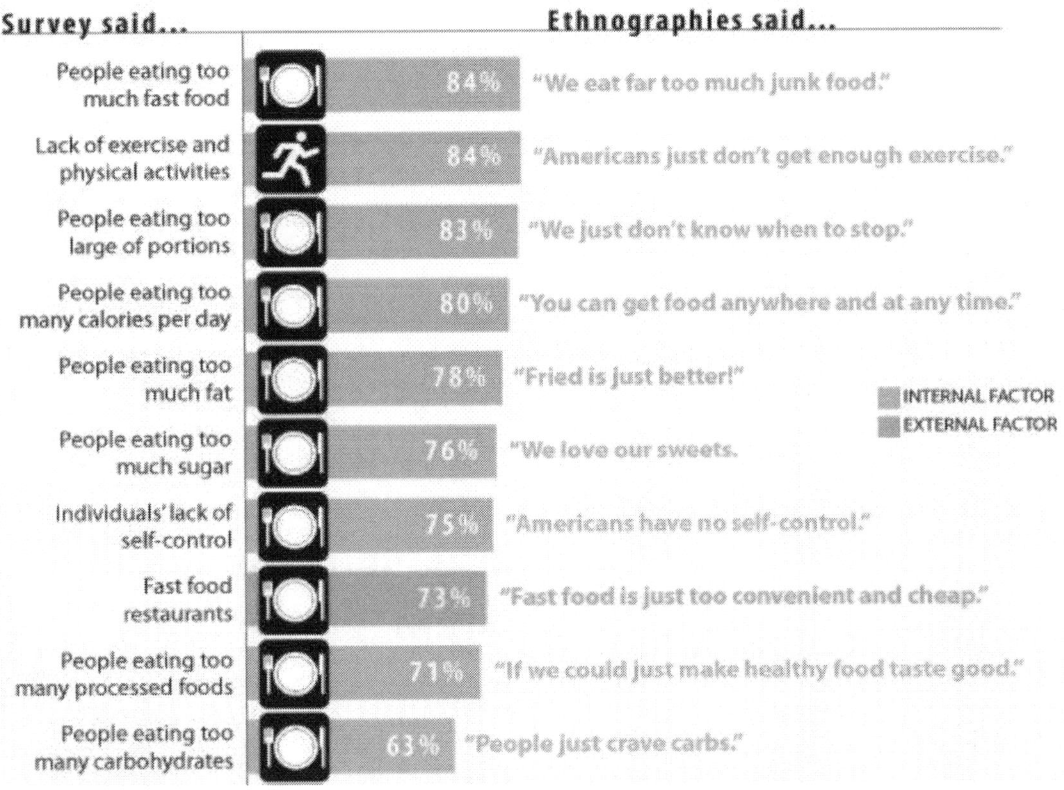

Read this article by Jill Weisenberger, who is the Lifescript Nutrition Expert: http://tinyurl.com/9w9wfa8.

It presents a number of unusual reasons why people don't lose weight, along with recommendations on what to do about it. An example:

You don't have enough muscle. The more muscle you have, the more calories you burn. Fat and muscle tissues consume calories all day long whether you're running, reading or sleeping. No matter what you're doing, muscle rips through more calories than fat. That's why men burn calories a lot faster than women; they have more muscle.

What to do: Lift weights. You don't have to get huge, but building and maintaining muscle week after week, year after year makes a difference in the long run. Registered dietitian and certified personal trainer Marci Anderson has her clients alternate between strength exercises and heart rate-raising cardio in each session. "That way, their strength training includes the calorie-burning effect of cardio."

"25 Reasons You Can't Lose Weight" at http://bodyandsoul.com.au is an excellent summary, and these six popped out at me as ones most people don't realize:

- You're drinking too much coffee. Caffeine stimulates the production of adrenalin which can elevate blood sugars.
- You need more fat. Fat and protein send "don't eat more" signals to our brain, so cutting out all fat can actually retard the process.
- You eat on the run. Picking up whatever is available means you're stuck with what's available – usually junk.
- You eat in the dark. Eating when it's light leads to signals going to our livers to start metabolizing fats.
- You eat with the TV on. Watching TV distracts you from concentrating on what you're eating, so it's easy to forget what you've eaten and just keep eating more.
- Your house is too hot. Reduce your heat by 5 degrees and that will lead to more calories being burned!

Finally, for a steady stream of tips that will help you lose weight, check out Dr. Lazarus' blog: http://tinyurl.com/ldoengp.

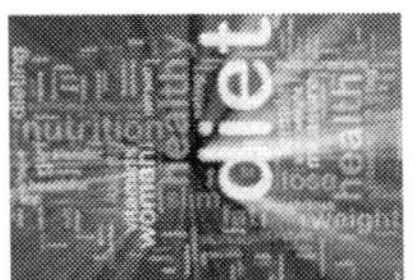

Belief #3

Believe in the Power of Words

This section has three major parts as it relates to words. One is the words we use when we talk or write about losing weight. The second is the words used to describe food that can often mislead us. The third are words used in diet advertising. Finally, there's a bonus list of words commonly substituted for sugar to throw you off track.

Words Used in the Weight Loss Process

The words we use in the weight loss process are often very revealing. Most people (and I was no exception) say "I'll try to lose weight" or "I'll take a shot at it" or "I'll start dieting and see what happens."

These are all **defeatist** phrases, dooming you to failure. Dieting is the one area where people use these phrases most often. For example, you would never say:

- "I'll try to do a good job."
- "I'll take a shot at marriage."
- "I'll take a vacation without planning for it and see how it goes."

What you should be saying is: "I will absolutely, positively, definitely, without fail and without hesitation, do everything in my power, every single day, to lose weight and keep it off permanently."

You should be repeating a phrase like this one, plus others like "I can't wait to go for my daily walk" or "I'm so pleased at the way I'm beginning to look" or "The heck with that buffet, I don't need all that food!"

Repeating positive thoughts to yourself and saying them out loud is an important top-level strategy that really works. I have done that every day since I started, and will do it every day for the rest of my life!

The power of words goes beyond what to say to yourself and others. It includes a variety of tools to help keep you on track and be more educated about the weight loss process.

Keeping a food diary has been shown to help people learn more and prevent themselves from eating bad foods. Diaries have been made even easier to keep as you can do so on web sites and cell phone applications (apps). While I didn't keep a diary, I wrote down a lot of information which ultimately became *The Mind Diet* collection of guidebooks.

Finally, it is quite common to view the word "diet" as a short-term fix for weight loss. Other terms like "lifestyle change" have become popular in an attempt to position weight loss as a long-term process. Once you've made up your mind, reached your Moment of Truth and have begun the serious weight loss process, what you call the process of losing weight is irrelevant.

I was certainly not afraid to use the word "diet" in the title of *The Mind Diet* because it's not important what you call it but how you get your mind around it.

Words Used to Describe Food That Can Mislead Us

As you pay more attention to the food you eat, read labels and think about product names and advertising slogans, you begin to realize that you need to question everything. It is not just words, but photos, drawings and TV commercials that influence our desire to buy and eat certain foods.

All too often people see or hear that a specific food is "home-made" and assume that it's good for you, and don't investigate further. Similar phrases include "Grandma's recipe" and "A recipe handed down for generations."

Words like these create visions of a grandmother or mother in a white apron, making home-cooked meals with amazing aromas that waft throughout the house. While whatever she's cooking will probably taste great, no one is asking for exactly the ingredients she's putting into the pot. Since every grandmother I know wants to get people to eat a lot of what she prepares, it would not surprise me if the ingredients are not the best healthy choices. So while it may be a home-made meal by grandma, there are usually better choices.

Another misleading word-play is "granola." We are led to believe that it is healthy for us. All the advertising and media coverage of granola leads people to assume that granola is good for you. Well, maybe some brands of granola are OK, but many are loaded with sugar. Take a look at the labels of foods that have healthy sounding names or healthy sounding ingredients to see if they are really healthy for you. Here's a list of words that raise a red flag when I see them:

- Wholesome
- Natural, nature
- Light
- Organic
- Healthy
- Heart Healthy, Heart Friendly
- Imitation
- Made with whole grain

- Made with real fruit
- Lowers/Helps Lower Cholesterol
- Fortified
- Low Fat (often has a lot of sugar), No Fat, Fat-Free
- No Trans Fat
- Only 1%
- No preservatives
- No artificial flavors
- Only 100 calories
- Locally grown
- Whole grain
- Omega-3
- Fresh
- Smart
- Balanced
- Optimal
- Ultra, Plus
- Baked, kettle baked
- Real food
- Breakthrough
- Miraculous
- Beverage, drink, cocktail and "ade" – these are clever ways of talking about juices that are not 100% juice and likely are packed with additional calories

Two of the most misleading words are "all-natural" and "organic." Three of "13 Things You Didn't Know About Organic Food" (rd.com) are critical to understand:

- "All-natural" is meaningless. The FDA does not regulate products with the all-natural claim, while foods labeled as organic must adhere to strict standards.
- Organic junk food is still junk food. Organic junk doesn't have artificial ingredients but it still has all the fat, sugar and calories.
- When buying produce, an easy way to determine if the food is organic is by looking for a 5-digit code beginning with "9" (while "4" indicates that the food was likely treated with herbicides and/or pesticides.

Generally, foods that are contaminated with the most pesticides, according to the Environmental Working Group, are those where you eat the skin: apples, celery, cherry tomatoes, cucumbers, grapes, hot peppers, imported nectarines, peaches, potatoes, spinach, strawberries, sweet bell peppers, kale/collard greens and summer squash – for these, consider buying organic.

Clean foods, typically protected by skins, where you don't need to buy organic, include: asparagus, avocado, cabbage, cantaloupe, corn, eggplant, grapefruit, kiwi, mango, mushrooms, onion, pineapple, sweet peas and sweet potatoes.

Finally, pay attention to serving size, for that often is a sleight of hand. While it doesn't involve words, it does involve numbers.

In order to be able to claim the **least** amount of calories, saturated fat, sugar and other ingredients that are not good for you, they play with the serving size. If the serving size listed is greater than one, then you need to do some math to determine your actual caloric intake.

If the "servings per container" is two, that means there are two servings in the package. **It also means that the numbers quoted for calories, fat, etc. must be multiplied by two if you plan to eat the entire package of food**. Many people don't look at the serving size and **assume** that the entire candy bar, bag of chips or whatever contains the percentages and amounts listed. And you know what they say about that word "assume!"

Another misleading concept is the 100-calorie packets or bite-size pieces. While on the surface this may seem like a good thing, you may be tempted to eat twice as many of something that's half the size – not a good idea!

The most important word to be on the lookout for is hydrogenation and its alternate forms: hydrogenated and partially hydrogenated. One of the most common ingredients used in food is "partially hydrogenated" oil, also known as trans-fat. Many experts think of trans-fat as being poisonous to the body.

When you eat fats other than trans-fat, it's important to know that it takes your body 18 days to metabolize (produce energy) half the fat eaten. With trans-fat, it takes 51 days, almost three times as long. The hydrogenation process that food manufacturers utilize is unacceptable, especially when there are substitutes for trans-fat that it makes no sense to even consider eating foods with trans-fat in them. The point here is to look for what has become a synonym of trans-fat: hydrogenation, and make sure you don't buy anything with those words on the label.

Bottom Line's *Food Lies & Dirty Labeling Tricks* reports that some labels that show 0% trans-fat actually contain partially hydrogenated soybean oil, which they call "hidden trans-fat," which is just as bad for you. Michael Jacobsen of the Center for Science in the Public Interest, refers to trans-fat as a "metabolic poison."

Studies conducted at two universities reported in the *WellnessLetter.com* showed that dieters rated a dish called a "salad" higher than a "pasta" dish even though the ingredients were identical! Dieters ate more candies when they were named "fruit chews" than "candy chews." Don't be misled by names that companies and restaurants dream up that might be misleading.

Do you know the difference between "reduced sugar," "low sugar" and "no sugar added?" Most people don't. Here's the scoop, writes Stacey Colino in Real Simple:

- Reduced sugar means that product contains 25% less sugar than the original one.
- Low sugar isn't even a regulated term so it can actually mean anything.
- No sugar added means that no sugar was introduced during the production of the food item, but does not always mean the product is low in sugar.

Registered dietician Kari Koo at the Methodist Hospital in Houston in a *HealthDay* article, explains that another side effect of misleading terminology is the "health halo." The health halo effect occurs when people consume more foods marketed as healthy than they should, not realizing that these foods are not as healthy as they think.

Koo says that "We need to educate consumers on how to read nutrition labels so they can avoid falling prey to the 'health halo' effect." Examples of the halo effect:

- Vegetable chips: very similar to regular potato chips; however many of the vegetables' nutrients are lost in the processing of the chips.
- Nutrient-enhanced water: it's more like sugar-enhanced drinks with minimal if any nutritional value.
- Muffins: they are basically cupcakes without the icing; large ones can contain 500 to 600 calories each!
- Premade smoothies: loaded with sugar and calories. They may be smooth, but not very healthy because they don't have much nutritional value.
- Frozen yogurt: while they may be fat-free, they are loaded with sugar. Plus, the cultures can't survive freezing, so you won't get any probiotic benefits.

Words Used in Diet Advertising

The Federal Trade Commission (FTC) has targeted diet product marketers that use false or misleading claims in their advertising. They fall into seven categories:

1. "Causes weight loss of two pounds or more a week for a month or more without dieting or exercise." This claim is usually found in ads for supplements. FTC advises that no supplement causes substantial weight loss by itself.
2. "Causes substantial weight loss, no matter what or how much the consumer eats." Obviously totally false.
3. "Causes permanent weight loss, even when the consumer stops using the product." No evidence that this is true.
4. "Blocks the absorption of fat or calories to enable consumers to lose substantial weight." FTC doesn't believe over-the-counter fat blockers work.
5. "Safely enables consumers to lose more than three pounds per week, for more than four weeks." Rapid weight loss like this is risky, sometimes fatal. A bad idea to buy a product that claims this.
6. "Causes substantial weight loss for all users." Even the best prescription weight loss drugs are only effective for ⅓ to ½ of consumers.

7. "Causes substantial weight loss by wearing it on the body or rubbing it into the skin." FTC believes patches and creams do not work at all.

Alternative Names for Sugar

It is also imperative to be knowledgeable of alternate names for sugar as this list (from www.dietblog.com) defines. Many of these are designed to make you think you're actually eating something healthy. "Turbinado" sounds like it might be healthy, right, but in reality it is just another name for sugar like these:

- Galactose
- Brown sugar
- Molasses
- Treacle
- Maple syrup
- Corn syrup
- Demerara sugar
- Dextrose
- Free flowing brown sugar
- Fructose
- High fructose corn syrup (HFCS)
- Honey
- Muscovado sugar
- Barbados sugar
- Invert sugar
- Lactose
- Malt, maltodextrin
- Panocha
- Powdered sugar
- Confectioner's sugar
- Rice syrup
- Granulated sugar
- Florida crystals
- Hyrolyzed starch
- Polydextrose
- Evaporated cane juice
- Beet sugar
- Grape sugar
- Caramel
- Raw sugar

Test your knowledge about sugar and sweeteners with this short quiz from WebMD: http://tinyurl.com/l8r6h2n.

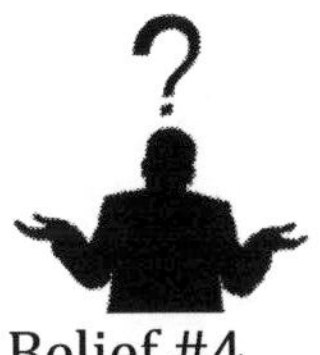

Belief #4

Believe in Discovering Why You Eat

Sometimes we eat for the sheer joy of the taste of the food. In those cases, we have not a care in the world, and we eat for no other reason than for taste.

In most cases, however, this is not the case. For most people, unnecessary eating is something we do as a reaction to something else that happened or didn't happen. In a society where food is plentiful and easy to get, food has become a band-aid, a short term fix, for a wide range of reasons, mostly negative. While we all celebrate special occasions, milestones and other good events, too many people turn negative happenings into excuses for eating.

Understanding why you eat is a critical strategy, for once you recognize them, you'll be able to resist food. You've got to get to the point where food is not used to cope with a problem. Here are a bunch of examples:

- **People problems**. Your boss reamed you out, or your best friend lied to you, or your mother/father/sibling/child did something that upset you. The answer is to resolve the problem, not eat a quart of ice cream.
- **Money problems**. You're having financial issues and you eat to take your mind off those issues. While resolving money issues can take a long time, recognizing that eating food is not the answer is relatively easy. Spend the time you spend over-eating investigating solutions to your money dilemma.
- **Anger issues.** You're mad about something: the economy, violence around the world, politicians or even how your team is performing. Food isn't going to help. Focus your energy on aspects of your life that make you mad that you can actually impact. You're not going to be able to do anything about a war across the globe, so eating to feel better about it is pointless.
- **Pressure problems.** You feel intense pressure to perform on the job, in your relationships and can't seem to deal with this pressure, so you eat. This happens all the time. Eating doesn't solve the core problem, which is something you need to do.
- **Stressors.** Quite possibly the most common reason people eat is stress, whether it be stress from people, work or any other aspect of life. Why do you think it's called "comfort food?" A big part of weight loss success is dealing with the actual stressors and not using food as a band-aid.

All of these issues can change one's mood. When that happens, often the result is eating in an attempt to improve the mood, which, of course, never works.

In fact, an interesting study from the U.K.'s Open University and reported in *Prevention* proved that chocolate and alcohol are not effective at improving peoples' moods long-term. What is effective and has zero calories is looking at personal photos. That's right! Look at photos to improve your mood instead of scarfing down food!

Even worse, the CDC states that 85% of disease is caused by emotions. Get your emotions and stress under control and you'll lose weight much easier and reduce your risk for contracting a wide range of diseases.

Dr. Roger Gould, author of *Shrink Yourself* (ShrinkYourself.com) has identified 12 types of emotional hunger, which he has used to help people break the emotional bonds of emotional eating for decades. They are:

Type 1. Dulling The Pain With The Food Trance.

If you get hungry when you feel angry, depressed, anxious, bored, or lonely, you suffer from Type 1 emotional hunger, and you use food to dull the pain that these emotions cause.

Type 2. Sticks And Stones May Break Your Bones, But Cake Won't Heal What Hurts You.

If you react by getting hungry when others talk down to you, take advantage of you, belittle you or take you for granted, then you suffer from Type 2 emotional hunger. You eat to avoid confrontation.

Type 3. A Full Heart Fills An Empty Belly.

If you crave food when you have tension in your close relationships, you suffer from Type 3 emotional hunger. You eat to avoid feeling the pain of rejection or anger.

Type 4. Hate Yourself, Love Your Munchies.

If you tend to become hypercritical of yourself, if you label yourself "stupid," "lazy," or "a loser," you have Type 4 emotional hunger. You eat to "stuff down" your self-hatred.

Type 5. Secret Desires Have No Calories.

If your hunger gets activated because your intimate relationships don't satisfy some basic need like trust or security, you suffer from Type 5 emotional hunger and you use food to try to fill the gap.

Type 6. Forty Million Big Gulps And The Well Is Still Empty.

If you stuff yourself to make up for the deprivation you experienced as a child, you have Type 6 emotional hunger

Type 7. It's My Pastry, and I'll Eat If I Want To.

If you eat to assert your independence because you don't want anyone telling you what to do, you have Type 7 emotional hunger.

Type 8. I Can't Come To Work Today – I'm Too Fat.

If your appetite kicks in when you're faced with new challenges – if you use food to avoid rising to the test, or to insulate yourself from the fear of failure – you have Type 8 emotional hunger.

Type 9. Aroused by Aromas, Not by the Chef.

If you eat in order to avoid your sexuality-either to stay fat so that nobody desires you or to hide from intimate encounters--you suffer from Type 9 emotional eating.

Type 10. I'll Beat You With this Eclair.

Type 10 emotional eaters stuff themselves to pay back those who have hurt them, often in the distant past. They use their bodies as battlegrounds for working out old resentments.

Type 11. Peter Pan and the Peanut Butter Cookie.

If you eat to make yourself feel carefree, like a child, you have Type 11 emotional hunger. You eat to keep yourself from facing the challenges of growing up.

Type 12. That Stranger In Lycra Wearing Your Face.

If you overeat because you fear getting thin, either consciously or unconsciously, you have Type 12 emotional hunger.

The more you understand why you eat, the faster you'll be able to solidify your Moment of Truth and be successful losing weight and keeping if off permanently.

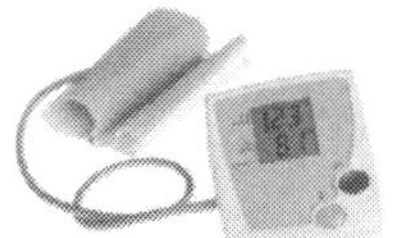

Belief #5

Believe in Knowing Your Numbers

There are several numbers established by the medical and nutritional communities that you should to know as they are generally accepted benchmarks. I suggest you print this section and keep it with you, so that you can consult it on a regular basis. Knowing these numbers is critical to your success, and seeing where you stand in relation to recommended values will help you identify weaknesses. Of course, this is not meant to replace advice from your doctor and dietician.

NUTRITIONAL DAILY VALUES

Based on a 2,000-calorie per day goal, these nutritional values may vary based on your particular caloric needs. These are found on most food labels.

Ingredient	**Maximum Intake**
Total Fat	65 grams
Saturated Fat	20 grams
Cholesterol	300 milligrams
Sodium	2400 milligrams
Potassium	3500 milligrams
Total Carbohydrates	300 grams
Dietary Fiber	25 grams

COMMON NUMBERS FROM BLOOD TESTS

Total Cholesterol	< 200 mg/DL
LDL "Bad" Cholesterol	< 129 mg/DL
HDL "Good" Cholesterol	> 60 mg/DL
Triglycerides	<150 mg/DL
Blood Sugar	<72 mg/DL

BODY MEASUREMENT

Body Mass Index (BMI)

Normal:	18.5 to 25
Overweight:	Above 25 to 29.9
Obese:	30 to 39.9
Morbidly Obese:	40 to 49.9
Super Obese:	50 and over

You can find an excellent BMI calculator here: http://www.webmd.com/diet/calc-bmi-plus

There is plenty of discussion about the validity of BMI. It's just one factor, reliable in certain situations (over 30) and not in others (athletes). Use it as a general guideline, in addition to your total weight and general health.

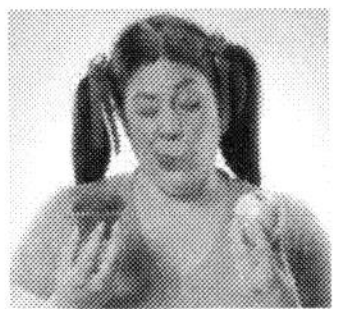

Belief #6

Believe in the Power of Substitution

Ever since I was a young adult, I have only consumed diet soda. This came after I became aware of how much sugar is in regular soda. But, several years ago, I came across studies that showed that the ingredients in diet sodas are just as bad for you.

I looked for an alternative to regular and diet sodas – I love the carbonation and taste – and discovered flavored seltzer. It's been years since I've had diet soda, and switching to flavored seltzer has been easy, healthy and has saved me a lot of money. I figure I save at least $1 a day over diet soda, which is about $365 per year! That's one great example of the power of substitution. And if you haven't had seltzer in a while, there are numerous natural flavors: orange, lemon lime, vanilla, cherry, mandarin, pomegranate and many more!

Another example of substitution is the Muscle Maker Grill. I came across the sign in the window of their store, reproduced below. Besides being a great marketing concept, it highlights the art of substitution and how important it is for our diets. They figured out how to make healthy food taste great, and that's why they are very successful chain. It's critical to adopt this "substitution mentality" as you plan your weight loss strategies.

What Sets Muscle Maker Grill apart from Fast Food Restaurants?

Muscle Maker Grill	Fast Food
No Deep Fryers	Deep Fryers
Whole Wheat Bread	Heavily Processed White Flour
Zero Fat Sour Cream	Full Fat Sour Cream
No Butter - 0 Carb 0 Fat 0 Calorie Spray	Fatty Butter
Zero Carb Signature Sauce	Secret Sauces Full of Hidden Carbs
Salad Dressings - Fat-Free or Zero Carb	All Dressings Full of Fat and Carbs
Whole Wheat Pasta	Processed White Flour Pasta
Brown Rice	Regular Cheap White Rice
Fresh, Never Frozen Lean Chicken Breast	Always Frozen Chicken "Parts"
Chicken Trimmed Lean / No Heavy Batter	Can't Tell It's Chicken From Heavy Batter
USDA Choice Steak	From "Somewhere?" Steak
All Cheese Lower Fat Portions	Every Cheese Full of Fat
Low Fat Turkey Meatballs and Turkey Bacon	Full Fat Beef, Pork and Veal
No Cream Vodka Sauces	Heavy Creams Full of Fat
Low Carb Wrap Available	Full Carb Wraps

Substitutions have been one of the easiest and most practical ways of losing weight. Once you get the hang of it, it's really simple to carry out on a daily basis. Here are a slew of examples:

Food Substitutions

- Replace steel cut oats for instant oatmeal.
- Use salad dressings where you mix ingredients vs. readymade – off-the-shelf dressings usually contain trans fats, denatured fats, excessive sugar and/or HFCS, artificial colors, preservatives and sweeteners – none of which are healthy.
- Drink black coffee with a little skim milk vs. "fancy" coffee drinks loaded with calories from whole milk, whipped cream, sugar and sugary syrups.
- Replace bottled tea with brewed tea and get 85mg more antioxidants and eliminate added sugar.
- Take your coffee with a few shakes of cinnamon instead of milk.
- Use flavorings, such as low-sugar sauces, salsa and seasonings to replace butter, cream-based and sugary sauces.
- Switch from regular milk to 2%...or from 2% to 1%...or 1% to skim. Every step downward cuts calories by 20% or so.
- Get protein from plants instead of animals, as animal protein diets will have saturated fat vs. unsaturated fat found in plant proteins, which include beans, Brussels sprouts, couscous, lentils and almonds.
- Replace unhealthy fats (butter, whole milk, fatty beef cuts, hydrogenated vegetable oils) with healthier fats found in nut butters, seeds, avocados, oils, canola, flaxseed and walnuts (women who eat walnuts are less likely to develop type 2 diabetes).
- Eat fresh fruit instead of fruit juice, which typically has sweeteners added. *I came across a fascinating fact in Prevention that underscores this substitution suggestion. In an 18-year study of 70,000 women, researchers found that for every 3 servings of fruit that they ate per day, they slashed their diabetes risk by 18%. But for those who drank one cup of fruit juice a day, their risk increased by almost the same amount!*
- Eat fresh fruit instead of processed and canned/bottled fruit, unless they are marked as not sweetened.
- As a change of pace, use ground turkey instead of ground beef.
- Instead of all great tasting high-fat cheese or all not-so-tasty low-fat cheese, mix the two types together.
- When eating out or at home, substitute organic eggs for regular eggs.
- Eat fresh fruit instead of dried fruit.
- Buy fresh food instead of frozen.
- Drink 100% fresh fruit juice, not concentrate from cans.
- Eat strawberries instead of other less nutritious fruits – strawberries have the highest total antioxidant power among major fruits.
- Replace half-and-half and 3 sugar packets with your coffee to skim milk and 1 sugar (you'll save 27,700 calories, equal to 8 pounds in a year).
- Same with vegetables – eat fresh instead of processed and canned/bottled.

- Choose white meat (fish and fowl) instead of red meat (beef and pork).
- Change from regular butter to cholesterol-free butter.
- Instead of mayo made with bad oils, use mayo made from good oils that are low in saturated fat and has no trans-fat.
- Instead of frying foods with oil or butter, try baking them, which requires lesser or no oil or fat.
- Cook only with coconut oil instead of other oils as heat damages them.
- Replace bad fats (saturated, trans) with good fats (polyunsaturated and monounsaturated).
- Replace bad carbs (simple) with good carbs (complex).
- Replace salt (which is no good for you and retards the weight loss process) with any of 50 different spices, such as cinnamon, garlic, onion and pepper, many of which are available in dry form, so you can bring a small bottle to a restaurant and sprinkle spice on your steak instead of salt.
- Replace movie theater buttered popcorn with, well, almost anything else, or better yet, eat before you go to the movies, or just buy a big water or seltzer and stay away from food altogether – if you can't resist a snack at the theater, check out iVillage's "Which Is Worse? At The Movies" quiz at: http://tinyurl.com/m7hh7s6.
- Dark vegetables are generally better than green and light veggies.
- Dark green lettuce (i.e. romaine) is better than light green (i.e. iceberg).
- Replace white bread with whole grain bread.
- Eat brown rice instead of white rice.
- Eat an orange instead of orange juice, because OJ has had all the fiber squeezed out of it, making the natural sugars more dangerous.
- Alternate oatmeal with eggs.
- Replace a milkshake with a smoothie without any sugar added to it.
- Instead of onion dip, use hummus.
- Eat applesauce instead of pudding.

Noted author, Registered Dietitian and advisor to sporting teams, Cynthia Sass points out in www.health.com that if you eat one blueberry muffin a week, and replace it with one cup of fresh blueberries, you'll save almost 20,000 calories over a year, enough to lose 5 pounds just with this one substitution!

For thousands of food swaps that can help you lose weight, check out David Zinczenko's book, "Eat This, Not That!" which goes into great detail about swapping good foods for bad ones.

Clever Substitutions

You can get really creative and practical when making food substitutions. Here are a few from eDiets:

- Try pureed cauliflower for mashed potatoes – great taste and texture.

- Replace 2oz oil with cooking spray and save 540 calories and 60g of fat.
- Do away with rice by pulsing raw broccoli in a food processor until the pieces are about the size of rice grains – then stir-fry or steam.
- Replace sour cream with plain non-fat yogurt and save 803 calories and 89g of fat (one pint).

Portion Substitutions

- Order wine by the glass, not the bottle, so you drink moderately, and add seltzer to make a spritzer and reduce the amount of alcohol.
- Order a cup of mushroom soup instead of a bowl (cut calories in half) and order non-cream-based soup as well.
- When you're in a restaurant, ask your server to put half of your meal in a doggie-bag BEFORE it's brought to your table; not only does it help you lose weight, but you get two meals for the price of one; and be very specific on how you want your food to be prepared – i.e. grilled chicken without any sauces or seasonings (which often contain sugar) – tips from BioTrust Nutrition newsletter.

Pantry Substitutions

- Replace anything in your pantry that's made with white flour (white bread, rolls, cake and pancake mixes, pasta, noodles, etc.) with whole grain alternatives (wheat and other whole grains).
- Replace vegetable oils with olive oil.
- Get rid of margarine in favor of unsalted butter and other healthy spreads.
- Get rid of all the candies and cookies and replace them with nuts, fresh fruit, crisp breads, yogurt and natural peanut butter.
- Replace any drink sweetened with sugar with unsweetened, diet, or simply water.

Cooking Substitutions

- Keep serving platters/bowls of fattening food OFF the table where you eat and keep bowls of salad, veggies and fruit ON the table.
- Replace larger plates with smaller ones (we have two size dinner plates, so we use the smaller ones).

Activities Substitutions

- Have a light dinner and go dancing (or whatever) instead of a heavy 4-course meal and watching TV or a movie.
- Cook at home instead of going out to eat – you control what goes into the food, not a chef or cook in a restaurant.

"Zero Substitutions" – Become a "Food Purist!"

I've become a food purist. I don't put ketchup that contains high fructose corn syrup on a hamburger. I enjoy the pure taste of the burger without adding anything. Other examples: no salt on steak, no bacon on eggs, no high-sugar marinade on chicken. Food tastes better when it's pure...try it!

One of the most fascinating companies I've come across is NuVal. They have developed a scoring method that takes into account numerous factors and assigns one number to each food. The higher the number, the more nutritious it is for you. At NuVal.com you'll find a wealth of resources including their "Trade Up" section that follows my philosophy on substitutions as described in this section. I think this is one of the best and easiest ways to know which foods are best. A few examples from the Trade Up area on their site:

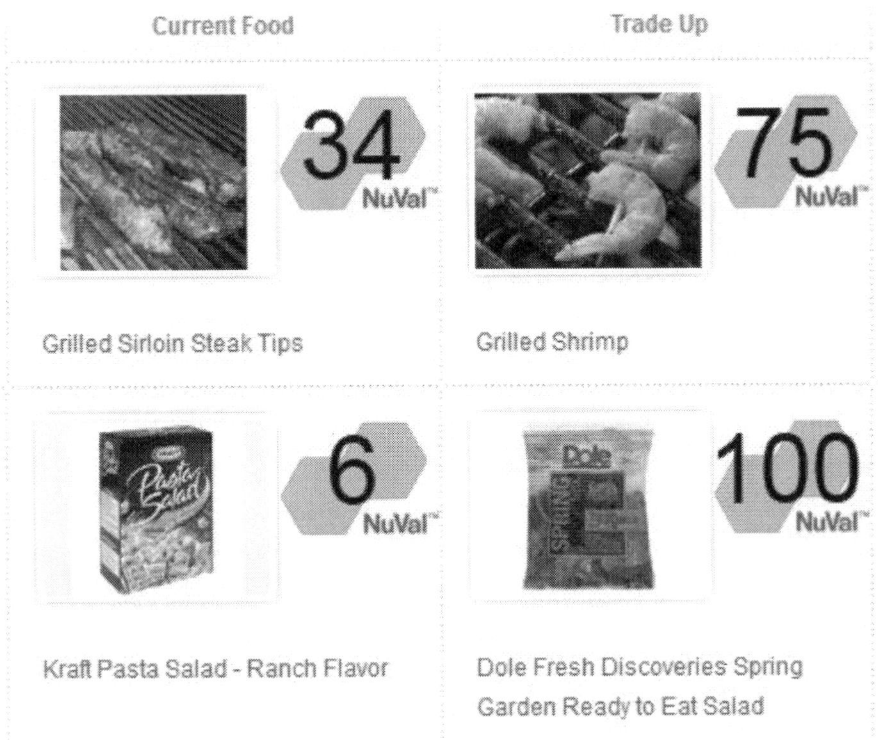

I hope the NuVal system is embraced by every store in the world that sells food!

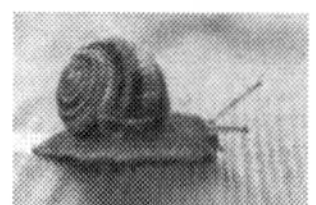

Belief #7

Believe in Going Slow and Going Small

Slow

These two "S" words are among the most important when it comes to losing weight. Slow is better than fast. Small is better than large.

Eating food slowly, losing weight slowly and eating small portions are hallmarks of successful weight loss and will enable you to keep it off permanently.

Conversely, eating food fast, losing weight fast and not watching portions are hallmarks of weight loss failures. We all know that when you lose weight fast, the likelihood is very high that you will put it all back on, and then some. Our bodies are just not built to deal with rapid weight loss.

Another benefit of eating slowly is chewing longer. The result is that your food is digested more effectively. Most of your digestive enzymes are in your mouth, not in your stomach as most people believe. The longer you chew, the better the breakdown of that food will be! Digestion is also aided by the saliva in your mouth – the longer you chew, the more the saliva can interact with your foods.

One of my favorite bloggers, Darya Rose (www.SummerTomato.com) presents 12 tips to help you eat more slowly:

- **Practice eating slowly**. Constantly remind yourself that eating slow is critical to losing weight.
- **Sit at a table**. When you eat "on the run," you quickly forget how much you have eaten. At a table, you're more focused.
- **Serve small portions**. We tend to clean our plates, a habit that's been passed down from generation to generation. If you start with a smaller plate, you'll eat less food.
- **Remove distractions**. Eating while watching TV takes your mind off the food, and you tend to eat more. For a 15-20 minute meal, turn off the tube.
- **Chew**. The more you chew each piece of food, the longer it takes to eat, the fuller you become and the greater the taste sensation.
- **Drink.** Constantly drinking during the meal will make you feel fuller and consequently you'll eat less food.
- **Put your fork down**. By putting your fork or spoon down, you'll take more time to eat and you can focus on chewing slowly, instead of focusing on getting the next forkful ready to eat.

- **Have a conversation**. The more you talk, the less you'll eat, because it will add time to your meal, resulting in a feeling of being full faster.
- **Eat with other slow eaters**. We tend to imitate other people, consciously or unconsciously. If you have a friend that is an eating speed-demon, don't eat with her/him if possible.
- **Don't eat when you're starving**. When hunger pangs strike, grab a healthy snack like nuts instead of scarfing down a big meal. A little food will help the pangs subside.
- **Dim the lights**. Dim lighting induces an inner calm, leading to slower eating. Bright lights can lead to faster eating.
- **Play mellow music**. As with light, mellow music enhances your mood to eat slower.

Eating slowly means avoiding the "quick fixes" that are heavily promoted, including starvation, extremely low calorie intake, magic pills, cleanses, detox plans, purging, extreme exercising, drugs and tobacco. AARP.org suggests taking at least 30 minutes to eat, because it takes your brain about 20 minutes to have a sensation of feeling full.

Eating slowly is a common recommendation by experts. Registered dietician and author Cynthia Sass urges people to eat slowly because "eating too quickly curtails the release of hormones that induce feelings of fullness, which can trigger mindless overeating."

Tens of millions of people try rapid weight loss programs with minimal success. Nia Shanks writes on her blog (www.niashanks.com) that rapid weight loss programs fail for five reasons:

- The method required to achieve drastic immediate results can't be sustained long-term.
- The plan is too stressful and complicated, so people give up soon after starting it.
- You always expect and refuse to settle for anything less than immediate results.
- The program doesn't teach you how to achieve and maintain results long-term.
- Some of these programs can lead to obsessive compulsive and harmful eating habits.

As I like to say, anyone can lose weight. **Hardly** anyone can keep it off. Rapid weight loss always results in the weight coming back on. This is a critical lesson!

To understand the "why" behind eating slowly, this article is well worth reading: http://tinyurl.com/l9g6anj.

In medical programs with proper medical supervision, lab monitoring, EKG monitoring, nutritional monitoring, significantly quicker weight loss results are achievable and safe. But, do-it-yourself rapid weight loss without medical and nutritional monitoring is not advised at all!

Small

Most of us eat too much food, that's obvious. How and why we eat too much can be directly linked to **portion size** and **cleaning our plates**.

Restaurants discovered a long time ago that by having overflowing plates and "all you can eat" stuff-you-face buffets, their businesses thrived. After all, who doesn't like to pay a relatively low fixed price and eat whatever they want and as much as they want.

Clearly you won't lose weight if you eat everything on a buffet. What about when you order a la carte or eat at home? The same sort of thing happens, but it involves eating every morsel on your plate.

"Cleaning your plate" has been an order from moms and dads for decades, and it has resulted in the continuance of that practice as adults, and possibly even for our kids.

In fact, an AICR (American Institute for Cancer Research) survey showed that 69% of us say that we finish all of our restaurant entrees all or most of the time; 30% say they based the amount of food they eat on the amount of food that they are served; and 42% determine their portions by the amount they are used to eating.

For excellent tips on how to easily remember portion sizes, read "11 Tips for Controlling Your Portions" from iVillage, here: http://tinyurl.com/ku3fnzr. To see portion sizes in a nifty graphical way, see this from WebMD: http://tinyurl.com/l34dqgl.

To boil it down, we eat whatever is put in front of us, and we repeat those behaviors over and over again, in restaurants and at home. Clearly that's not a very good idea. Back in 2013, Los Angeles county ran ads designed to encourage people to simply eat less food with the slogan "Choose less, weigh less" according to L.A. County Supervisor Zev Yaroslavsky. L.A. county officials point out that 70% of adults in the county are overweight.

One of the most valuable lessons I learned from my dietician was what portions look like. She had food models that made it easy to visualize how a portion of steak or chicken looks. Because portion sizes are so important, you need to know how to estimate them accurately or you'll retard your weight loss activities.

There's something else you need to know. Back in 2003, NYU compared the maximum allowable size of foods and drinks when they were introduced vs. 2003. Because of changes in these rules, food and drink producers can produce larger and larger sizes in order to entice us, and most people tend to eat all of what's put in front of them or what they order. This is one of those "hidden" things you never think about. Examples:

Product	Year Introduced	Maximum Allowable Size Then	Now
Bottled Beer	1976	7oz	40oz
Chocolate Bar	1908	0.6oz	8oz
French Fries	1954	2.6oz	6.9oz
Fountain Soda	1954	12oz	64oz

And here's a visual way to look at how dramatically food portions have increased in the last 60+ years:

The New (AB)normal

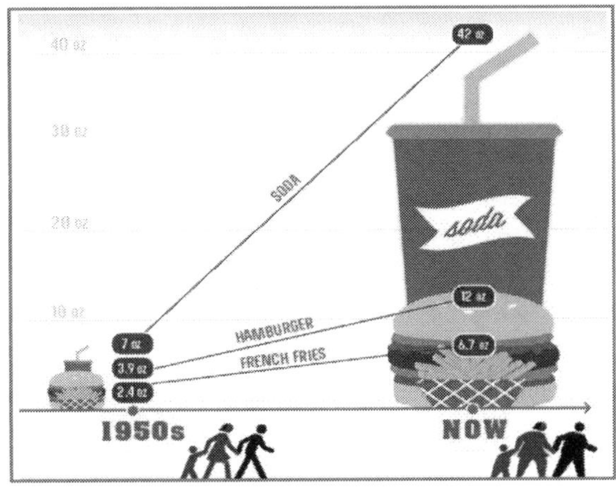

In terms of going small, I'm reminded of a quote by Robert Collier: "Success is the sum of small efforts, repeated day in and day out."

As reported in BlissTree.com, the city of Los Angeles embarked on an anti-obesity campaign that featured great ads designed to get people to understand how much food they should be eating to lose weight:

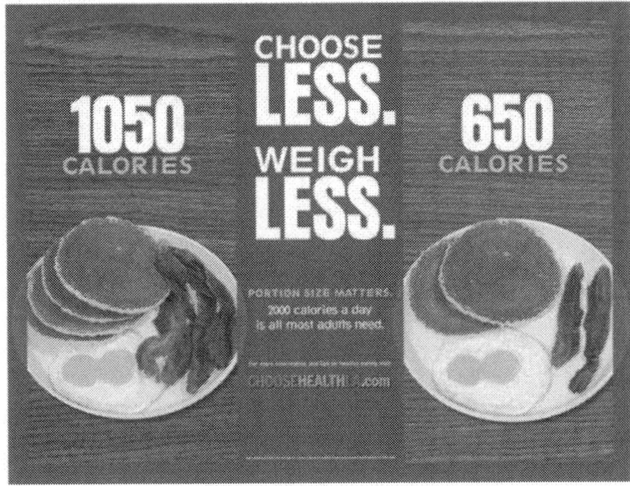
1050
CALORIES
CHOOSE
LESS.
WEIGH
LESS.
650
CALORIES
PORTION SIZE MATTERS.
2000 calories a day
is all most adults need.

Choosing less can be as simple as understanding what kinds of dishes at restaurants are good or bad for you. The Center for Science in the Public Interest underscored this with a comparison of two dishes from Long John Silver's restaurant:

- "The Big Catch" is a piece of fried haddock, hush puppies and the choice of a side. Lab tests showed 33 grams of trans fat, 19 grams of saturated fat, 3700 milligrams of sodium and 1,320 calories in this meal.
- On the same menu, you can order "Hold the Batter Shrimp" or "Hold the Batter Cod" which has zero trans fat, zero saturated fat and both are about 100 calories.

That's an astounding difference, but making the right choice is in your hands!

There's another aspect to "slow," and that is something that Dr. Ethan Lazarus pointed out while reviewing this book. He noted that "small changes often lead to large changes in health." The Diabetes Prevention Program found that a 7% reduction in weight reduces diabetes by a whopping 58%. The Centers for Disease Control is basing recommendations on this, and other agencies and organizations are behind the fact that small amounts of weight loss (5% to 10%) provide the greatest risk reduction for health problems.

For a 200 pound person, 7% is only 14 pounds, a goal that is realistic and attainable. So don't think that you need to lose an enormous amount of weight to get any benefit – the opposite is true in reality!

While the percentage of body weight lost is one measure of progress, there are others which I address in Strategy #63. It's really all about changing your behavior, which results in actual weight loss.

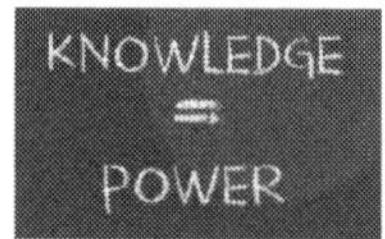

Belief #8

Believe in the Importance of Knowledge

The more you know about every aspect of losing weight, the more weight you will lose and keep it off. There are so many misconceptions, misinformation and misunderstandings about food, dieting and health. Key points of knowledge you need to understand:

- We have a tendency to eat when we <u>see</u> food, even if we're not hungry and even if we've eaten recently. Hence the joke "I'm on the see-food diet" where I see food and eat it. All kidding aside, stick to the game plan in terms of when you eat, and don't be tempted by food just because it's there.

- When we sit down to eat, our brains are looking for **nutrients**, not calories. The more empty calories without nutrients you eat, the more your brain will want you to eat more until it gets the nutrients it needs.

- Ever wonder what's actually in the fast-food burgers and other "meat" dishes you eat? The U.S. Department of Agriculture (USDA) requires that for products that are labeled as "ground beef" it must contain a minimum of 70% beef and no more than 30% fat.

- If you knew how much exercise it really takes to work off calories from snacks, you'd be shocked. Here are a couple examples from *Nutrition Action Healthletter:*
    - One Crumbs Bake Shop cupcake: over 2 hours strength training
    - One Panera chocolate chip cookie: brisk walking for 1 hour, 30 minutes
    - One piece Starbucks banana nut loaf: swimming for 1 hour, 15 minutes

- Do NOT skip meals. They are all important, especially breakfast and lunch, which is when your body needs nourishment. Skipping meals only leads to overeating when you finally do eat. The National Weight Control Registry found that successful dieters who have kept their weight off never skip breakfast, get an hour of exercise almost every day and they keep a food journal and monitor their weight.

- There are a lot of myths floating around, and I always cringe when I hear someone say, "I heard that organic milk is better for you" or "they said that eat anything you want in moderation." I always ask who is the "they" that they are referring to? Who did you "hear" this from? You can't simply take one's word for it, and you need to investigate whatever people tell you, no matter how close you are to them or how well-intentioned you are.

- When you're faced with choices at a restaurant, it's helpful to have a good idea what dishes are the worst for you. Examples from *Nutrition Action Healthletter*:
    - Cheese ravioli has fewer calories than spaghetti and meatballs, lasagna, eggplant parmesan and chicken parmesan.
    - Tiramisu has fewer calories than a brownie sundae, plain cheesecake, apple crisp a la mode and chocolate lava cake.
    - General Tso's chicken has more calories than beef and broccoli, eggplant in garlic sauce, mu shu pork and combination lo mein.

- One of the most interesting things I learned was that certain oils, when used in cooking, and heated up, wind up being very bad for you. So while olive oil is typically good for you when cold, it is not the best choice for cooking. In terms of oil that is OK to cook with, pure virgin coconut oil is the best. The **worst** oils to cook with are corn, soy, safflower, sunflower and canola.

- Most people think of soy products as being healthy, as a result of advertising and press. But, like with oils, there is a hidden story. There are two kinds of soy products: fermented (good) and unfermented (bad). Fermented soy products include tempeh, miso, natto and soy sauce. Unfortunately, most of the popular soy products are unfermented and not very healthy: soybean oil, soymilk, soy cheese, soy ice cream, soy yogurt, soy "meat," soy protein, edamame and soy infant formula. Soy also happens to be one of the top 8 food allergens. Says Dr. Russell Blaylock, an expert on soy and excitotoxins, and author of several books, "I think people ought to avoid soy products as if they were poison."

- There are three other foods that people believe are healthy for you:
    - Sugar Free Cookies – many have a lot of butter and starch to make up for the lack of sugar.
    - Lowfat Granola – lowfat yes, high sugar yes – even worse!
    - Fat Free Muffin – once again, high in sugar and starch.

- There's been a debate for as long as I can remember about red meat. In a major data from 20 studies involving 1.2 million people, researchers found that those who ate 1 serving of red meat per day were at no greater risk for heart disease than those who ate less than 1 serving per week. However, and this is critical: they also found that 1 serving of **processed meat** (bacon, salami, hot dogs, etc.) eaten every day increased the risk of heart disease by 42% and diabetes by as much as 50%. They found that eating just one sausage a day increases risk of bowel cancer by 20%, and other cancers by 38% to 67%.

- Another debate involves chicken breasts vs. thighs. The facts, according to prevention.com are that thighs are more nutritious, with twice as much iron and three times as much zinc as breasts...and skinless thighs only contain one more gram of fat per serving than skinless breasts. Plus, thighs cost less too!

- Alcohol can make you feel hungry. Alcohol increases your serotonin levels just like carbs. Order a low-calorie drink or something else.

- In a report about food marketing to children, The Yale Rudd Center for Food Policy and Obesity indicates that cereals targeted at children have 57% more sugar and 52% less fiber than cereals marketed to adults.

- It gets worse when it comes to cereals, according to MedicalNewsToday.com. Shredded Wheat has hardly any sugar – but these comparisons with other more popular cereals are pretty dramatic:
    - Fruit Loops has 106 times more sugar than Shredded Wheat
    - Cocoa Krispies has 96 times more
    - Frosted Flakes has 89 times more

  In fact, most cereals aimed at kids have 40 to 90 times more!

- Mercola.com's list (http://tinyurl.com/oq57rsb) of 9 foods you should never eat is worth reading:
    - Canned tomatoes
    - Processed meats
    - Margarine
    - Vegetable oils
    - Mircowave popcorn
    - Produce and foods known for high pesticide contamination
    - Table salt
    - Unfermented soy products
    - Artificial sweeteners

One extremely important conclusion that I've reached is that it is critical to cut through all the information and advice clutter and find a handful of sources of information and advice that you can trust. This "short list" includes a medical doctor, nutrition specialist, possibly a therapist and a couple of Internet sources with reliable and accurate information. My "golden resources" are included as part of the *Mind Diet Collection.*

You see, most diet books are written for the masses. The authors can't possibly know your individual situation. They don't know your medical history, food allergies, predisposition to any number of conditions, etc. Same with things you hear from other people who typically say "I've heard that soy is great for you" or "they say butter is bad for you." We tend to trust people close to us, so when we hear things like this from friends and family, we often don't bother to ask for the source or who "they" is.

Only your doctor can take and read the results of blood tests, which is an important starting point. A nutrition specialist is the key person to help you create a diet that's individualized for you, educate you about nutrition, and dispel myths that you might have.

When I reached my Moment of Truth, my first two stops were my doctor and dietician. Between the two of them, I got my game plan, which I have followed religiously to this day. I supplemented their advice with information I found online at two trusted sources: WebMd.com and Mercola.com. When I read something online that I think is pertinent to myself, I check it out with my doc or dietician. For example, I checked out the two articles below and my dietician said they were right on. This sort of confirmation of what I read or hear is important, so that I don't believe information that turns out to be false or just not appropriate for me.

We are hit with so much information on a daily basis, from food ads, news items, Google alerts, friends and family, TV and radio, and information from other online sources including web sites, blogs and more. Also, food names and packaging are enticing, so much so that anything with "granola" in it is always thought to be healthy, even though most granola cereals are loaded with sugar.

Take these two articles from Mercola.com. Over the years, we have become conditioned to the notion that butter is no good for us and that soy is good for us. The titles of these stories suggest otherwise:

- This Vilified Daily Food Slashes Heart Attack Risk in Half.
- Eating This "Healthy" Food? It Could be Slowly and Silently Killing You.

The first article, talking about butter, actually shows how much better butter is than margarine and other spreads, giving the reader a litany of reasons for this conclusion. The second talks about how soy-based products are bad for you, also giving numerous reasons, despite the "healthy" qualities advertising for soy products has conveyed.

While butter may not be recommended for some people, and while soy may be recommended for some people, these articles conclude that for most people, rethinking butter and soy is important. Discussing it with your doctor and nutrition specialist is the best way to determine if conclusions reached in articles like these are relevant to your personal situation.

While a lot of what I talk about pertains to your mind, you've got to understand the role of your brain. Here's one amazing example, from the Oak Ridge National Laboratory:

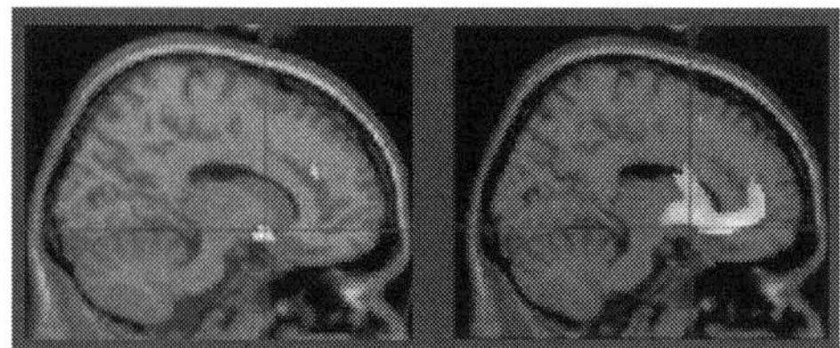

This brain scan shows that when people view images of appetizing foods (right photo), there is more activity in the part of your brain associated with reward, than with distasteful foods (left photo). This is directly related to leptin, the hormone that controls your appetite, which I'll discuss later.

At the online *Big Food* exhibit of the Yale Peabody Museum of Natural History (peabody.yale.edu)they have a great interactive game called "Smash Your Food" that teaches you what's in 10 common foods in a fun way. You actually get to smash pizza, burgers, fries and others. Here are some screen shots that shows how this works!

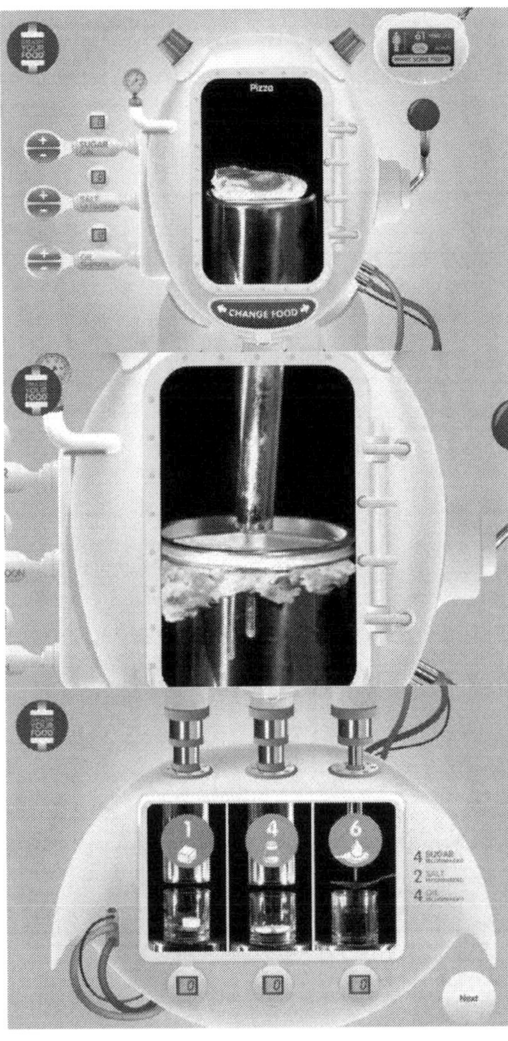

The more I read and researched this book, the more scary statistics, facts and information I discovered. "The 7 Nastiest Things Lurking in Your Supermarket" is a good example of why you need to become knowledgeable about everything you eat and drink. Author Judy Molland of www.Care2.com, a consumer action site with over 22 million members, reveals these gems:

- The toxic flame retardant chemical BVO is found in many soft drinks.
- Many candies and other foods with bright colors contain petroleum-based dyes.
- The FDA allows mold to be present in canned or frozen blackberries and raspberries.
- Many salad dressings contain titanium dioxide, which is also used in paints and sunscreens.
- Your milk may contain rBST, a synthetic hormone used to increased milk production.
- Find out if meat in your supermarket contains staph bacteria.

- Less than 2% of all imported seafood is inspected. If the shrimp you eat comes from farmed shrimp pens, it could contain a number of nasty things.

Read the entire article at: http://tinyurl.com/k4opyff.

Back in 2013, Google introduced nutrition facts for foods when you search on foods like apple, donut and soda. The search results return a listing like this – kudos to Google for doing this – especially by highlighting the "% Daily Value" percentages:

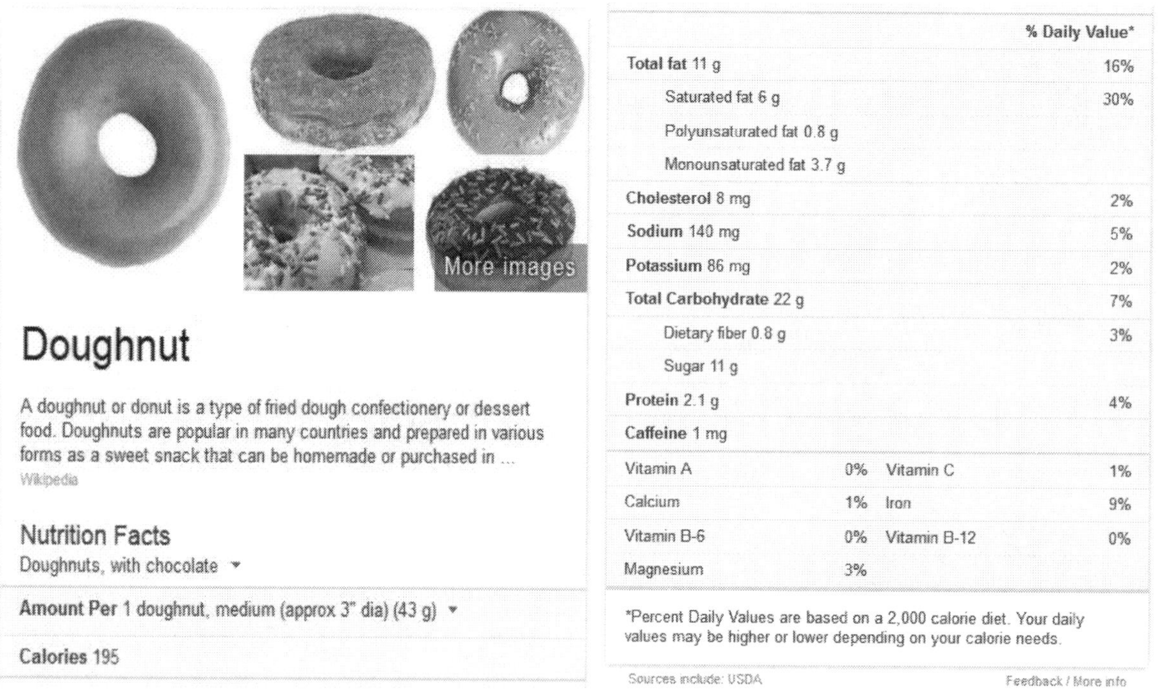

More images

Doughnut

A doughnut or donut is a type of fried dough confectionery or dessert food. Doughnuts are popular in many countries and prepared in various forms as a sweet snack that can be homemade or purchased in ...
Wikipedia

Nutrition Facts
Doughnuts, with chocolate

Amount Per 1 doughnut, medium (approx 3" dia) (43 g)

Calories 195

			% Daily Value*
Total fat 11 g			16%
Saturated fat 6 g			30%
Polyunsaturated fat 0.8 g			
Monounsaturated fat 3.7 g			
Cholesterol 8 mg			2%
Sodium 140 mg			5%
Potassium 86 mg			2%
Total Carbohydrate 22 g			7%
Dietary fiber 0.8 g			3%
Sugar 11 g			
Protein 2.1 g			4%
Caffeine 1 mg			
Vitamin A	0%	Vitamin C	1%
Calcium	1%	Iron	9%
Vitamin B-6	0%	Vitamin B-12	0%
Magnesium	3%		

*Percent Daily Values are based on a 2,000 calorie diet. Your daily values may be higher or lower depending on your calorie needs.

Sources include: USDA Feedback / More info

Milk is another tricky one. Reduced-fat chocolate milk, according to Dr. David Ludwig, is a real culprit, especially among kids. "The worst possible situation is reduced-fat chocolate milk: you take out the fat, it's less tasty. So to get kids to drink 3 cups a day, you get this sugar-sweetened beverage." Milk is generally fine but not when it has flavors in it.

Here's good news about peanuts, one of the cheapest nuts and also the nut that has the most protein than any other nut, according to the Peanut Institute. Author David Spero, writing in *www.DiabetesSelfManagement.com*, says that a study out of Purdue University and the Federal University of Vicosa (Brazil) showed that eating peanuts or peanut butter with breakfast limited the rise in blood sugar after both breakfast **and** lunch. Eating peanuts in the morning reduced blood glucose levels, reduced appetite and food consumption for most of the day. And natural UNsweetened peanut butter tastes great. Basically a grand-slam home run, as long as you're not allergic to peanuts.

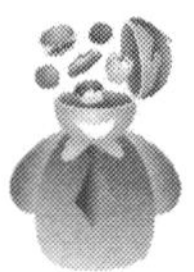

Dr. Ludwig suggests alternatives to milk that contain plenty of calcium: kale and spinach. See the Ingredients Awareness Chart (Guidebook #9) to learn about other foods that are high in calcium. To further drive home the importance of knowledge, www.takepart.com brings us this comparison of an entire stick of butter (not that we'd ever eat one in one sitting) vs. popular restaurant desserts:

Item	**Calories**	**Grams of Fat**
Stick of butter	810	91
Cheesecake Factory Brownie Sundae Cheesecake	1368	61
Applebees Chocolate Chip Cookie Sundae	1550	74
TGI Friday's Whiskey Cake	1270	54
Olive Garden Zeppoli	920	35
Ruby Tuesday Italian Cream Cake	990	56
Outback Steakhouse Chocolate Thunder Down Under	1550	106
PF Chang's Great Wall of Chocolate	1520	72

Yikes!!!

Your knowledge of food wouldn't be complete without understanding that some foods that you think are good actually are not. This chart, taken from a www.mercola.com article, shows ten foods that are actually banned in other countries:

Food	**Countries Banning It**
Farm-Raised Salmon	Australia, New Zealand
Genetically Engineered Papaya	European Union
Ractopamine-Tainted Meat	160 Countries
Flame Retardant Drinks	Europe, Japan
Processed Foods with Artificial Colors and Dyes	Norway, Austria
Arsenic-Laced Chicken	European Union
Bread with Potassium Bromate	European Union, Canada, China
Olestra/Olean	UK, Canada
Preservatives BHA and BHT	European Union, Japan
Milk/Dairy with rBGH	Australia, New Zealand, Israel, Canada, EU

Learn more at: http://tinyurl.com/l4zmm3m.

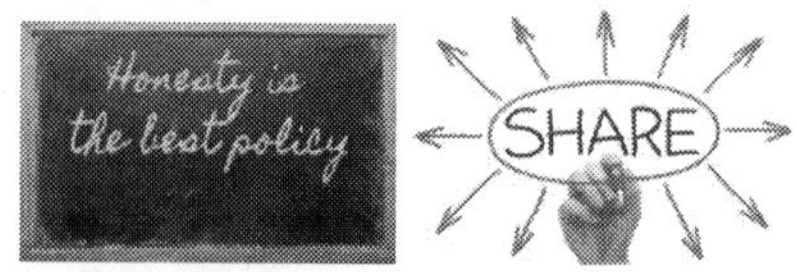

Belief #9

Believe in Honesty and Sharing

When it comes to how we perceive our weight, we are either in denial or not very honest with ourselves. In one of many polls I've come across (Meridian Health Magazine, 3/2011), 33% of Americans who **are** overweight said that they were not!

Almost 75% of those who **are** obese said they were merely overweight! And 39% of those who **are** morbidly obese (more than 100 pounds too heavy) said they were just overweight! Call it what you want, but denying that you are fat is one thing you need to stop doing. You have to recognize exactly what your situation is, and then deal with it. Minimizing it or denying it is not progress.

As you know, it's hard to lose weight and keep it off. But I discovered is that it is harder to lose weight alone, and easier when you share what you're doing with others. I can tell you first-hand that by getting friends and family involved, you dramatically increase the likelihood that you will be successful. It's all about two things: support and feedback.

When you share the weight loss process with people, they will be much more supportive than if you do it in secret. My wife and I lost our weight together, and we provided a lot of support, encouragement and tips. We cooked healthy meals for each other. Whether you do it with a partner, sibling, co-worker or friend, you will find that cheering each other on is a great part of the process. And people in your circle of friends represent people you can talk to whenever the need arises.

There are practical reasons as well. People who know that you are extremely serious about losing weight will respect you that much more when you've taken them into your confidence. They won't push food on you. They will be considerate when planning a meal out. They'll share recipes and their own weight-loss success stories.

And, they'll give you feedback. They'll be among the first who notice you've lost weight. They'll brag about you to others. They'll pat you on the back and some of them might even join you in the process once they see how successful you are. It's a win-win, no-lose proposition, sharing your weight-loss journey with others who care about you.

But don't take only my word for it. Studies have shown that positive feedback is an important part of weight loss. In a study of 179 people taking part in the "Shape Up RI" program, they found that people who had computer-generated feedback lost the most weight. This finding is similar to other studies that show that online weight loss support groups are an important tool in losing weight. *Health* magazine reports that when a woman tries to lose weight on her own, the average weight loss after one YEAR was 2.9 pounds.

The loss for those women who joined a diet support group was 9.5 pounds, more than three times better.

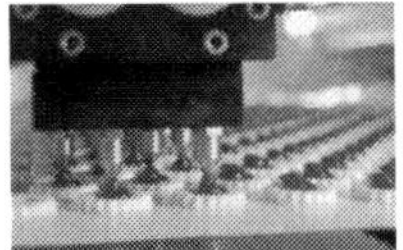

Belief #10

Believe in Learning About Processed Foods

A really good way to look at what you eat is to understand food vs. food products. Foods grow on trees and in the ground, live in the water and on land, and include:

- Meat
- Fish
- Chicken
- Fruits
- Berries
- Nuts
- Vegetables
- Water
- Milk
- Eggs

Food products, on the other hand, are basically man-made, almost always involving some sort of machinery and added ingredients. The most commonly used word to describe food products is **processed**, which means that some machine process is used to make the food product. Typical examples include:

- Cheese Spread
- Soda
- Luncheon Meats
- Cakes
- Candy
- Syrup
- Sauces
- Hot Dogs

Food products, or processed foods, are quite possibly the single most important reason for the obesity epidemic in this country and in many places around the world. With ingredients like High Fructose Corn Syrup, Sugar, Hydrogenated Oils, MSG and Trans Fat (all of which earn my “skull and crossbones” designation), it’s no wonder that we’ve all become addicted to foods that are not natural.

Processed foods are very similar to sugar (next belief) in that both are really, really bad for you. In fact, here are 9 reasons why you should never eat processed foods again, distilled from an article on www.NaturalNews.com.

#1: Processed Foods are Highly Addictive. Processed foods over-stimulate the production of dopamine, which gives you pleasure when you consume these foods, leading to an endless cycle of eating what gives you pleasure.

#2: Processed Foods Often Contain Phosphates. Phosphates and other additives cause health problems like rapid aging, kidney deterioration and weak bones.

#3: Fresh Foods are Actually Cheaper than Processed Foods. Numerous studies show fresh food alternatives end up costing less per serving. Want to save money? Give up processed foods! A reader adds: “Cheaper medical bills too!”

#4: Processed Foods Cause Chronic Inflammation. Ingredients found in processed foods are largely responsible for inflammation, which leads to heart disease, dementia, neurological problems, cancer and more.

#5: Processed Foods Ruin Digestion. Because they have been stripped of their natural fibers, enzymes, vitamins and nutrients, processed foods wreak havoc on your digestive tract.

#6: Processed Foods Destroy Your Mind. Junk foods can cause people to become angry and irritable. Too much processed food could lead to your acting in an inappropriate manner, difficulty concentrating and thinking.

#7: Processed Foods are Loaded with GMOs. Genetically modified organisms created in a laboratory have been linked to infertility, organ damage, cancer and more bad things.

#8: Processed Foods are Loaded with Pesticides. Breakfast foods alone have been found to contain as many as 70 different types of pesticides, chemicals and other residues that have zero value for your body.

#9: Processed Foods are not Actually Food. Created in labs, manufactured in factories and lying on supermarket shelves for long periods of time, processed foods are essentially synthetic, using unhealthy methods to make these creations taste like real food, even though they’re not.

Check out this graphic that shows what’s in some of the processed foods you eat:

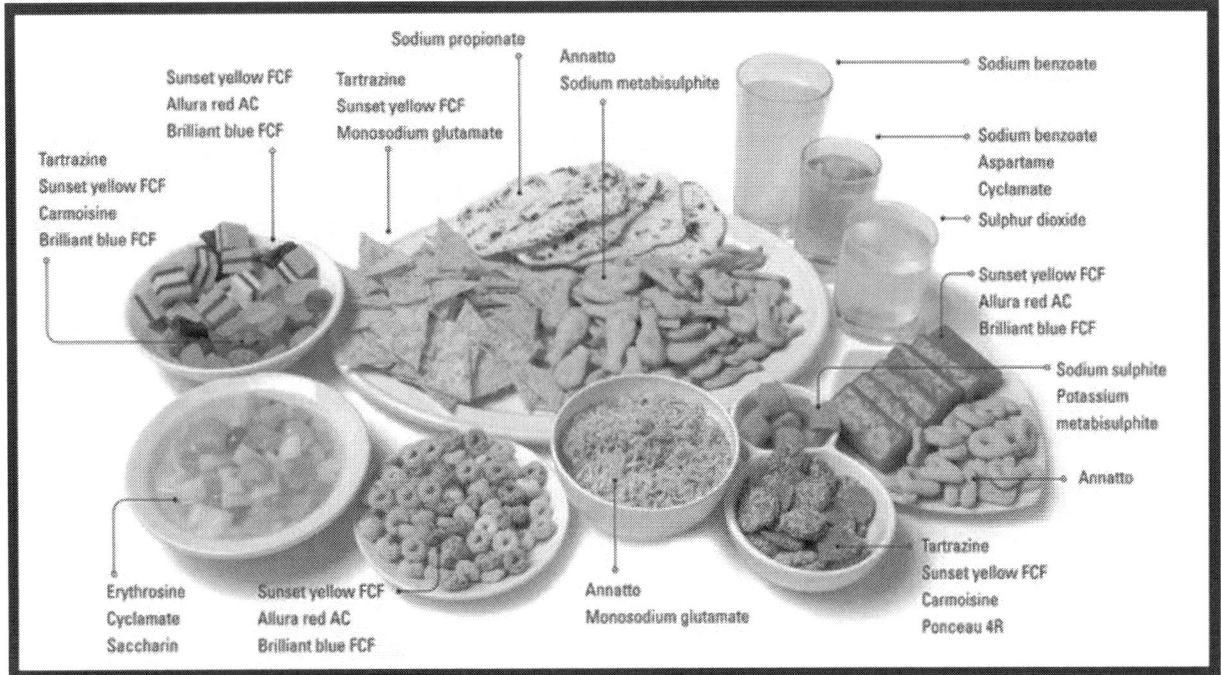

Not eating processed foods should be an easy decision for you. If it's not, re-read this section until it is.

Obesity expert Dr. David Katz likens obesity to drowning, which I think is a very good analogy. www.DietDoctor.com says: "Our entire food supply is full of sugar and starch – it's hard to find a processed food item without it – and it's making us too hungry." The faster you eliminate added sugar and processed food, the faster you will lose weight safely and keep it off permanently.

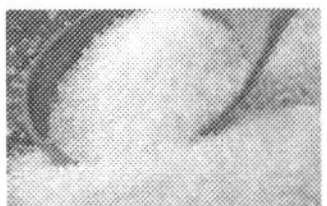

Belief #11

Believe That Added Sugar is Deadly

Fructose may be the single most important food ingredient to understand, for it can do the most damage to your weight loss endeavors. Fructose can be both good for you and horrible for you.

Fructose is a dietary carbohydrate that is one of the primary sources of a substance called Glycerol-3-Phosphate, that causes fat to become fixed in your fatty tissue. Fructose also raises insulin levels, which in turn, prevents fat from being released from your body.

Key point: fructose, especially **high fructose corn syrup (HFCS)**, is one of the most patently bad food ingredients for you, requiring your liver to work extremely hard to digest it. To make matters worse, in an article in www.preventdisease.com talking about how HFCS can cause reactions in people similar to cocaine, almost half of HFCS samples tested contained mercury.

How fast can you run from HFCS? Run fast, because American's consumption of HFCS between 1970 and 1990 rose 1,000% which paralleled the rapid rise of obesity (*Are You Suffering from Fructose Poisoning?* in Life Extension Magazine, 10/13).

The Center for Science in the Public Interest reports that in 2010, each American consumed an average of 78 pounds of added sweeteners. Doing some quick math, that's about 6 ounces every single day!

If you only ate fruits and vegetables, you'd get 15 grams per day, which is OK. But when you start adding in regular soda, processed foods, juice drinks and other products made with HFCS, your daily intake of fructose shoots through the roof to 75, 100 or more grams per day. Fructose is almost single-handedly responsible for the teenage obesity epidemic.

This belief is based on your understanding WHY fructose is so bad for you, so that you immediately dramatically reduce your intake of it. Here are a handful of scary facts about fructose:

- 100% of metabolic burden rests on your liver after you eat fructose.
- Fructose is turned into fatty free acids, bad cholesterol and triglycerides, all of which are stored as fat.
- 33% of calories found in fructose are stored in fat.
- Fructose actually stimulates overeating in your brain.

The worst fructose offenders include regular soda, other sugary drinks, most processed foods, ketchup, soup, salad dressing, bread and crackers. See several tools that are in this collection that makes it easy for you to identify foods that are high in sugar. Even some "natural" sweeteners such as agave syrup should be avoided as it is almost 100% fructose!

For a really good (and scary) infographic about how much sugar we eat, from Forbes, created by www.OnlineNursingPrograms.com and reported by Alice G. Walton, go to: http://tinyurl.com/8jc9mxj.

I came across a post on Blake Hagen's blog *The Fight for Fitness* (blakehagen.com) where he presented a pie chart developed by the United States Department of Agriculture's Center for Nutrition Policy and Promotion. What's fascinating about these sources of added sugars in your diet is that they come from so many different sources:

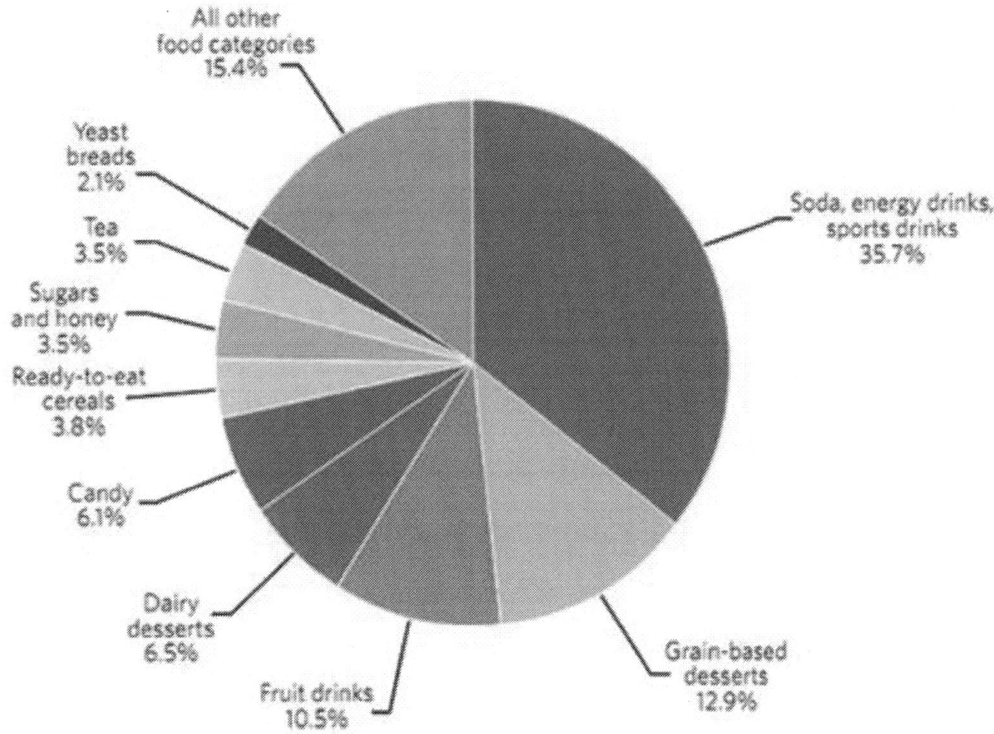

What stands out is that almost 50% of added sugar comes from drinks, including soda, energy drinks, sports drinks, fruit drinks and tea. Watching what you drink is just as important as watching what you eat!

If you're still not convinced that added sugar is truly evil, one of the *Mind Diet Guidebooks* is devoted solely to this topic. And I'm not the only one. One of the most outspoken anti-sugar pioneers is author Dr. Nancy Appleton, who wrote *Suicide by Sugar* and *Lick the Sugar Habit.* Dr. Appleton has developed a list of 141 reasons why sugar is ruining your health, available here: http://tinyurl.com/2wn79aw.

I've read the entire list and picked out 25 of the most serious conditions that sugar directly or indirectly causes (in addition to obesity):

- Suppresses your immune system
- Loss of tissue elasticity and function
- Reduces high density lipoproteins (HDL) the "good" cholesterol
- Interferes with absorption of calcium and magnesium
- Hypoglycemia
- Premature aging
- Alcoholism
- Arthritis
- Asthma

- Gallstones
- Heart disease
- Appendicitis
- Multiple sclerosis
- Decreased growth hormone
- Food allergies
- Eczema in children
- Impair DNA structure
- Ages your skin (just like cigarettes and UV rays do!)
- Cataracts
- Pancreas damage
- Gastric cancer
- Indigestion
- Reduces learning capacity
- Dizziness
- Induces salt and water retention

After reading these and the other 116, I don't know how anyone could not recognize the toxicity of added sugar. Want more? Check out Connie Bennett's Sugar Shock! Blog at www.sugarshockblog.com and her books *Sugar Shock* and *Beyond Sugar Shock* – you will be shocked. And this may be the most important takeaway from this section: researchers have found that when people taste sugar, brain scans reveal that their brains light up in the same regions as it does with alcohol. Think you can't get addicted to sugar? Think again!

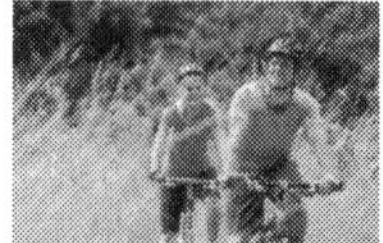

Belief #12

Believe in the Value of Exercise

I lost my first 20 pounds with just weekend casual walking. Everyone told me that would happen, and that in order to continue losing weight, I'd need to get serious about exercise. On day #97, I reached my second Moment of Truth. I made up my mind once and for all that I will embark on a consistent exercise program that would not only help me lose more weight, but help my overall health as well.

I hate "working out," because as you know, using machines feels like work. Plus, you're indoors, whether at home or at a facility, and it gets very boring very fast.

So let's start with a simple question: can everyone find 20 to 30 minutes a day to take a nice brisk walk?

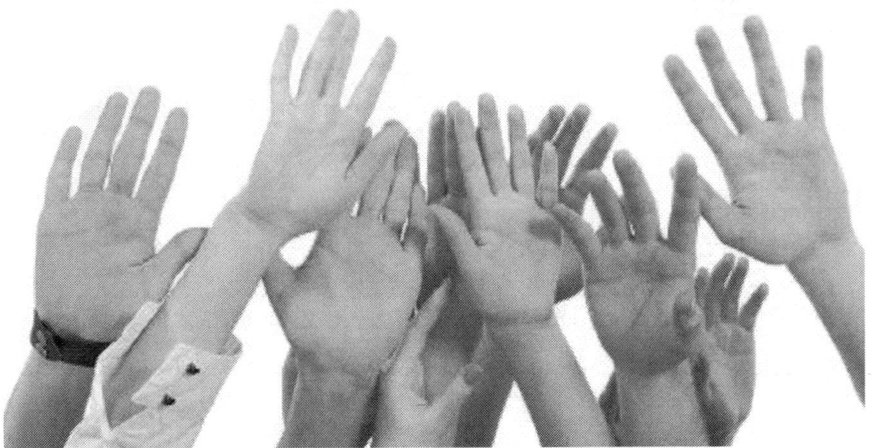

I thought so. Everyone can.

Experts say that you only need to walk 20-30 minutes a day at a decent pace to help your weight loss efforts.

You don't have to kill yourself at a gym.

You don't have to run marathons.

You don't have to bench press 300 pounds.

Walking to and from work counts, as long as it's a brisk walk.

Instead of spending an hour eating lunch, walk around the block for a half hour and eat during the other half hour.

I decided to spend 30 minutes per day walking briskly, outdoors. The Centers for Disease Control and *Prevention* Magazine recommend 20 minutes per day. Sometimes it would be before working, sometimes as a short lunch hour, and sometimes after work. On weekends, it would be any time.

Fortunately I live five minutes from a park with a big lake. I've decided that's going to be my weekday stomping grounds. I walk three laps around this very large lake, which is about half a mile, in about 25 minutes. That burns about 200 to 250 calories, depending on how fast I'm moving.

A study of 12,000 people by the Harvard School of Public Health found that walking inhibits genes that promote weight gain...and conversely, sitting in front of the TV results in a rise of the same gene, as summarized in *Bottom Line Personal.*

More importantly, moving your body on a daily basis is instrumental in faster weight loss and in warding off a variety of diseases.

The best choice I made was to exercise outside, especially when it's sunny. I get fresh air, lots of sunshine, a nice breeze blowing in my face, nice scenery and lots of wildlife including geese, dogs, birds and others to look at.

There are absolutely no downsides to exercise, if done in moderation and according to what your doctor says is OK. And walking isn't the only exercise there is that is fun. You can get plenty of valuable exercise jogging, riding a bicycle, bowling, playing tennis and other sports, ice skating, roller blading – the list goes on and on. To see how many calories you burn, go online and use any of the free calculators. There are other ways to get exercise throughout the day:

- Have a desk job? Get up and walk around every 30 minutes. Adding 50 steps twice an hour is an extra 800 steps. Every bit helps.
- Split your lunch hour (or however long it is) into part exercise and part food. Take a brisk walk in the park, followed by a box lunch on a park bench.
- Take the steps instead of the elevator.

And, a couple of final tips:

- Exercise as much outdoors as you can, so you get sunshine and fresh air, and get away from the indoor environment.
- Get an "exercise buddy" so that you keep each other committed and support each other.
- When your body tells you it's had enough, stop. Don't fall into the "no pain, no gain" school of thought. This is not Olympic training here; it's exercising to aid weight loss.
- If you have a dog that can run, let the dog lead you which gets you walking/jogging faster. When I had my dog, I really enjoyed walking with him.
- In addition to walking and jogging, think of other activities where you get exercise, but they are not typically associated with exercise, such as dancing, bicycling, swimming or mowing the lawn, just to name a few.
- Always warm up and cool down for 5-10 minutes.
- If you walk steadily as I do, add some "interval training" where you speed up your walking (or other exercise) for a couple of minutes every so often.
- In addition to aerobic exercise (walking, running, etc.), make sure to add weight and strength training, which includes sit-ups, push-ups, pull-ups, lifting weights, etc. Consult a trainer or fitness expert so you don't do too much or do exercises that are not good for you.

And remember, consistent, regular exercise is the key. You don't have to kill yourself; just get exercise 5-7 times a week without fail. Exercise does a lot more than help you lose weight. Daily exercise lowers the risk of:

- Heart disease
- Stroke
- Type II Diabetes
- Breast cancer
- Colon cancer
- Osteoporosis
- Depression
- Anxiety
- Cognitive decline

Exercise lowers:

- Blood pressure
- Blood sugar level
- Body fat
- Bad LDL cholesterol

Exercise increases:

- Muscle
- Good HDL cholesterol
- Self-esteem

And maybe best of all: exercise can help people experience better sex – greater frequency, better orgasms and greater satisfaction. Do you need any more reasons to start exercising every day?

One caveat about weight loss: my conclusion after extensive research is that exercise **alone** is not sufficient to lose weight. My gut tells me that exercise is about 20% of the equation and diet is 80%. Exercise and weight loss expert Dr. John Britta writes that a study found that people who believe that obesity is the result of inactivity are heavier than people who believe that obesity is the result of an unhealthy diet.

Bottom line – exercise for overall health and as a small contributing factor to weight loss.

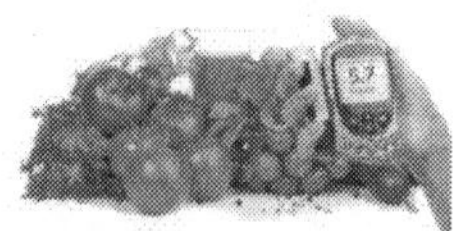

Belief #13

Believe in Understanding Carbs, Insulin, Glycemic Index/Load and Leptin

Carbs

Carbs have a direct impact on insulin levels. Understand this fact, what carbs are OK for you, and which ones can mess up your insulin levels, is critical. Diabetes expert Johanna Burani (jcburani.mydiabeteseducator.org) has coined what I think is an easy way to understand what goes on inside your body to visualize the difference between good and bad carbs.

She divides carbs into two groups: **gusher** carbs and **trickler** carbs.

Gusher carbs release glucose into the bloodstream very quickly, causing a blood glucose spike (not a good thing). If there isn't enough insulin available to move this glucose out of the blood and into the cells, the glucose will stay in the blood too long (also not a good thing). Gusher carbs include candy, sugar-laden juices and drinks, processed foods and cereals, tropical fruits, etc.

On the other hand, trickler carbs release smaller amounts of glucose into the bloodstream (a good thing), making it easier for your body to process the glucose and does not result in the kind of spikes you see with gusher carbs. Examples of trickler carbs are cooked oatmeal (not instant), heavy grainy breads, beans, sweet potatoes, vegetables, apples, oranges, berries, etc.

Glycemic Index/Load

The gusher and trickler carbs together have been profiled in what's called the Glycemic Index (GI). Carbs with high GI scores are gushers and low scores are tricklers. A more advanced measure is the Glycemic Load (CL) which some think is even better than GI by itself (GL contains a GI component).

Without getting too technical, the higher the GL of a food, the greater the expected rise in your blood glucose and the greater the adverse effect the food has on your insulin levels. Foods with the highest GL include:

- Many pastas (linguine, macaroni, spaghetti)
- White and Asian rices
- Couscous

- Baked russet potatoes
- Corn and corn flakes
- Cranberry juice
- Cream of wheat (instant)
- Dates
- Pop Tarts
- Rice Krispies
- Shredded Wheat
- Risotto

Go here to read more on GI and GL: http://tinyurl.com/l66wccf.

Here's a great graphic (thanks to Massive Health) that shows which foods are likely to lead to a sugar crash and which are not:

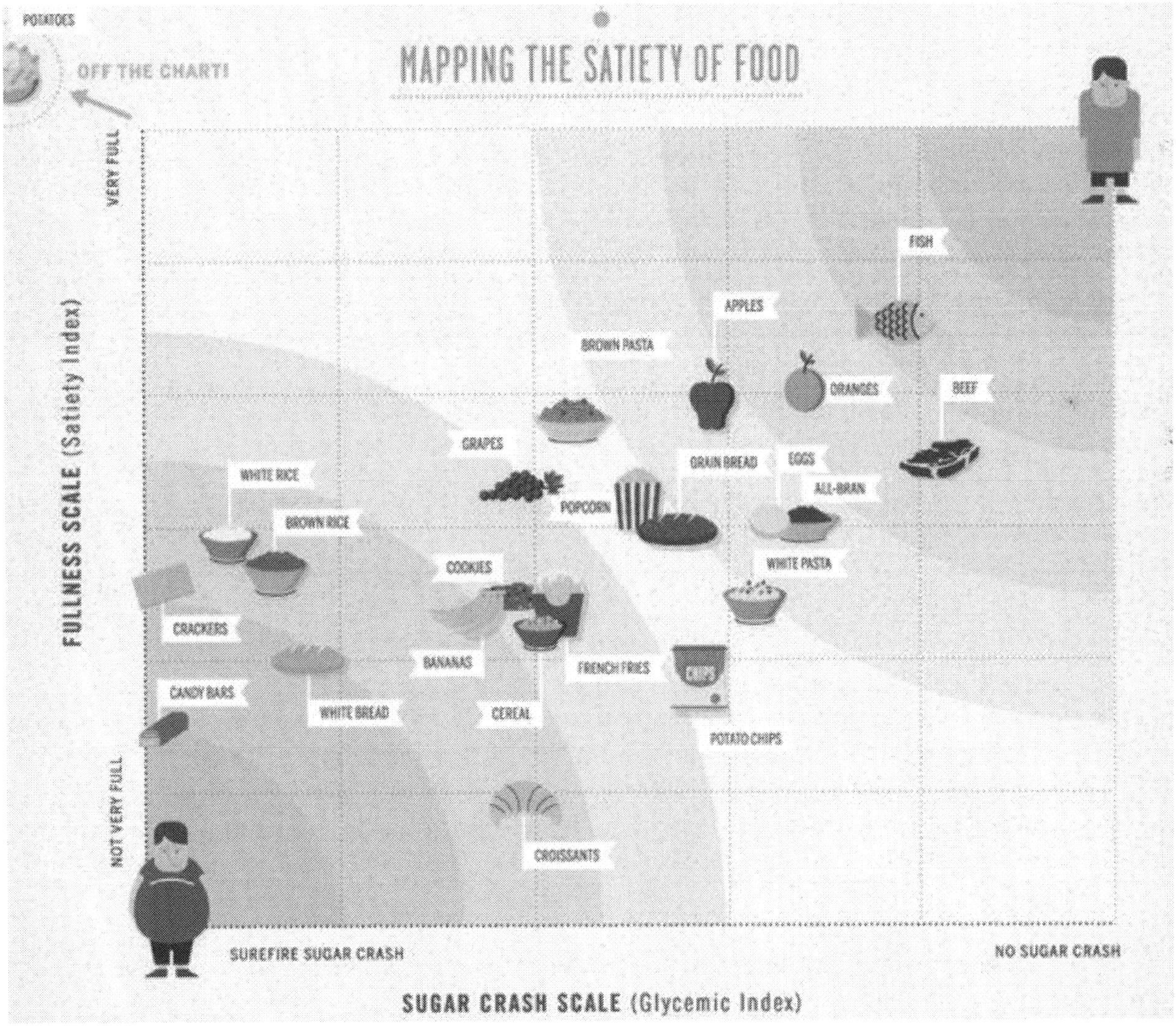

Insulin

Insulin is a topic that many people don't understand. Many people think having too little insulin is bad, and having too much is good. They, like me, also didn't understand just how important insulin is to obesity, diabetes and other chronic conditions. Basically, insulin is a hormone that regulates carbohydrate and fat metabolism. When you eat many types of food, insulin increases, but once glucose has been safely sent to energy producing cells or stored, insulin levels usually drop. When insulin doesn't drop, it's a warning sign.

People think that insulin is evil. It is not – it is necessary for our survival. The key is the amount of insulin that is present.

According to Dr. Mark Hyman, author of *The Blood Sugar Solution,* in an interview in Life Extension Magazine (5/13), "type II diabetes and diabesity are diseases of too much insulin, not too little insulin. Insulin is the real driver of problems with diabesity." Here's the key takeaway: **"When your diet is full of empty calories and refined carbohydrates, your cells become resistant or numb to the effects of insulin."**

Dr. Hyman calls insulin "the fat storage hormone," and says that too much insulin is likely the cause for:

- Inflammation
- Oxidative stress
- High blood pressure
- High cholesterol
- Low LDL
- High triglycerides
- Poor sex drive
- Infertility
- Thickening of the blood
- Increased risk of:
    - Alzheimer's
    - Cancer
    - Depression

Clearly, having too much insulin is not a good thing. If your diet is filled with empty calories, talk to your doctor about having your insulin tested.

Leptin

I never heard of leptin until I started researching this book. And I think most people have not either. I've come to learn that an understanding of leptin is critical to weight loss.

Leptin is a hormone that tells your brain when you are full – that it's time to stop eating. In this "leptin feedback loop" from www.hollandclinic.com, author Dr. Mark J. Holland explains how leptin affects weight gain and loss.

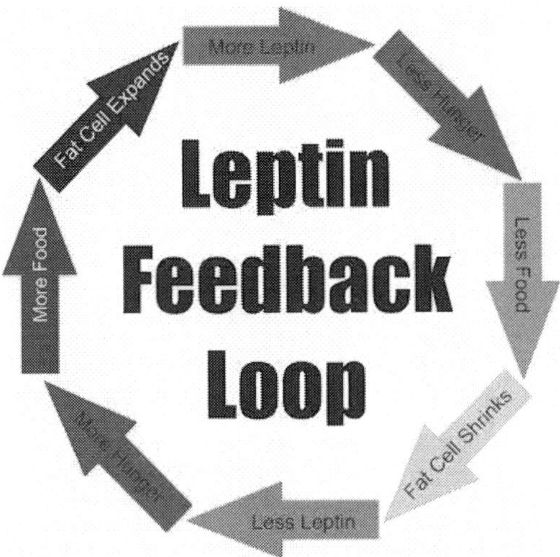

Basically, the more leptin in your system, the less hungry you feel and the less you eat.

The less leptin in your system, the hungrier you feel and the more you eat.

Leptin is made in our fat cells, enters the bloodstream and travels to the brain, sending a signal that we're no longer hungry.

Many experts believe that consuming fructose causes leptin resistance, which leads to us feeling hungry when we're not. Reducing fructose intake makes a lot of sense.

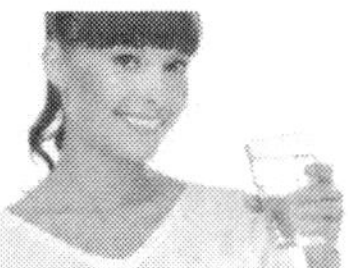

Belief #14

Believe in the Value of Water

Water is the purest liquid on the planet. It has no calories, no carbs, no fat, no sugar, pretty much no nothing. It's refreshing and it has numerous benefits for us in general, and for weight loss in particular. And in case you don't remember your elementary school biology, our bodies are mostly water.

A study out of Virginia Tech (WebMD, 8/23/10) indicates pretty convincingly that "Water may be a secret weapon in weight loss." Those people in this study (and this is one we should all pay attention to) who drank two cups of water before meals lost almost 50% more weight than those who did not.

Further, they also kept "the weight off for a full year after the weight loss study" was completed. The reason, explains study senior author Brenda Davy, is that water makes people feel fuller, and they consequently eat less food. Drinking regular soda will defeat the purpose because it is loaded with sugar. In fact, people who drink just one 12-ounce serving of regular soda a day are 26% more likely to develop type 2 diabetes than those who drank less than one serving a month, or none at all (*Diabetes Care*).

Generally, the more water you have in your body, the better you will feel, and the faster you will lose weight. Drink 6-8 tall glasses a day: when you get up, and before and during each meal. A really easy secret to getting more water and losing weight faster is to eat foods that have a high percentage of water...examples:

- Lettuce: 90% to 96% water content
- Watermelon: 97% (but also high in sugar)
- Cucumbers: 97%
- Tomatoes: 95%
- Zucchini: 95%
- Eggplant: 92%
- Red Kidney Beans: 77%
- Roasted Chicken Breast: 65%
- Baked Salmon: 62%

While we're on the topic of drinking water, not everything that contains water, such as fruit juices, wine and beer, is good for you. You've heard of the proverbial "beer belly" right? Take the time to learn what is in everything you drink and you'll quickly learn that nothing is better for you than H2O! For an excellent presentation of good and bad juices, check out WebMD's slideshow: http://tinyurl.com/78blkzt. *Bottom Line Health* reports that just ONE sip of beer increases levels of the brain chemical dopamine, which is associated with alcohol abuse!

Here's a great graphic that depicts the health value of water: http://tinyurl.com/n898h8v.

One of the crazes in the early part of this decade was vitamin-enriched waters, sold by numerous companies. And while there's nothing wrong with adding vitamins (if you even need them), look at some of the labels and you'll see added sugar as well – something you don't find in vitamin-less water!

There's one caveat to water. Many people, consumers and professionals alike, believe that fluoridated water is not good for you. In fact, the citizens of Portland, OR voted no to fluoridation. Your tap water may adversely affect you if it's fluoridated – read more here: http://tinyurl.com/kzhdapp.

Well, there you have it. About as close to a magic potion as you can get, one available for free at the nearest faucet at home or drinking fountain at work.

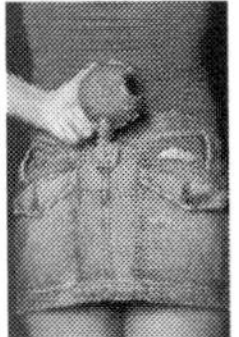

Belief #15

Believe That Cheating Never Works

Most people (including myself at one time) who want to lose weight search for the "magic bullet," which is almost always promoted as a "quick fix" or some monumental weight loss in a ridiculously short period of time.

Perhaps this is because we live in an "instant gratification" society, where just about anything we want is immediately available, whether it's gas for our cars, fast food at 2am, information via the Internet, etc.

Any type of magic bullet that you come across where the end result is to achieve a significant weight loss in a short period of time is what I call a trick or a cheat. Weight loss tricks and cheats take many forms, the most common being crazy diets and pills.

I once made a $1,000 bet with my business partner to see who could drop 20 pounds the fastest, hoping that would be my motivation. It was, and we pretty much got there at the same time, so no money changed hands. But we both gained the weight back – that's a good example of a trick that worked in the short-term but had no lasting power.

33% of U.S. companies offer or plan to offer some sort of financial incentive to get employees to lose weight, via their wellness programs. Not surprisingly, the results aren't very good, and they don't generally help the companies reduce costs resulting from overweight and obese workers. While well-intentioned for sure, offering people money to lose weight is just another cheat, especially when the amount of money is very low.

Look around you. There are tricks and cheats everywhere. Don't fall for them and keep your wallet or purse closed. They are just a waste of money. Hopefully by now you realize there is only one way to lose weight, and it does not involve tricks and cheats.

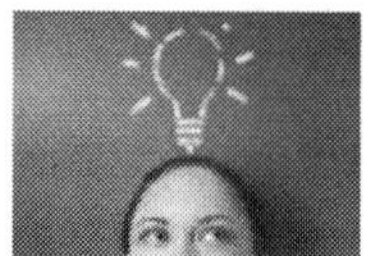

Belief #16

Believe in Visualizing Your Way to Success

I've often found that visualizing food portions is very helpful to remind me just how much food I can eat. While you can easily find lists of recommended amounts of food, they are usually in grams or other measures which most of us can't translate while we're standing at a salad bar or looking at a menu.

For key foods, spend a little time to understand how to visualize what you can eat. For example, a daily serving of almonds can be visualized like this:

- A handful
- ¼ measuring cup
- Empty mint tin
- Two wells of an ice cube tray

In addition to visualizing food portions, try visualizing two other things in relation to how you look. Visualize how you look when fat (look in the mirror) and when you're thin (look at old photos when you were thin). You'll be surprised, even shocked, at the difference!

Visualizing is a great technique to create visual snapshots in your mind, which in turns helps you lose weight and keep it off.

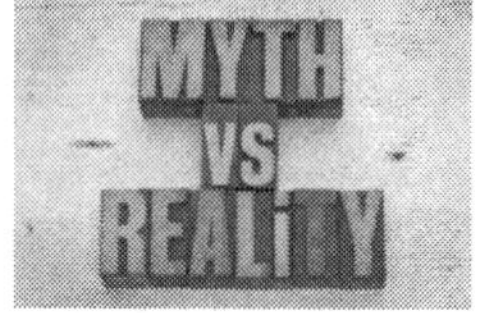

Belief #17

Believe That Myths and Misinformation Can Derail You

There is so much misinformation floating around as well as myths that continue to persist. I constantly hear people say things like "they said it was OK to eat anything in moderation" or "I heard you can lose 20 pounds in one month easily." And I always respond by asking who the "they" are and where they heard these things. They never have a good answer.

People tend to believe what they want to, even if the information defies logic. And in many cases, they just take the word of a friend, family member or even a total stranger as truth, without checking it out.

The answer is simple: NEVER take anyone's word (except your doctor and dietician) for anything regarding your health and weight loss. They are likely to be wrong. Check everything out online at reputable web sites and with your doctor and nutrition specialist.

For example, many of people have purchased HCG weight loss products, which contain a hormone made by the placenta during pregnancy. The FDA calls this product targeted for weight loss as fraudulent and illegal. And like many supplements and other "magic pills," they are not effective and are a waste of money.

It gets even worse. People who refuse to lose weight naturally and in a healthy manner opt for injections of HCG and even get the shots from people who aren't even licensed to give them.

Another myth floating around is that low fat means low calorie. Nothing could be further from the truth. Food tastes good because it has either fat or sugar. Reduce one, and typically you find more of the other. Always look at the first 5 ingredients on the nutrition facts label to see what's in a low fat product you're considering...in many (but not all) cases you'll be surprised, even shocked, at how much sugar and/or carbs and/or starches have been added to make that product taste good.

Eggs have been demonized for decades as raising cholesterol. But an article in NaturalNews.com based on research by the journal *Food Chemistry* indicates that eggs:

- Are loaded with antioxidants, which help prevent cardiovascular disease.
- Have about the same amount of antioxidants as a serving of cranberries (one egg).
- Contain peptides that actually help lower cholesterol.

The question is no longer whether to eat egg yolks or not. Finding organic, pasture-based eggs is now what's recommended, overcoming a long-time myth held by millions of people.

Adds Michael Pollan, author of *Cooked*, "Eggs are great and always were. Nutrition researchers used to think that cholesterol in eggs raised cholesterol in the blood, but this turns out not to be the case for most people." Your doctor and nutrition specialist can advise you if eggs are not OK for you.

Writing in AuthorityNutrition.com, Kris Gunnars calls eggs a "perfect food" for humans, loaded with protein, healthy fats, vitamins, minerals and Choline, a nutrient important for brain health. He says that 90% of us are not getting enough Choline.

In fact, a study from the *International Journal of Obesity* found that people who ate two eggs for breakfast lost 65% more weight (and a 61% greater reduction in BMI) than people who ate a bagel and no eggs.

Want more? Serving sizes for some foods are unrealistically small, which means that most people go over the listed serving size, and wind up eating a lot more sugar, fat, calories, etc. A few examples:

- Ice Cream: serving size is ½ cup (4oz), which looks like the size of two golf balls. Can you eat just that? Or do you wind up eating three, four or five times that amount?
- Pasta: serving size is 2 ounces uncooked. Cooked it winds up being the size of a baseball. Have you ever seen a serving of pasta that small?

One more: people tend to think that over-the-counter diet pills have been approved by the Food and Drug Administration (FDA). Wrong again. After they are in stores and sold online, they are monitored by the FDA, but they don't have to be approved in advance like prescription medicines. There's no guarantee that they are safe.

Nutritionist Josh Bezoni in the *BioTrust Nutrition* newsletter, outlines seven deadly sins of diet pills:

- They sound like medicines, which they are not.
- They make you feel jittery, anxious, depressed and/or hungry.
- They often come with questionable endorsements.
- Some make outrageous claims that can't be supported.
- They are often not backed by a 100% money back guarantee.
- They don't contain enough of the key ingredients to be effective.
- They are often not tested by independent, third-party labs.

Registered dietician and diabetes expert Hope Warshaw identifies four myths about carbohydrates and diabetes:

- People with diabetes need to drastically reduce their carb intake. Wrong – it's not the number of carbs – it's the **type** of carbs.
- Reducing carb intake improves blood glucose levels. In people with diabetes, normal carb intake had better levels than those consuming a low percentage of carbs.
- Carb restriction eliminates the need for medication. If you have diabetes, this is not likely to be true as it's a matter of when you'll need medicine to deal with Type-2 diabetes.
- A low-carb diet decreases chances of other diseases. People on low-carb diets tend to eat more saturated fats and protein, pushing organs in our bodies to work harder.

Some people think that fruit can make you gain weight because of the sugar content. Well, for one thing, the sugar in fruit is natural sugar, not added sugar. Registered Dietitian Cynthia Sass points out five reasons why fruit should always be part of a healthy eating and weight loss strategy:

- The more fruit you eat, the less you'll weigh.

- Fruit is packed with water and fiber, so the sugar in fruit is much less concentrated than sugar found in other sweetened foods.
- Fruit has great vitamins, minerals, nutrients and antioxidants.
- Due to the antioxidants, fruit eaters often have healthier skin.
- Fruit is a great fuel for those of us who are active.

People often ask, "fruit has sugar so should I stay away from it." All fruits except watermelon contain huge amounts of fiber that dilute the fructose in fruit so that they are absolutely safe to eat...but NOT as juice (in most cases) where the fiber has been stripped out (www.HollandClinic.com).

For an in-depth article published in the respected New England Journal of Medicine and written by *The Mind Diet* contributor Dr. Ethan Lazarus, read this 4-part series here:

- http://tinyurl.com/n7b6l4x
- http://tinyurl.com/lsu77zp
- http://tinyurl.com/nymdops
- http://tinyurl.com/ks4uedr

Bottom line: don't put anything in your body that your doctor and dietician have not approved, especially if you are pre-diabetic or already have diabetes. Question everything that people say, even if well-intentioned. Make informed decisions only after you've thoroughly educated yourself.

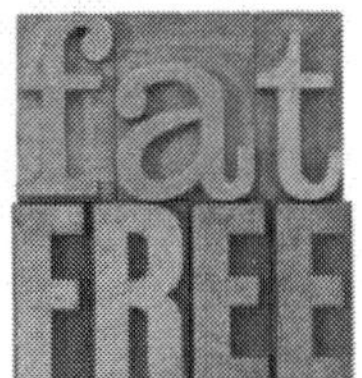

Belief #18

Believe That You Must Understand Fat

One of the most misunderstood things about food is fat. In talking with hundreds of people of all walks of life, most do not understand these two very important facts:

- Not all fat is bad. There are good fats and bad fats.
- Low or no fat typically means higher added sugar.

In this infographic (blog.friendseat.com)it's very easy to see which fats are good for you and which are not:

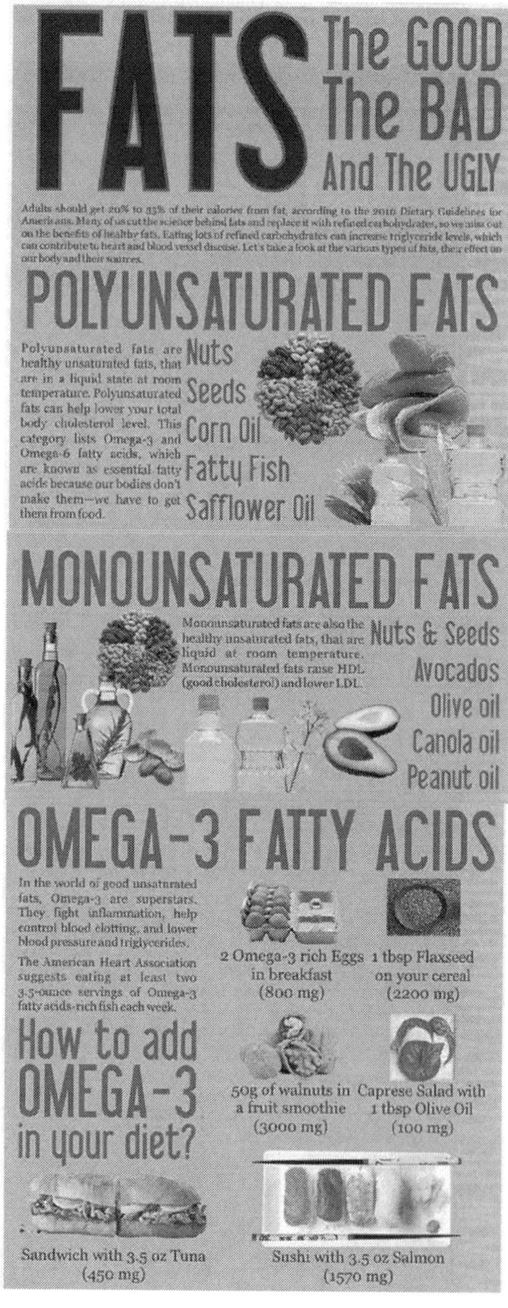
FATS The GOOD The BAD And The UGLY
Adults should get 20% to 35% of their calories from fat, according to the 2010 Dietary Guidelines for Americans. Many of us cut the science behind fats and replace it with refined carbohydrates, so we miss out on the benefits of healthy fats. Eating lots of refined carbohydrates can increase triglyceride levels, which can contribute to heart and blood vessel disease. Let's take a look at the various types of fats, their effect on our body and their sources.
POLYUNSATURATED FATS
Polyunsaturated fats are healthy unsaturated fats, that are in a liquid state at room temperature. Polyunsaturated fats can help lower your total body cholesterol level. This category lists Omega-3 and Omega-6 fatty acids, which are known as essential fatty acids because our bodies don't make them—we have to get them from food.
Nuts
Seeds
Corn Oil
Fatty Fish
Safflower Oil
MONOUNSATURATED FATS
Monounsaturated fats are also the healthy unsaturated fats, that are liquid at room temperature. Monounsaturated fats raise HDL (good cholesterol) and lower LDL.
Nuts & Seeds
Avocados
Olive oil
Canola oil
Peanut oil
OMEGA-3 FATTY ACIDS
In the world of good unsaturated fats, Omega-3 are superstars. They fight inflammation, help control blood clotting, and lower blood pressure and triglycerides.
The American Heart Association suggests eating at least two 3.5-ounce servings of Omega-3 fatty acids-rich fish each week.
How to add OMEGA-3 in your diet?
2 Omega-3 rich Eggs in breakfast (800 mg)
1 tbsp Flaxseed on your cereal (2200 mg)
50g of walnuts in a fruit smoothie (3000 mg)
Caprese Salad with 1 tbsp Olive Oil (100 mg)
Sandwich with 3.5 oz Tuna (450 mg)
Sushi with 3.5 oz Salmon (1570 mg)

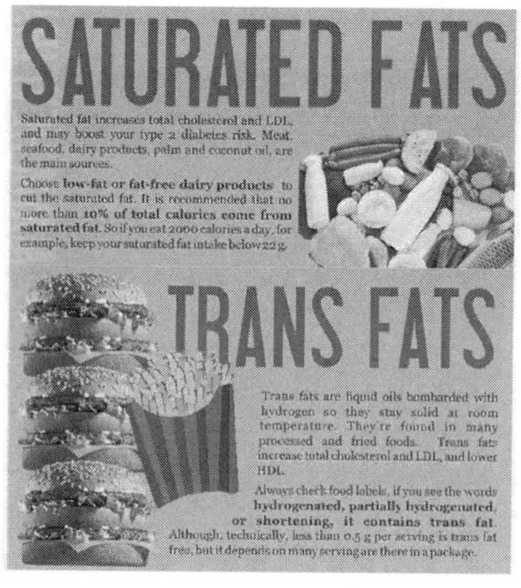

Instead of embracing the notion that "all fat is bad," you need to learn which are acceptable and which are harmful. We've been conditioned to think that all fats are going to make you fat, which is simply not true.

Even worse, most products labeled "low fat" or "fat free" often have a lot of added sugar. As you'll remember from Belief #11 about added sugar, there's nothing worse than assuming that all fat is bad and downing unnecessary added sugar. It's even worse than that. When natural fats are stripped out of foods (in order for manufacturers to say "fat free"), they are replaced with not only added sugar, but also salt and thickeners, none of which are good for you. You're left hungrier as well.

To delve further into this topic, check out WebMD's quiz, "How Much Do You Know About Fats and Oils?" at: http://tinyurl.com/le56hct.

This is pretty much all you need to know: seek out and eat good fats and stay away from bad fats. Plus, check labels on low/no fat foods to see if sugar has been added.

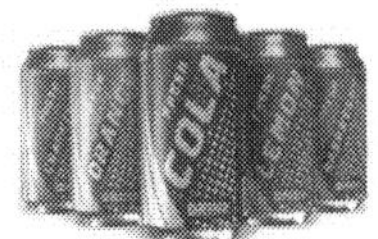

Belief #19

Believe That Regular and Diet Soda are Very Bad for You

Regular, non-diet soda may be the single largest contributor to obesity around the world, especially in children and teens. These mind-boggling statistics prove that soda is not just bad, but it's about as close to poison as you can get…cleverly disguised as something that tastes good. And the sad part is, it's very easy to wean someone off regular, sugar-laden soda to naturally flavored seltzer or water. Take a read:

- The average worldwide consumption of soft drinks is 89.8 liters per person per year (and the U.S. is at 216 liters per person per year!).
- 21% of all the sugar in the average American diet comes from soda.
- Drinking two sodas per week increases your risk of pancreatic cancer by 87%.
- Drinking one soda per day increases a child's risk of becoming obese by 60%.
- Drinking two sodas per day increase gout risk by 85%.
- One can of soda per day can easily add 15 pounds in a year.
- One can of soda contains as much as 10 teaspoons of sugar, which is ALL the sugar you should consume in an entire day.

Soda has been directly linked to these diseases:

- Obesity
- Liver damage
- Tooth decay
- Kidney stones and kidney disease
- Diabetes
- Heartburn and acid reflux
- Osteoporosis

- High blood pressure
- Heart disease
- Impaired digestion

In a massive study involving 264,000 people aged 50-71, those drinking four cups of regular soda per day were 30% more likely to develop depression, and those who drank diet soda were at a greater risk. And it's not just soda. Those who drank fruit juices had a 38% higher risk for depression (*Bottom Line Personal)*.

Soda has been linked to 25,000 deaths per year in the U.S., and 180,000 worldwide, according to research from the Harvard School of Public Health, and reported in www.HealthDay.com. Here's what happens when you drink a can or bottle of regular soda:

- Within 20 minutes, your blood sugar spikes and your liver responds by converting massive amounts of sugar into fat.
- Within 40 minutes, your blood pressure rises, and your liver dumps even more sugar into your bloodstream.
- You'll start to have a "sugar crash" after about an hour, which often leads people to craving and eating even more sugar, followed by crashes, in a horrible "sugar cycle."

Want to know how much sugar is in 20oz of cola?

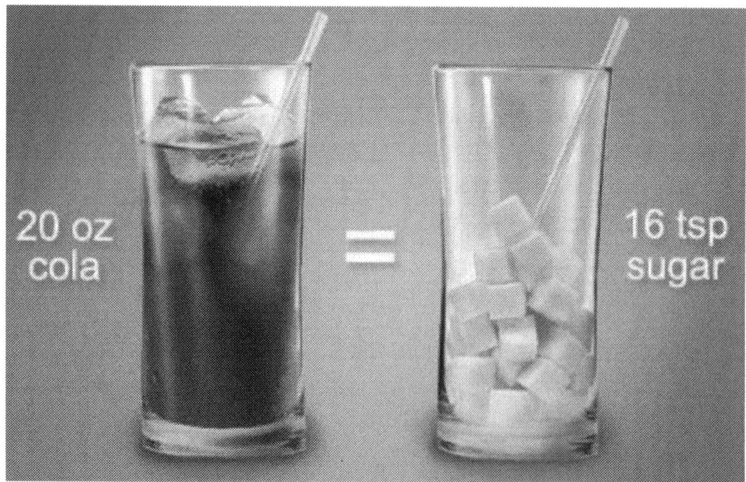

You should also know that Nobel Prize winner Otto Warburg way back in 1934 clearly demonstrated that cancer cells require more sugar to thrive. Let me phrase that in another way: eat more sugar, increase your chances for cancer. Any questions?

Two excellent articles about just how bad soda is for you:

- http://tinyurl.com/y8mfgoy
- http://tinyurl.com/7xwngme

Studies reported at Tufts.com also show a direct link between sugar and high blood pressure. The more regular soda and sugar-sweetened drinks you consume, the higher your blood pressure can be. Just get off sugar!

In terms of diet soda, they are not much better than sugared sodas. Numerous studies show that diet soda has additives that negatively impact your body. Now, I never drank regular soda, but drank diet soda for decades. I recently switched to fruit flavored seltzer (cheap, delicious and healthy), a brand of healthy no-sugar soda Zevia, and more water. For a well-written article on diet sodas, check out this article on Authority Nutrition: http://tinyurl.com/lwlkdfe.

The Tufts University Health & Nutrition Letter reports that a 12-ounce serving of regular soda has 39-41 grams of sugars (more than an entire day's allowance by a wide margin), 38mg of caffeine and zero protein. They report that in several studies, people who consume either regular or diet soda were more likely to develop metabolic syndrome, a precursor to heart disease and type-2 diabetes.

You might be shocked to know how much regular soda kids consume (www.mercola.com):

- Soda pop provides more added sugar in a **toddler**'s diet than cookies, candy and ice cream **combined**.
- 56% of 8-year olds drink soft drinks daily.
- 33% of teen boys drink three or more cans of soda every day.
- 60% of all public and private middle schools and high schools sell sugar-laden soda.

The Douglass Report (www.DouglassReport.com) reports that aspartame, the sweetener in most diet sodas, has been linked to at least 92 symptoms and side effects, and migraine headaches are high on the list.

There's more. Unless kids drink caffeine-free soda (hardly likely), they are getting plenty of caffeine. Do you really want your kids hooked on caffeine when they are toddlers, kids or teens?

As unbelievable as this seems, kids as young as five years old have kidney stone issues – soda consumption is a major contributor to this trend.

I think Dr. Richard Besser, ABC News' chief health and medical editor, summed up the issue of drinking soda very well, saying "It may not be easy at first, but your body will thank you."

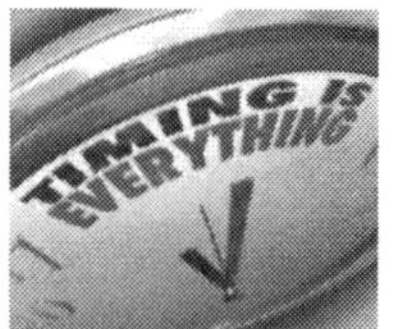

Belief #20

Believe in the Power of Timing

Quite possibly the most important thing I've learned in my weight loss journey is that *when* you eat is just as important as *what* you eat. In fact, I developed a 50-40-10 plan that defines how much food I eat throughout the day. I have found this to be extremely important in losing weight and keeping it off.

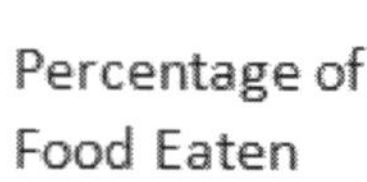

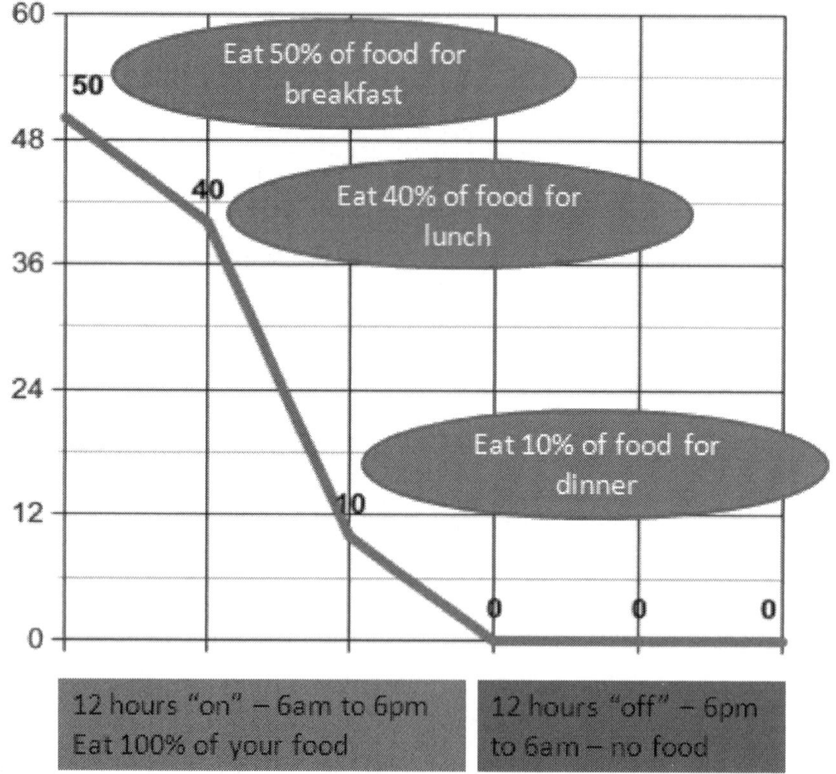

On most days, I eat 90% of my daily food for breakfast and lunch, and have usually fruit for dinner. Since we're all more active during the day than at night, it makes sense to eat food while you're active vs. watching TV or reading a book.

Eating all your food for breakfast and lunch and skipping dinner and snacks is called "intermittent fasting," which gives your body 12 to 18 hours to shift into what Dr. Mercola calls "fat-burning mode." It takes about 6 to 8 hours for your body to burn off carbs and sugar, which it does before it burns off fat. The more you can go without food (and not be

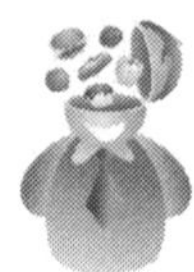

hungry), the more time your body has to get past the sugar/carb burning phase and into the fat burning phase. A well-written and researched piece on this topic is at:

http://tinyurl.com/cx6wfm8

Of course, it isn't possible to eat this way every single day, but if you can eat this way 5 days a week, you'll be way ahead of the game. It worked for me!

Dr. Steven Sisskind writes that people who eat lunch before 3pm lose significantly more weight and at a faster rate, that those who ate a later lunch. The early lunch eaters also had significantly better insulin sensitivity as well. More evidence that eating most of your food early in the day works.

This pattern of eating is certainly not new. Remember this quote from American author and nutritionist Adelle Davis:

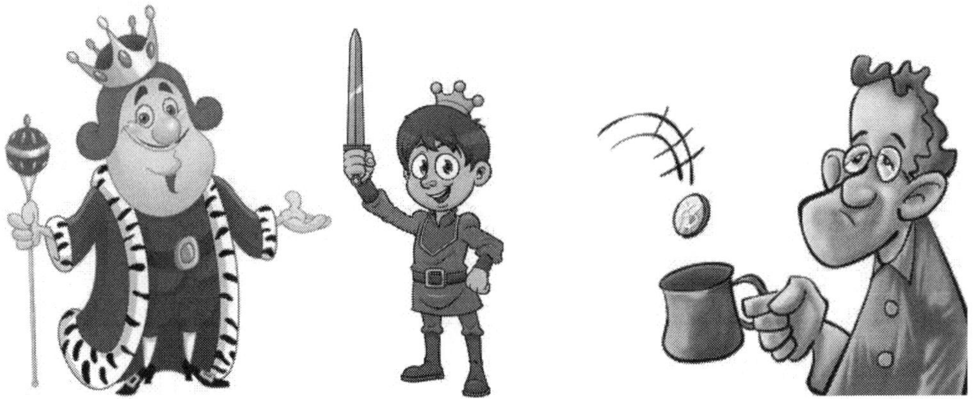

"Eat breakfast like a king, lunch like a prince and dinner like a pauper."

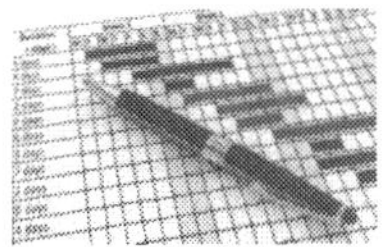

Belief #21

Believe in Frequent Milestones

This is one of the most powerful beliefs I've embraced. Most people recommend weighing yourself once every week or two. For many reasons, I think this not a good idea. For one, it gives you time to go off your diet and then get back on and starve yourself so you lose or don't gain at the next weigh-in. Clearly that's not a good strategy.

There are two really good reasons to weigh yourself every day, completely naked, in the morning. These are really, really, really, really important. You need to run out and get a digital scale that measures your weight in tenths of a pound, if you don't already have one.

Next, do some quick math. Let's say you weigh 150 and want to lose 30 pounds over 9 months, which is a good rate of loss – about 3 pounds per month. Convert your monthly goal (i.e. 3 pounds) into ounces (i.e. 48 ounces). Then divide the number of ounces (48) by 30 days in a month. That works out to 1.6 ounces you need to lose per day to lose 30 pounds in 9 months.

Now what sounds easier, losing 30 pounds in 9 months or losing a mere 1.6 ounces per day? I can tell you without a doubt that losing weight, even in small chunks on a day-in and day-out basis is something that kept me 100% motivated throughout my weight loss process. All those little losses – an ounce today, 3 ounces tomorrow – all added up to a lot of weight lost. Plus it was great motivation.

A great by-product of a daily weigh-in is what I call "frequent milestones." A frequent milestone occurs when you lose a nice amount of weight (i.e. 5 or 10 pounds), you're doing well for a specific amount of time (i.e. 90 days), and others.

The cool thing about this is that you will hit frequent milestones very often – they will make you feel good and you can brag about them to those who support you. Using our 30 pounds in 9 months example, here's what a frequent milestone chart would look like:

Pounds Lost	**Milestone**
3	On track for first 30 days
5	First of six five-pound losses
6	Two months and going strong
7.5	5% of body weight lost
9	Three months into the program
10	Second five-pound loss, first ten-pound loss
12	120 days into the program
15	10% of body weight lost, third five-pound loss, halfway point!
18	Six months of success
21	Seven months "on the wagon"
20	Down one clothing size, second ten-pound loss
22	BMI down 10%
24	30 days to reach goal
25	Fifth five-pound loss, only 5 pounds to go
30	Goal, 9 months of successful weight loss

Get the point? You'll have milestones to feel good about very often, and I'm sure you can add some of your own. Frequent milestones make you feel great about your progress. You can make a chart like this or not – that's up to you.

But make sure to embrace the concept of losing a little bit each day and feeling good (and bragging!) whenever you hit a new milestone!

It really, really, really, really works!

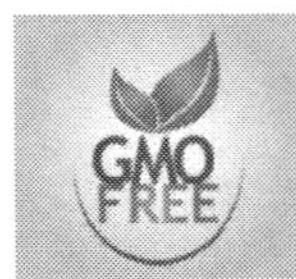

Belief #22

Believe in Learning About Genetically Modified Food

If you want to freak out about some of the food you've been eating for years, even decades, you need to take the time to learn about genetically modified (GM) food. Just Google "dangers of genetically modified food" and see what comes up. One of the best articles I've read is on mercola.com, and titled "Engineered Poison Lurking in Your Everyday Food?" and get the best-selling book on the topic by Jeffrey Smith, "Seeds of Deception."

The NonGMO Project writes that GMOs (Genetically Modified Organisms) "are made by forcing genes from one species, such as bacteria, viruses, animals, or humans, into the DNA of a food crop or animal to introduce a new trait."

Several of my doctors have talked about avoiding GM food. And Smith and Mercola are not the only ones who write about GM food and how harmful they can be.

Scary? Absolutely. Can you do something about it? Absolutely.

I'm not going to go into a long explanation of GM/GMO and the litany of problems it has and can cause, but urge you to simply spend 10 minutes reading this article. If you want to go further, doing more research (there's plenty of info online) and/or buy Smith's book.

But what I will get into is the importance of eliminating GM food as one of your weight loss and healthy eating beliefs. You should know that over 90% of U.S. corn and soy crops are genetically modified, and these two foods and their many derivatives (soybean oil, corn oil, high fructose corn syrup, cornstarch, tofu, etc.) are the most common ingredients in all processed foods. Other GM foods include canola, cottonseed, sugar beets, most Hawaiian papaya and small amounts of zucchini and yellow squash. Plus, about 80% of packaged and processed foods contain GMOs (www.CaltonNutrition.com).

"Big Bad Corn" is a scary infographic all about corn. What lurks behind the bright yellow ears of corn will surprise you. Find it here, courtesy of Found Health: http://tinyurl.com/98d9qox.

Mercola.com also has a related article "How to Wean Yourself Off Processed Food in 7 Steps" which you should read when you're ready to swear off GM foods.

There's a website devoted to this entire issue, where you can find a GMO-based shopping guide: www.NonGMOShoppingGuide.com. And you can look for this seal in addition to buying products labeled "100% organic," "organic" or "made with organic ingredients."

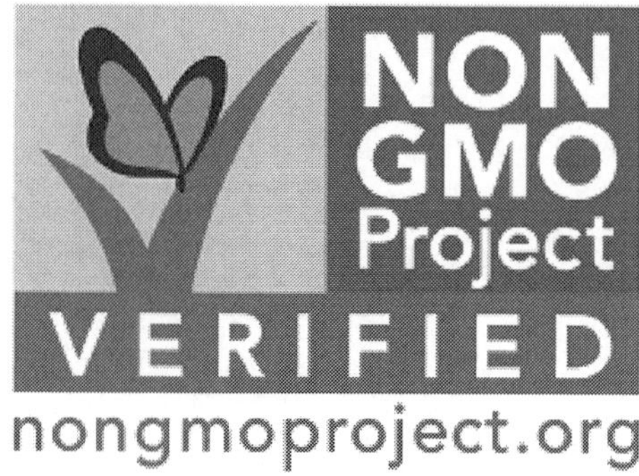

According to *Prevention* Magazine (4/12), the top 8 food crops containing GMOs are:

- Corn
- Soybeans
- Canola
- Cottonseed
- Sugar beets
- Hawaiian papaya
- Some zucchini
- Some yellow squash

Bottom line: get rid of as many GM foods from your diet as possible. Eating fresh foods (i.e. salads every day as I do) is a good start!

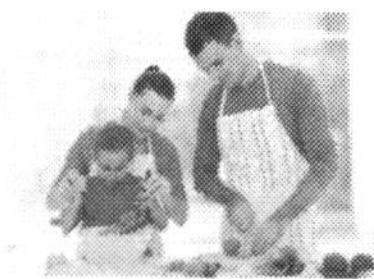

Belief #23

Believe in Teaching Your Children Well

I remember the hit song "Teach Your Children" by Crosby, Stills, Nash & Young, and the message that it talked about: teach your children well (obviously!). There's nothing more important when it comes to raising kids than teaching them well about food, and the earlier you start the better.

If one or both parents are fat, there's a very good chance the child will grow up to be fat. And that's just plain sad. This *Newsweek* Magazine cover from 2000 says it well:

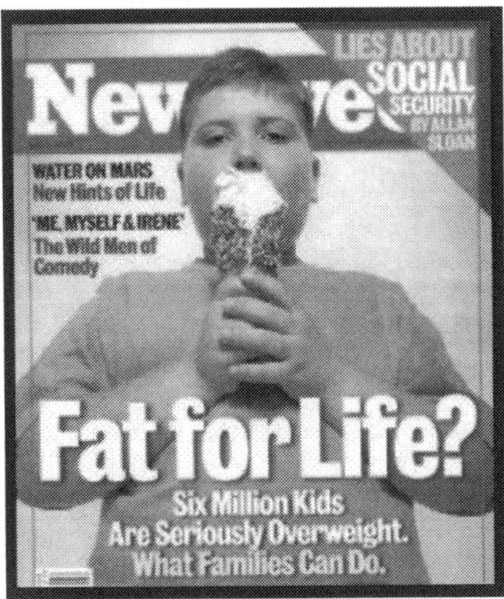

It's one thing to let yourself go, but to directly and negatively impact the life of your children is another. They don't deserve to be behind the 8-ball in life because their parents didn't care enough to educate them about the dangers of food.

From www.geardiary.com, here's an idea of complications that are brought on by childhood obesity:

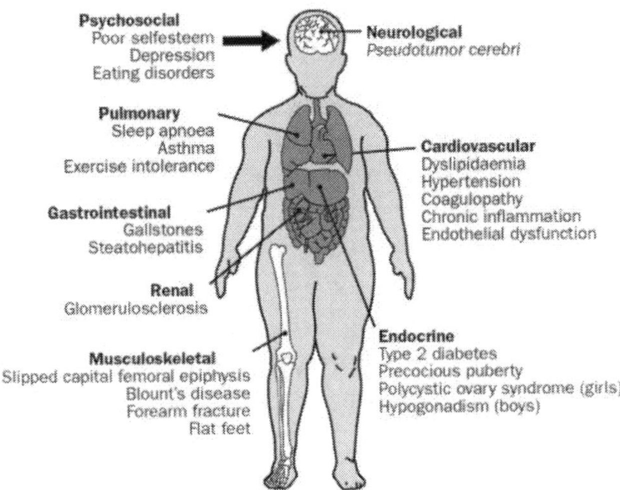

For those of us parents who are at an acceptable weight, we all have an ongoing battle with our kids in trying to get them to eat good foods and avoid the junk. One of the best articles I've ever read on this topic is from WebMD.com titled "10 Ways to Help Your Child Develop a Positive Relationship with Healthy Food." Starting as young as your child can comprehend, here is a condensation of the 10 techniques:

- When banning bad foods, educate your kids about why you're doing so and focus on the nutritional and health value of good foods, and see the next tip.
- Keep only healthy food in your home. Kids eat what is in the fridge or pantry, so stock it with the good stuff.
- Tie food into the things that your kid enjoys, such as sports, singing, acting, etc. Explain how certain foods are good for stamina, energy, etc.
- Praise your kids when they make healthy choices.
- When your kids eat or want to eat junk, steer them to better alternatives
- Never use junk food as a reward. If you do, this is something they will carry with them, even as adults. I know, I did that. Not a good plan.
- Strongly encourage light family dinners at night. Families that have dinner together and not "on the run" have better nutrition, eating habits, and less likely to get into food troubles as they grow up.
- Prepare the plates in the kitchen instead of serving buffet or family style where the kids take their own. You control their portions, not them.
- Get your kids involved in a positive way. Play one or more food games with them (see the article for a cool one).
- Talk with your child's pediatrician before starting any weight loss regimen. Never diagnose your child as being too heavy or too thin without doctor input.
- Some kids are easily caught up in an addictive/allergic craving cycle. This is something to explore if your child craves something he/she is allergic to!

Another wonderful article (from HelpGuide.com) with more tips on getting your kids to eat healthy is here: http://tinyurl.com/cbv95n.

When your kids say they're hungry, instead of just reaching for food, find out if they are truly hungry and what food or drink they want. Try to determine if they are truly hungry, or they are asking for food for another reason. Kids need to recognize as early as possible that many times when they think they are hungry they actually are not.

A study in the journal *Pediatrics* reports that kids and parents who received instruction on how to make good food choices ate more "go" foods (good, nutritious foods) and less "whoa" foods (junk), and the educational value stuck with the kids for years after the classes. Getting kids into the right habits when coupled with education so they understand **why** is a pretty powerful combination!

A British study reported in *The Atlantic* concluded that kids are prejudiced against fat people by age 4 – "kids are cruel and quick to reject those who are different from them" – so at a very early age, fat kids are likely to be rejected and ostracized. Don't let that happen to your child!

When your kids are old enough, teach them to read food labels, and tell them to watch out for the "bad guys" – see the *Mind Diet Guidebooks* section that gives you a detailed explanation of nutrition labels.

"Children subconsciously mimic what they see and hear from the adults around them, so parents and other adult role models play an important role in promoting a positive body image," writes Jacqueline Silvestri Banks on Foxnews.com.

One expert nutrition coach and frequent guest on TV shows like Dr. Oz, Dr. Ro (Rovenia Brock, PhD), -- has created FitKidz™ -- an interactive series that empowers kids to take charge of their own health. Dr. Ro has devoted much of her life working on stemming childhood obesity, and this program is worth checking out: http://everythingro.com/fit_kidz.html.

In a very well-written and emotional piece in www.CelebrateWomanToday.com, Boyd Jentzsch talks about how the current generation has been born into a mean world. He's not talking about wars, crime, poverty or disease. He's referring to the "first full generation to be born into a world of plenty…a place of advertised, appetizing enchantment wrapped around an abundance of food that will kill them. And you, and I, and the whole lot of us are unknowingly doing the poisoned feeding." A litany of depressing stats makes this article a must read if you have kids or are planning to start a family:

- One out of every three kids will get Adult Onset (Type 2) Diabetes. If they are Hispanic, African American or Pacific Islander, it will be 50%. For Native Americans, it's already over 80%.
- A child that is overweight by age 8 has triple the risk of being an overweight teen. An overweight teen is three times more likely to be an overweight adult.
- Children with diabetes are often not diagnosed, and have a high risk of permanent small blood vessel damage.
- Obese children are 53 times more likely to have the risk factors for diabetes.
- Dieting in pre-teens and early teens is leading to eating disorders.

There's much more in this article, and I strongly recommend reading it, at: http://tinyurl.com/knpgcy7.

Parents may be unwittingly contributing to their kids' obesity, according to food comparisons highlighted in BET Health News (http://www.bet.com/news/health.html): Some parents who stop their kids from drinking sugar-laden soft drinks and substitute apple juice may not realize that 8 ounces of sodas have the same 27 grams of sugar as apple juice.

This comparison goes deeper, according to "Black and Latino Kids Drink More Sugary Juice Drinks" author Kellee Terrell:

- School districts in California label these sugar-laden juices as "healthy" and include them in lunches.
- There is a lack of literacy programs to educate parents that drinks that "sound good" are often not any better than regular soda.

"Contrary to the common perception that chubby babies are healthy babies and will naturally outgrow their baby fat, excess weight tends to persist," says Leann Birch, professor of human development and director in the Center for Childhood Obesity Research at Pennsylvania State University. "This is a national concern because weight-related conditions such as diabetes and high blood pressure once occurred almost exclusively in adults but are now occurring at rising rates among teens and young adults," Birch said.

My research for this section led me to www.kidshealth.org, the most visited site on the web for information about health, behavior and development from before birth through the teen years. I'd strongly suggest spending some time on it!

This is hardly a U.S. problem. A survey by the Schools Health Education Unit in the U.K., reported at www.dailymail.co.uk, revealed that in a survey of 68,000 10-15 year olds, nearly two-thirds said they would like to be slimmer, indicating that they are concerned with their weight and have fallen into bad habits, such as skipping breakfast and/or lunch. Since kids **want** to eat healthy, parents need to make that happen with prudent guidance.

A very good rule of thumb is the 5-2-1-0 formula developed by the National Initiative for Children's Healthcare Quality (www.nichq.org), defined as:

- 5 servings of fruits and vegetables daily
- 2 or less hours of non-homework screen time
- 1 or more hours of physical activity
- 0 sugar sweetened beverages

Lots of additional good information on this site. Like so much misinformation, parents need to be vigilant about their babies' weight so their childhoods and teenage years are not filled with health problems that usually befall adults.

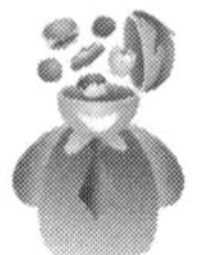

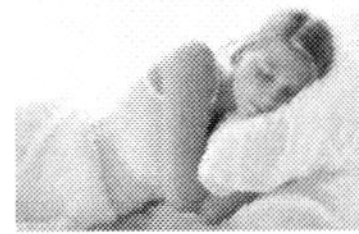

Belief #24

Believe in Sleep's Important Role in Weight Loss

The finding that most people don't realize is the important role sleep plays in obesity. Quite simply, the more you sleep, the better it is for your body in terms of losing weight. Conversely, the less you sleep, the easier it is for your body to pack on the pounds.

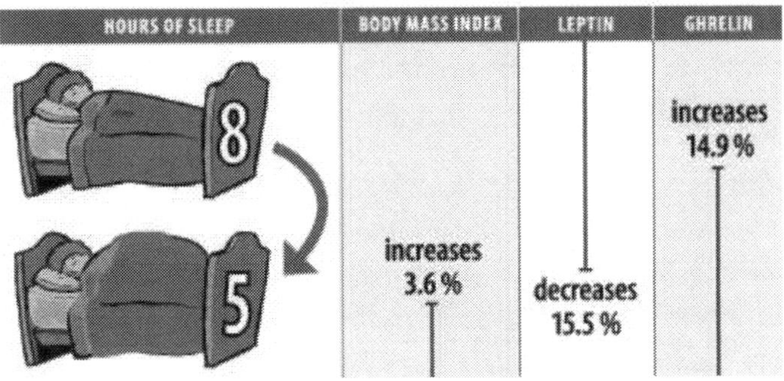

As you can see from this infographic from SixStepsToSleep.com, getting 5 or so hours of sleep instead of 8 results in an increase in Body Mass Index, a decrease in leptin and an increase in ghrelin. *Prevention* Magazine reports that night owls consume 248 more calories than those who go to bed early. The Endocrine Society showed that sleep deprivation appears to prompt the production of higher levels of a molecule in the blood that is responsible for the feelings of reward and enjoyment that comes from eating.

Getting more sleep may be the easiest and fastest change you can make to help you lose weight. Count 8 hours back from the time you need to wake up for work to determine when you need to go to sleep. If you need to get up at 6am to get ready for work, then you need to be in bed by 10pm.

When you are sleep-deprived, it throws off your metabolism, which directly controls weight gain and loss. The hormone ghrelin tells you to eat, and when you're sleep deprived, more of it is produced. Leptin is the hormone that tells you to stop eating, and when you don't get enough sleep, you have less leptin. It's that simple. Aim for 7-8 hours of quality sleep every night.

Registered dietician, author and lecturer David Grotto suggests eating tart cherries one hour before going to sleep, as it is very high in melatonin, a sleep-inducing hormone!

Bottom Line Health reports that drinking plenty of water and eating a wide variety of foods including vegetables and fruits, leads to better sleep. So what you eat affects how you sleep.

One reader shares what she does: "I turn off all electronics, and read or meditate one hour before turning in for the night."

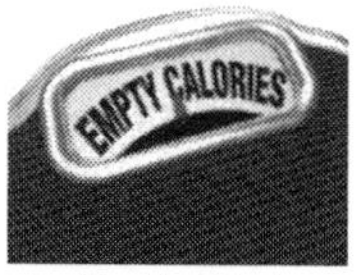

Belief #25

Believe That Empty Calories are Horrible for You

Perhaps you've heard of this term, maybe not. As it sounds, consuming foods that have empty calories is not a good thing. Basically, foods with empty calories have little or no nutrition to counteract the calories, usually from sugar. Foods that are high in empty calories include:

- Regular soda
- Fruit drinks
- Candy
- Cookies/Donuts/Pastries
- Margarine
- Butter
- Cream
- Bacon
- Deep-fried foods

The simple fact is, stay away from foods with empty calories. I talked extensively about the power of substitution earlier – and in this context, substituting for empty calorie foods is a great thing to do.

Barbara Rolls (nutritional expert, past-president of The Obesity Society and Chair of Nutritional Sciences at Penn State) is a pioneer of "calorie density." She has found that the more water in the food you eat, the more food you can eat with the same calorie count as foods with empty calories. A small handful of jelly beans has 100 calories as does a big apple. The big apple will leave you full while the jelly beans won't. Her scientific proof is yet another reason to ditch empty calories.

The UCLA Division of Geriatrics publication HEALTHY/Years recommends that empty calories should be no more than 10% of your total caloric intake per day.

One question you should ask yourself before eating foods high in empty calories is, "Is it worth it?" Stack.com has a great graphic of what it takes to burn off a variety of junk foods at http://tinyurl.com/lr4b4qb. Examples:

- Slice of cheesecake and large movie popcorn: 6.8 hours of walking
- 4 slices of pizza plus double gulp of regular soda: 2.93 hours cycling
- Double cheeseburger plus French fries: 7.1 hours of yoga

Is it worth it? Simple question you should ask every time you eat!

To give you an idea of what 500 calories looks like, for both junk and healthy food, here's a great resource – and you WILL be surprised: http://tinyurl.com/mc8g79u (LifeHack.com).

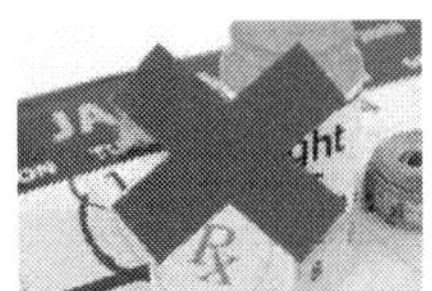

Belief #26

Believe that You Need to Forget Most of What You Know About Weight Loss

There's a very, very good chance some of what you believe about weight loss and dieting is wrong. So much of what we think is true comes from hearsay, misinformation, misinterpretation and folklore handed down from generation to generation.

Take the cliché "everything is OK if taken in moderation." Some people interpret this to mean "I can eat anything I want as long as I don't overdo it." Nothing could be further from the truth. The bottom line is this: some foods are so bad that even small amounts will retard your weight loss efforts. The better cliché is: "good foods in moderation are OK as long as they are a part of your overall weight loss game plan." Here are a few sayings you need to erase from your mind:

- "It's all in the genes. Some people just can't lose weight." Almost anyone can lose weight and genes play a small role in a small percentage of the population.
- "All fats are bad." There are two main types of fats: saturated and unsaturated. In general, stay away from most saturated fats. The truth is, many foods high in "good" fat is actually good for you, like many types of nuts.
- "Eat whatever you want as long as you exercise." For this to be true, you'd have to be working out 4-5-6 hours a day. Exercise is only one component of weight loss. It helps, but not to the exclusion of eating right."

Onward and upward!

At this point in time, two things should have happened.

First, you should have reached your Moment of Truth. Congratulations if you have. If not, you MUST go back to square one (the first guidebook) and reach your Moment of Truth. Failure to do so will result in failure to lose weight and keep it off.

Second, you should have embedded these 26 beliefs in your mind and understand why they are so important. If you have, wonderful. If not, reread this guidebook until you do.

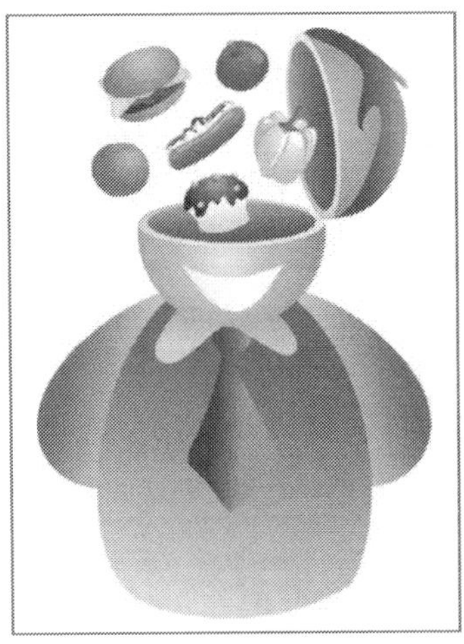

Guidebook #3
Strategies

How to Use this Guidebook

This guidebook presents 122 "bite size" strategies (each usually no more than a page long), asking you to think about how weight impacts you in a specific situation. They are all real-life situations that we all encounter over time.

These "think about" strategies are organized into eleven sections:

The ideal way to use *The Mind Diet: Strategies* is to read it cover to cover first. Then, use the strategies as refreshers for specific situations. For example, you can brush up on strategies for eating at parties or when you're invited to a restaurant that has only a buffet.

Each strategy also has a **"what to do about it"** paragraph or more that are specific strategies you can immediately use in your daily life.

After each section I end it with **"Think about it. This is your life we're talking about here."** That line is a constant reminder that this is not a game, and if you want to have the best possible outcome, you need to think of this in terms of your life.

OK, let's get started!

Section I: Top-of-Mind

Section II: Get Practical

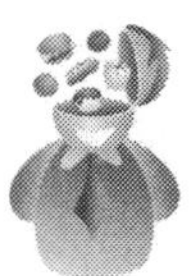

Section VI: Eating Situations

Section VII: Inconveniences

Section VIII: Exercise

Section IX: Ailments

Section X: What's In The Foods You Eat

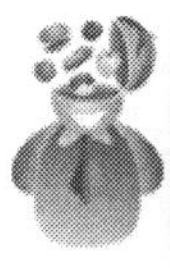

Section I: Top-of-Mind

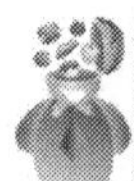

Strategy #1

Think About Why We Eat

My basic premise is real simple: there are only two **positive** reasons why people eat. I'm not talking about eating to celebrate, eating out of frustration or the need to pig out on a whim. No, I'm thinking at a higher level of defining why we eat.

One reason is **sustenance**. You need food to live. If this were the only reason to eat, we'd all be thin, because the body doesn't need all that much food to survive and be healthy.

The second reason is **taste**. We eat because food tastes good. Depending on your palate and pocketbook, we're talking about a $7.95 minute steak or a $35 Porterhouse. We spend time cooking up great tasting meals and finding delectable restaurants. In addition to spending lots of money on food because of the taste, we also will drive considerable distances just to please our palates. That's it. Those are the only two reasons to eat. Period.

There is a slew of what I call negative **excuses** for eating: frustration, depression, long-standing habits, peer pressure, parental pressure, boredom, previous failures and many others. We also tend to eat when good things happen (promotion, graduation, birthday, etc.), and while there's nothing wrong with that, for many, eating out has replaced other non-food-related activities.

There's a huge difference between a "reason" to eat and an "excuse" for eating, though most people think they are the same. Ideally, we all should only eat because we need food for survival and because it tastes good.

But most of us eat as an excuse resulting from those other factors listed above. Many years ago, my first job out of college was selling ads to local retail stores for a newspaper. I developed this "negative eating habit" of eating when I didn't make sales (out of frustration) and also eating when I did make sales (as a celebration). It was easy to justify eating, and I ended up eating a lot more than I should. Unfortunately, I sold ads in towns that had great bakeries and delicatessens!

What to do about it: you've got to fully embrace the thought that you eat to live, not live to eat. Other things in your life MUST take priority over eating. You need to focus on finding enjoyment from other activities, relationships, work and play.

Think about it. This is your life we're talking about here!

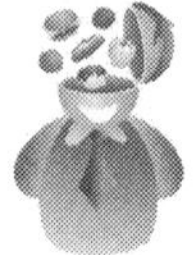

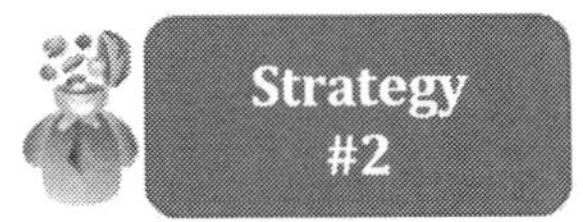

Think About How Taste Works

It's elementary – we have about 4,600 taste buds located on our tongues. If you buy into the premise (previous strategy) that there are only two good or "positive" reasons to eat (sustenance and taste), getting the maximum pleasure from taste would be a logical goal. We also know that foods have flavors, and when those flavors seep into the taste buds, there is either a positive or negative sensation sent to our brain: it tastes good or it doesn't. End of story.

But when you swallow, the food leaves your tongue on the way to your stomach, and the taste sensation fades pretty quickly. The obvious conclusion is that the faster you eat, chew and swallow, the least amount of taste sensation you get. In thinking about it in this manner, why would you want to rush the process?

If you get pleasurable taste sensations only when food is resting on your tongue and when it is being chewed (but not swallowed), wouldn't you want to keep the food in your mouth and on your tongue for as long as possible – and get as much taste sensation as possible? Especially when you've traveled many miles and/or are spending a bunch of money on dinner.

Think about it – a minor change in the way you "process" food can make a major difference in both taste and weight loss. **Chewing longer and letting food rest on your tongue results in a longer taste sensation.** We work hard to make tasty meals or spend good money eating out – so why not enjoy it two, three, five or even ten times as much as you do now, by simply tasting and chewing longer?

This same minor change will help a lot in the weight loss process. The more time you spend chewing, the faster you will feel full. If you eat fast, it will take longer for you to feel full, and as a result you will probably eat more.

What to do about it: kill two birds with one stone. Before you start chewing, let the food rest on your tongue and rub the food with the top surface of your tongue against the top of your mouth. You'll get a lot of flavor without chewing. After 5 to 10 seconds, start chewing, nice and slowly. You'll wind up eating less food because you'll feel fuller long before you've stuffed your face silly!

Think about it. This is your life we're talking about here!

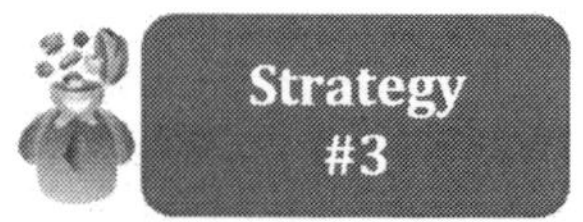

Think About Willpower

We all use this word in reference to weight loss. Either you've got the willpower to lose weight or you don't, people say. But what exactly is willpower, and how do you get it?

According to the American Heritage Dictionary of the English Language and online at www.dictionary.reference.com, willpower is defined as: *The strength of will to carry out one's decisions, wishes, or plans.*

In this context, I define "eating willpower" as **the strength of character to make decisions that will cause you to lose weight and keep it off.**

And what exactly is required to make these decisions? Without minimizing how hard it is, making a decision is simply a matter of making up your mind to take a specific course of action. That is actually the easy part. Carrying out that decision, under various pressures, is a lot harder, and that's what the heart of willpower is all about.

When you make a decision, any decision, you typically think about the pros and cons of that decision. It's no different in the world of weight loss. The overall decision "I want to lose weight" is actually supported by thousands of individual decisions at various points in time:

- I will not take a second helping of pasta at the party.
- I will leave over half of my potatoes.
- I will refuse to eat foods that are not on my diet.
- I will eat more slowly.
- I will chew food longer.
- I will choose water or seltzer instead of regular sugar-laden soda.

Notice the positive nature of these statements. Remember earlier I said that the word "try" should not be used in the context of losing weight? Well, wouldn't these statements all have been much weaker if I had inserted the words "try to" after "will?"

Every day you will be faced with many eating decisions, all of which derive from your primary decision to really get serious about weight loss. If you can make the right decision most of the time, the weight will come off, no matter what diet or program you're following (more on that later). You'll need to apply little "bursts" of willpower when these daily decisions arise.

What to do about it: when faced with these individual decisions, add a "because" to every decision:

- ***I will not take a second helping at the party because I'm full and don't need to eat any more.***
- ***I will leave over half my potatoes because it will lead to me looking great in smaller sized clothes.***
- ***I will refuse certain foods that are not on my diet because they make me feel sleepy and that affects my job performance.***
- ***I will eat more slowly because that will help me taste and enjoy what I am eating, and lead to feeling fuller sooner.***
- ***I will chew food longer because that's how I can really enjoy it.***
- ***I will choose water or seltzer because all the sugar in regular soda is just plain bad for me. A small sacrifice.***

Think about it. This is your life we're talking about here!

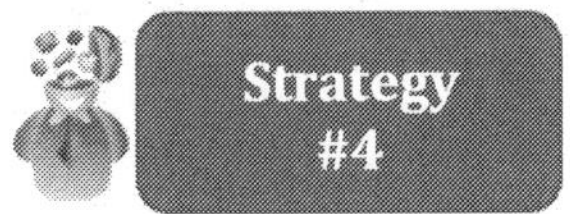

Think About the Time Paradox

In a previous section, I asked you to think about a small change in the way you eat food, one that will increase taste sensation and help you lose weight. There's some solid "math" behind that advice. Let's assume you eat like most people do. The amount of taste sensation pleasure you get might be 5 seconds per bite. Assume that you get 50 "taste sensations" per meal, you eat 3 meals a day, and have 2 snacks a day.

This looks like 200 taste sensations (50 x 3 plus 50 for snacks) per day at 5 seconds each = 1000 seconds or 1000/60 = about 17 minutes per day of taste pleasure.

That leaves 23 hours and 43 minutes a day when you have to deal with the after-effects of overeating: tight clothes, sweating, medical problems related to overweight, etc. Think about it: for the 17 minutes of eating pleasure you get per day, is it really worth it?

What to do about it: wouldn't it be better to cut down your food intake by 50% and get the same 17.5 minutes of pleasure (by chewing twice as long) and take a big step towards eliminating all the other problems? Of course it would!

Think about it. This is your life we're talking about here!

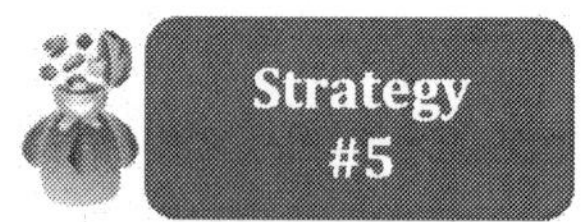

Think About the Ease of Dieting Today

It used to be that if you were on a low-fat, low-carb or most any other diet, you would have to sacrifice great tasting food for rabbit food or food that tasted like cardboard. I'm sure you've heard all the jokes – what's worse than airline food? Diet food, not even close.

The good news is that it doesn't have to be that way. Companies have developed really tasty food for whatever diet you're on. I've found a low-carb, low-sugar chocolate bar that tastes every bit as good (well not as good but very good) as its high-carb, high-sugar counterpart.

Major supermarket chains are stocking big diet food sections so you have a great selection of whatever you need. Cookbooks abound with recipes created for specific diet programs. It's no longer frozen TV dinners and not much else. And there are specialty stores and websites catering to most major diet programs. Michelob even has a low-carb beer for those of you on low-carb diets.

A warning from a reader: "Not all of these foods are good for you. Some are processed. Just because you have a lot of choices doesn't mean they are all healthy. Buyer beware!"

In the past, it was easy to say "I can't find good tasting foods, so I'm not going on a rabbit food diet" as a way to justify stopping one's diet. That excuse no longer exists – today diet food tastes great.

What to do about it: once you know which program you're going to follow, spend the time to find good sources of great tasting food. It's that simple.

Think about it. This is your life we're talking about here!

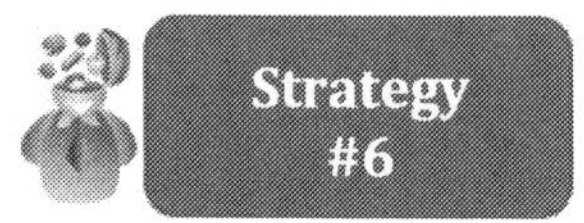

Think About Tomorrow

I would think that everyone who has ever contemplated a diet has said "I'll start tomorrow." And for most of us, tomorrow keeps being put off or it never comes. On a Friday, we might say we want to start tomorrow, but then tomorrow is the weekend, and who wants to start dieting on the weekend. So Saturday becomes Monday.

The problem gets even worse when tomorrow becomes next week, or next month, or some date in the future. Let's say you're going on vacation in August, and here it is April. You say, "I'm going to lose 20 pounds by my vacation, so I'll look and feel great." But as the months go by, you never really start, figuring that you still have plenty of time to lose those 20 pounds. So in April, May and June, you don't diet, and gain weight. All of a sudden, you now need to lose 30 pounds in one month, a virtual impossibility.

In the Garth Brooks song "If Tomorrow Never Comes" he sings about what would happen in that event: *"If tomorrow never comes, Will she know how much I loved her?"*

In this song, tomorrow means that something happens and you're not around tomorrow. How does that fit in with weight loss?

Flash forward 20 or 40 or 60 years. Someday, all of our tomorrows will come. Do you want to be in this position (my words):

If tomorrow never comes, would I have enjoyed life more if I had lost weight? "This is my new mantra!" writes one of my readers.

What to do about it: think of tomorrow as today. Losing weight, exercising and enjoying life should never be put off, even one day.

Think about it. This is your life we're talking about here!

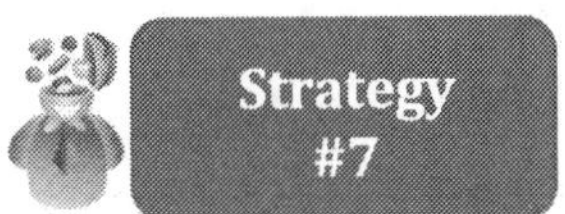

Think About Rationalization

We all rationalize, about a lot of things. But I don't think we rationalize more about food and weight loss than any other topic. So what exactly is rationalization, and how can we put an end to it?

The American Heritage Dictionary's definition is one of the best I've seen, for it relates to weight loss perfectly: "To devise self-satisfying but incorrect excuses for one's behavior." To put it another way, you fool yourself into doing something that isn't good for you. Examples:

- "One more French fry isn't going to hurt me."
- "I had a bad day. I need ice cream." Or, "I had a good day. I want ice cream."
- "I read that dark chocolate can be good for you. I'm going to have a bar. The more the better, right?"
- "I'm OK being overweight; that's my choice."

- "I didn't get the job because I'm overweight; the other guy was more qualified."
- "I'm going to fast all day and then pig out at the party."

Get the point?

The mind is a wonderful but tricky thing. It can come up with rationalizations like these in order to help us fool ourselves into going off our plans or eating foods that we know are bad for us. Google Cynthia Sass' article "5 White Lies That Stall Weight Loss" and see if you're telling yourself any of them.

What to do about it: make your slogan "Rationalization is Wrong" and remember it every time your mind starts to play these games. Force yourself to remember the slogan when food that you know you should not eat is in front of you or in your hand.

Think about it. This is your life we're talking about here!

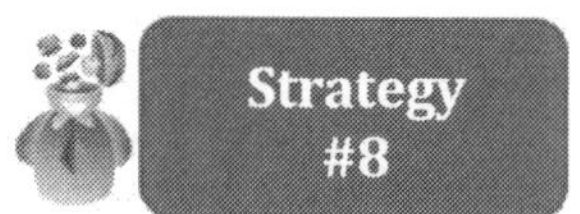

Think About Our Supersized Culture

The marketing geniuses at the fast food chains figured out that by asking if people wanted to "supersize" their meals for a small additional cost, many if not most people, would take it. After all, why wouldn't you want to get more fries for a pittance? And that's exactly what has happened – and the fast food chains are laughing all the way to the bank.

Look around – when it comes to food – supersizing is the name of the game.

- All you can eat buffets.
- Overstuffed, overflowing sandwiches.
- Unlimited refills on soft drinks.

And so on. Because food, at wholesale prices, is so cheap, offering a ton of food has become the staple of not only fast food joints, but just about every eating establishment. When's the last time you had an ice cream cone that wasn't overflowing and dripping down the sides?

If you're going to make any progress losing weight, you'll need to recognize this issue as a real problem. The temptation is to take as much as will fit on your plate and go back until you're ready to bust a gut because it's one price, or in the case of cruises, weddings and other institutional functions, the food is included or is free.

What to do about it: if you have a choice between a buffet and a regular restaurant, choose the restaurant, not the buffet. That's the most important choice you can make.

In a case where you have to attend a buffet, make up your mind in advance of how to deal with buffets. Never supersize, period. And if you get one of those overstuffed sandwiches, eat half and take the rest home. You need to stop falling victim to the marketing gimmicks used by establishments that sell food.

Think about it. This is your life we're talking about here!

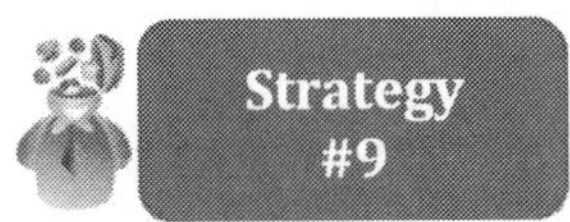

Think About Time

Let's do a simple exercise. I want you to determine, honestly, how much of each day is negatively impacted by your weight. You may be very surprised. Make a list like the one below. A "Y" under "Negative Impact?" means that activity is made more difficult by your being overweight.

Activity	Negative Impact?	Time Per Day
Sleeping	Y	6 hrs
Driving	Y	3 hrs
Eating	N	2 hrs
Watching TV	N	3 hrs
Working	Y	7 hrs
Walking	Y	1 hr
Preparing Meals	Y	1 hr
Using Your Computer	N	1 hr
Total		24 hrs
% negatively impacting your day – total all hours next to the Y's and divide by 24		67%

The definition of a negative impact is **any** of the following:

- You're uncomfortable
- You're in pain
- You have trouble performing an activity
- You sweat profusely when thinner people would not

Or any other inconvenience or annoyance that results from your weight.

Surprised? Shocked?

What to do about it: next time you eat any food that's not on the diet you've chosen, or you eat more than you know you should, think of all these hours that negatively affect you because of your weight.

Think about it. This is your life we're talking about here!

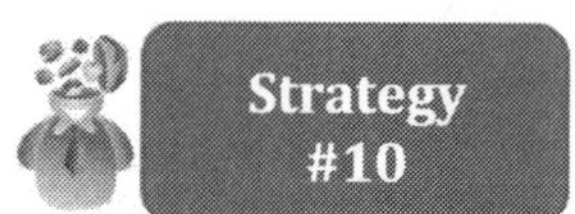

Think About Percentages

There are some foods that are so bad, that eating just one of them can account for a huge percentage of what you should have for the entire day. Let's look at a couple of examples.

- Suppose you're on a low-carb program, and your total allowable intake is 20 grams of carbs for the entire day. If you were to have just 10 small pretzels – not very much, right – that would account for over 45 grams of carbs! That's more than double what you're allowed! And you could easily eat those 10 pretzels in a few minutes!

- Suppose you're counting calories and your limit is 2,000 per day. Look how each of these foods accounts for a big part of that limit:

Food/Portion	Calories	% of Daily Limit
6 oz ribs	801	40%
5 crackers	393	20%
1 pc pecan pie	503	25%
6 oz duck	916	46%

It's so easy to blow your entire day's worth of fat, calories, carbs or whatever you count with just one or two small portions of foods that are bad for whatever program you're on. Yet, this is so easy to prevent!

What to do about it: this is going to require some effort on your part, but hey, that's why you're reading this book, and you only have to do this exercise once. Once you determine which plan you're going to follow, you need to learn which foods are terrible for you, and stay away from them. I know, that for my program, I have to stay away from pretzels, potato chips and other foods, because they are so high in carbs. Once you memorize those truly bad foods, you just avoid them. It's that simple.

Think about it. This is your life we're talking about here!

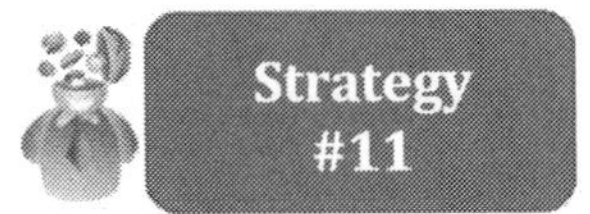

Think About The Importance of Eating

Are you a person who:

- Eats to Live

OR

- Lives to Eat

This question is at the heart of why we eat, and it's a critical one.

The person who "eats to live" is someone who eats the right foods in order to live and be healthy. He or she does not focus on food, but enjoys it in addition to other interests, hobbies, work and relationships.

The person who "lives to eat" is the opposite. He or she focuses totally on food, living for meals, and in some cases ignores the other parts of living that have nothing to do with food. When asked, "What is your favorite thing to do?" this type of person usually answers "Eat out" or some other food-related conversation.

What to do about it: if you are, or think you might be, someone who "lives to eat," think about how food has come to dominate your life. Think of what you're missing by concentrating on food to the exclusion of other pursuits. Think how much fun you're missing out on by "living to eat."

Think about it. This is your life we're talking about here!

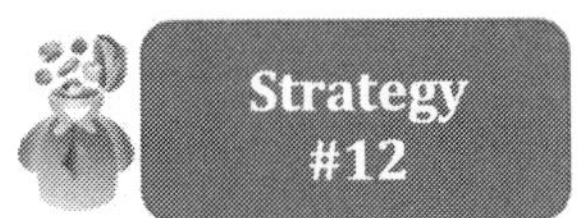

Think About Eating Out of Frustration

Earlier I talked about my belief that there are only two valid reasons to eat: sustenance and taste. The first of the many "negative" reasons we eat is when we're frustrated.

Someone at work annoys you. A family member does something you don't appreciate. Your favorite team keeps losing. You keep trying to achieve something but it never happens.

There are thousands of reasons why we get frustrated. And for those of us who turn to food as a response, it only makes matters worse. Eating, or should I say, the taste sensation you get from eating, is instantaneous. You get "eating pleasure" quickly, which, at least in theory, alleviates or lessens the impact of the frustration that resulted in eating in the first place.

But does it?

The frustration is still there after you've enjoyed the candy bar. Nothing has changed in the seconds or minutes it took you to get and eat the food.

So what you've done by eating in response to frustration is to give yourself a moment of eating pleasure and put on some more weight. You haven't solved the problem or even attempted to. You've taken the easy way out.

What to do about it: first, recognize and admit that you eat in response to frustration. Second, divide the things that frustrate you into two groups: those that you can change and those that you can't. You may be able to figure a way to deal with other people, but you can't find a way to help your favorite team win (unless you're the coach, and even then it might be impossible). Either deal with frustrations head-on or ignore them, but make sure not to eat in response to them.

Think about it. This is your life we're talking about here!

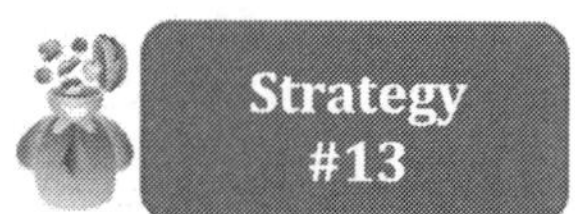

Think About Eating Due to Boredom

After thinking about it, if you conclude that you eat because you're bored, that's a big problem that you need to start working on immediately. The reason is that boredom usually is a feeling that covers up the root cause. You could be bored for dozens of reasons. Finding out **why** you're feeling bored is a must – not eating to take your mind off boredom.

Most people think of boredom as having nothing to do that's interesting. When you're bored, you often have no energy or desire to do much of anything. Eating becomes something real easy to do, a "crutch" and that leads to a cycle of boredom/eating that you need to break.

I'm not a psychologist, but I would think the best way to stop being bored is by making up your mind to do something that could be fun, interesting and not boring. The choices are endless – here are a few:

- Read a book
- Listen to music
- Play sports
- Call a friend or family member
- Join a club
- Write a letter or email
- Start a hobby or craft, like taking photographs or scrapbooking
- Play cards
- Go for a walk or jog
- Play a musical instrument
- Take a course
- Visit a museum
- Paint or draw

And so forth. The more you do that's interesting, the less you'll focus on eating as a replacement. As you are learning, making up your mind will be your key to success. Being wishy-washy will not work.

What to do about it: get off your butt! Get into the swing of things. Start trying lots of things until you find activities that you enjoy.

Think about it. This is your life we're talking about here!

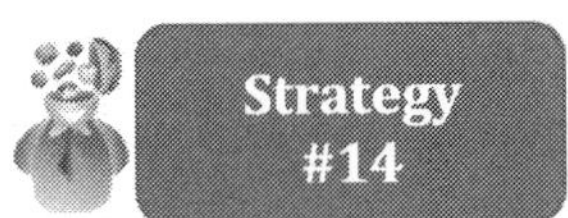

Think About Eating Because You Think You Can't Lose Weight

For most people, weight loss appears to be a daunting task. The more you have to lose, the more insurmountable a job it appears to be. This leads to thoughts like:

- "I can't lose that much weight."
- "This diet will never work."
- "This is a waste of time"
- "I'll never be thin again."
- "It will take years to lose all this weight."
- "I've never been able to lose weight and keep it off."

When faced with thoughts like these, it's easy to throw up your hands and start eating. But it doesn't have to be that way.

Like anything else in life, you can't get the job done overnight. It takes time to lose weight, and that's just the way it is.

In our society where everything is "instant" we have to recognize that some things just don't happen instantly. You can't become a great tennis player or actress without a lot of practice. Completing college takes four years and achieving success at work sometimes takes decades.

So it is with weight loss. The fact is, you <u>can</u> lose the weight, like millions of others have. If you choose a proven diet program, it will work. Weight loss is not a waste of time, because the benefits are so great. And you can become thin again. But it all comes back to making up your mind that weight loss comes in small steps, which happens to be the healthiest way to lose weight.

What to do about it: realize that you do have the ability to lose weight. It's simply a matter of making up your mind to do so and following the principles and practices in this book. People lose weight every day, and they realize that they can do it, that they do have the confidence. So do you...just find it from within you.

Think about it. This is your life we're talking about here!

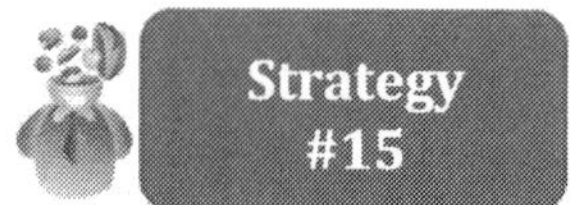

Think About Eating in Reaction to Past Failures

You've tried weight loss programs and they haven't worked. As a result, you may be feeling that there's no hope, that because it didn't work one or more times in the past, trying to lose weight now isn't going to work either.
Chances are your past attempts at dieting did not incorporate the three key elements that I outlined in the beginning of this book:

- A sensible diet that you follow religiously, one that is right for you and your personal circumstances, and one that is easy for you to follow.
- Exercise that you do regularly and that you will come to enjoy doing instead of dreading.
- A change in thinking that makes the other two possible.

Most people have tried dieting without exercising or a serious change in mind-set.

Others have tried diet and exercise, but without doing serious thinking.

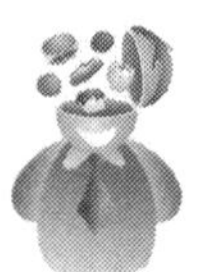

Very few people have tried and failed, in my opinion, when they followed all three of the "pillars" of successful weight loss listed above. A reader confirms this: "This was true for me. When I didn't do these together, I did not lose."

That's why the past is irrelevant; what you do from today onward has a much greater chance for success as long as you believe in and put all three principles into action.

What to do about it: think of the three pillars as a three-legged stool. Take any one away and the stool falls down. A sensible diet + exercise + a new mind-set = successful weight loss.

Think about it. This is your life we're talking about here!

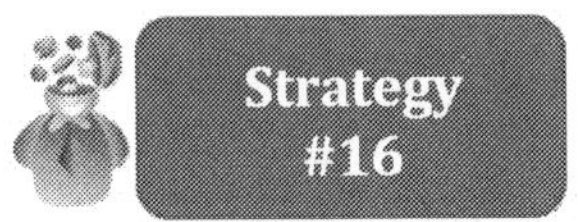

Think About Eating as Making a Pact with Yourself

How many times have you, or someone you know, said any of these phrases in relation to weight loss attempts:

- "I'll give it a try."
- "I hope it works."
- "I'll see if I can stick to it."

All these phrases are feeble attempts to start losing weight. In reality, they are what I'd call "future excuses" for when it doesn't happen:

- "I tried, and it didn't work."
- "I prayed but it wasn't meant to be."
- "I just couldn't stick to it."

If you're going to simply "see what happens" then you simply have not yet decided to get serious about losing weight. And you keep eating and stuffing your face. The goal of this book is to get you to make statements to yourself, and to others, like these:

- "I'm really serious about losing weight."
- "I know I can do it, and I will do it."
- "I'm ready to work hard at losing weight."
- I absolutely, positively am ready and will lose weight as my life depends on it."

See the difference? It's time to make a pact with yourself. It's time to actually make a promise to yourself that this is the "big push" at weight loss, the right way.

What to do about it: once you've truly decided to get serious about weight loss, make a solemn promise to yourself. Every time you're in a situation that could lead to eating food you shouldn't, repeat your promise to yourself: "I am serious about weight loss. I will not cheat. I will not eat foods that are no good. I promise this to myself."

Think about it. This is your life we're talking about here!

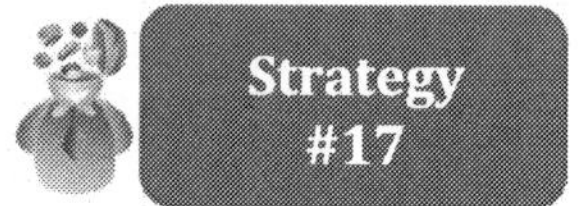

Think of Eating as an Escape

Yes, life can be tough at times. Yes, we all have problems and pressures. Some are worse than others.

From time to time, we all need an escape from our daily routines. Escapes can take many forms:

- Seeing a movie
- Going to a concert
- Taking a vacation
- Walking around the neighborhood
- Skiing, hiking, swimming, biking, etc.

And the one that's the worst is eating. An escape in this sense is when you do something positive or fun to get away from problems and pressures. At least for a short time, you've escaped into another world where these problems are not top-of-mind.

But if you eat as an escape, you're making a bad situation worse. **Think of your problems and pressures as a pile of bad stuff, and every bite of food you eat is more bad stuff added to the pile.** So when you eat to escape other problems, you're making your personal pile of problems greater.

What to do about it: make up your mind to do "positive" escapes that are fun, interesting and enjoyable and don't hurt your body. Look around you – positive experiences abound by the zillions.

Think about it. This is your life we're talking about here!

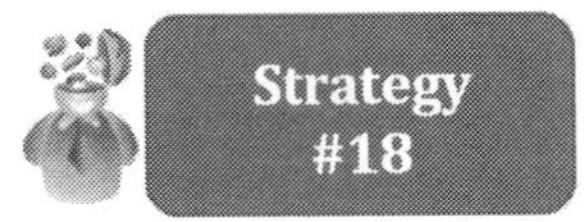

Think About Eating and Stress

It's a well-documented fact that people who are under stress almost always tend to eat more than those who are not. Whether you're under stress from work, watching after young kids, your relationships or any other reason, getting stress under control will lead to weight loss.

So what exactly is stress? I think everyone knows when they're **feeling** it, but how would you define it? Simply put, stress is a pressure or strain caused by some external (the outside world) or internal (you) force.

Now that we know what stress is, how do we deal with it? It should be quite clear that if you don't learn how to deal with stress, you will not lose weight, and you may continue to gain weight if the stress is not under control.

If you're eating because you're stressed, you need to realize that the time you spend eating is just a momentary break from stress, and that while it might make you feel good for a few seconds or minutes, the stress will be there when you're done eating. So in a very logical way, it makes absolutely no sense to react to stress by eating and putting on more weight.

As I see it, there are two kinds of stress: that which you can control or do something about, and that which you can't. First, think about stresses that you can work on -- those that are under your control. You may have to read more about dealing with stress or even seek the guidance of a therapist, but dealing with stress is the only real way to remove it or lessen it. And when you do, you'll eat less. Second, for stresses that you just can't control, find a way to let them roll off your shoulder, so they don't affect you.

You should also know that stress intensifies sweet and salty tastes, which can make junk food, processed food and other sweets more appealing when you're under stress (*Bottom Line Personal)*.

What to do about it: if stress is causing you to eat, spend the time to learn how to deal with it. It may be as simple as breathing techniques, yoga or other means of relaxation. Regular exercise is a great way to release stress – hit the boxing bag or the treadmill. For an interesting video on de-stressing at CafeMom.com, visit: http://tinyurl.com/l7qvatc. But if stress is still in your life, get serious about determining the cause and ways to deal with it. There's no way around stress except tackling it head on. Period.

Think about it. This is your life we're talking about here!

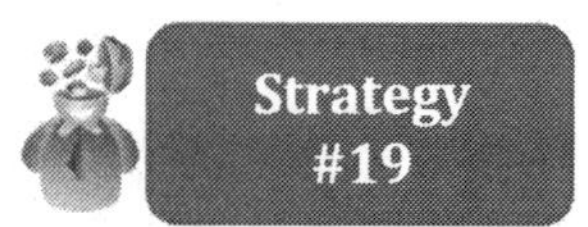

Think About Being Pressured to Eat

It's something most of us have experienced many times: you're at a family dinner or at a party, and the host or hostess seems to have one mission: to get everyone to eat as much as possible. They're continually asking you to eat more, to take a second portion. Depending on who is asking or even demanding that you eat more, this can be real pressure. Several comments about this issue:

"The hostess would say, 'If you love me you'll eat it. I made it for you."

And, "The more we'd eat, the happier she'd be. Usually I just give in so I wouldn't cause a scene or be in the spotlight."

And in many cases, it's very difficult to say "no" in social situations.

So you end up eating a lot more than you intended, and you're annoyed at them and yourself for doing so.

I have a couple of ways around this problem. They're easy to do and they won't annoy your host/hostess.

What to do about it: first, take a lot less food on your plate than you usually do – like half or one-third as much. Then, when the host or hostess wants you to eat more, you say "Sure, I'd be delighted" and take the other half or two-thirds that you didn't take in the first place!

If you don't have a choice of how much food is on your plate, eat extremely slow. Talk a lot. Chew slowly. If the host sees that you still have a lot of food on your plate, they probably won't bug you to take more!

Finally, when a hostess is persistent, here's another way to handle her – say: "I loved the meat-loaf, and while I'm stuffed, I'd love to take a piece home....would that be possible?" What you've done is give the hostess what they're looking for: validation that you liked her cooking, while not actually agreeing to eat it right then and there.

Think about it. This is your life we're talking about here!

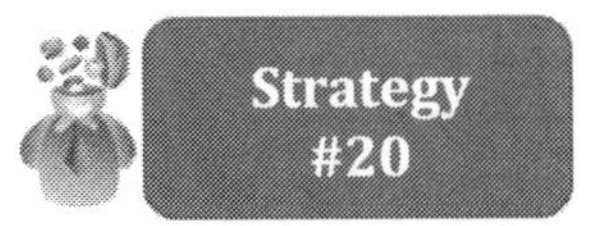

Think About Your Eating Habits

Another "negative" excuse why people eat is habit. We tend to do the same things every day: we wake up, shower, brush our teeth, grab the morning coffee or orange juice (with or without breakfast), drive or take the train to work, pick up something on the way, take a mid-morning break, etc. We are creatures of habit because those habits feel good to us.

Remember the habits I developed when I was selling advertising? Soon those habits became so ingrained within me that I did them automatically, and didn't even think about what I was doing.

Overeating simply because that's what you've always done is no longer acceptable. Snacking at 10:30am every day because everyone goes down to the cafeteria or out to the food truck needs to be revisited.

Destructive habits must be broken now.

It is also probable that you'll have a bad eating day once in a while. How you react to this is very important. In "Bounce Back From a Bad Eating Day" in www.QualityHealth.com, Laurie Saloman suggests six ways to recover. Perhaps the most important is eating breakfast the following day. You might be tempted to skip it, but that's not a good idea. You want to get right back on a good schedule, which always includes breakfast.

What to do about it: make a list of all the times during the day you eat or drink. Do this for a solid week, and carry the list with you so you don't forget. You'll be amazed at how much you eat and drink.

Next, analyze what you've eaten and drunk in terms of the diet program you're on. If you're on a low-carb, low-sugar program, you'll probably discover that many juices are loaded with sugar, which is not good for this kind of diet. Or that the high-fat, high-sugar donut you grabbed at the train station isn't good for your low-fat diet.

Make up your mind to consciously do away with the bad foods and/or substitute healthier foods for them. If you must have a mid-morning snack, for example, replace that donut with an energy bar, if the energy bar is permitted on your diet.

Think about it. This is your life we're talking about here!

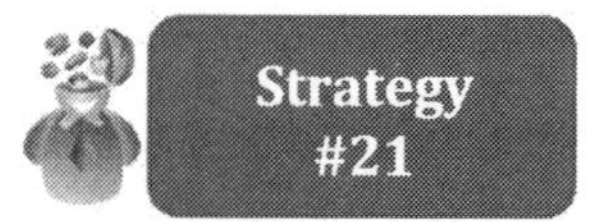

Think About Food Addiction & Food Allergies

According to leading doctors, many people are physically addicted to foods – some know this and many don't. Here are a few foods that actually have a biochemical basis for addiction based on what's contained within these foods:

- Chocolate (surely you already know that!)
- Meat
- Cheese and other dairy products
- Coffee
- Wheat
- Eggs
- Corn
- White potatoes
- Sugar
- Flour

For example, chocolate contains caffeine and other stimulants, and it releases chemicals into the brain that send the message "give me more!"

Meat and cheese break apart during the digestive process and one of the byproducts is opiates – a sedative narcotic containing opium! While eating meat or cheese is a lot different than using opium or other drugs, the result is somewhat similar: withdrawing from those foods is difficult.

Clinical ecologists, specialists dealing with food addiction and food allergies, believe that many chronic health problems, including migraines, fatigue, depression and arthritis – are caused by allergies to foods and chemicals contained within foods. Others believe food sensitivities can cause the body to retain both water and fat, leading to weight gain.

What to do about it: check with your doctor about getting tested for food allergies and addictions if you have an abnormal craving for certain kinds of foods. You may need to see a specialist like a clinical ecologist or a nutritionally oriented allergist.

Think about it. This is your life we're talking about here!

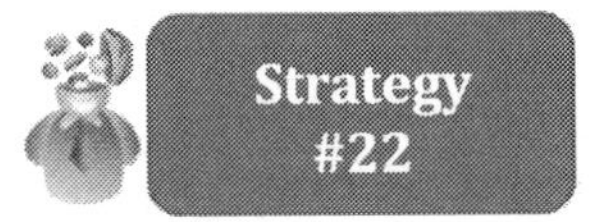

Think About Advertising and Eating

How many times have you seen a mouthwatering TV commercial or seen a print ad that makes you just want to eat the advertised food?

One of the best examples is the challenge by Lays: "Betcha can't eat just one!" Lays challenges people to eat just one, knowing they can't. Why? Because chips and other foods are so addictive that most people can't eat one, or two or five or ten.

Advertising is another stimulus to overeating that affects some people. Because the quality of the ads is so good, the food becomes almost irresistible. This effect is particularly evident among kids and their reaction to fast-food ads.

While suits by people claiming that fast-food chains' advertising has caused them to overeat have been dismissed, there is plenty of evidence that people are affected by advertising. After all, that's exactly what ads are supposed to do – influence people.

But the bottom line when it comes to advertising is that you have a **choice** to respond to the ad or not. You don't have to buy a car that's being advertised. You don't have to buy the paper towel brand that's in the ad. And, you don't have to eat the gargantuan cheeseburger that looks so good!

What to do about it: if you react to food ads by running out to get the food that's advertised, think long and hard about why you do that. Surely you're not hungry at the exact moment the ad comes on the TV or you see it in a magazine. When you see a food ad or commercial, close your eyes and visualize weight being added to your belly, your arms, your legs and your butt.

Think about it. This is your life we're talking about here!

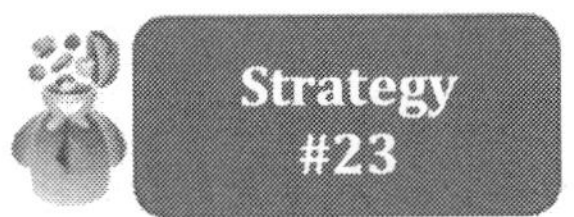

Think About Eating to Celebrate

One of the most common activities people do to celebrate special occasions is to go out to eat, or invite people to parties at home. Whether it's a reception following a wedding, going out with colleagues after work, celebrating a birthday with a family dinner or going to a restaurant after the game, eating out has become the focus for celebrations of all kinds.

And there's nothing wrong with this.

Except for one thing: when we eat out with others or go to parties with lots of food, we tend to eat more food. One reason is the popularity of buffets and the gigantic portions that many, if not most, restaurants dish out. With all that food, many people simply can't control themselves and wind up eating a lot more than they should.

Also, when we're in a group, some people are embarrassed to leave food over or "eat like a bird." And in many group situations, people order appetizers "for the table" that everyone can share...in addition to the main meal.

Granted, eating out is fun and we all love doing it. But if you're serious about losing weight, there are two ways to deal with celebrating by eating out.

What to do about it: first, plan ahead. If you've got a big brunch on a Sunday, by all means eat smaller meals the rest of the day. Practice some of the techniques in this book, such as filling up your plate half way, taking longer to eat and eating only foods that are on your diet.

Second, if you have some say in the activity, suggest something other than eating out, such as: going to a show or concert, dancing, going to a sporting event, etc. While you may end up eating something at these kinds of events, they are not the focus – that's the key point here.

Think about it. This is your life we're talking about here!

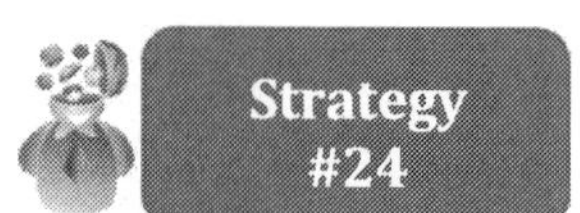

Think About Responsibility

Now that we've talked about the numerous "negative causes" of overeating, this is the perfect time to talk about responsibility.

We're all bombarded with the same food advertising, buffets and food choices. Yet some people can't lose weight and others can. Some people have the willpower and others don't. Why is that?

Excluding people who have fast metabolisms, those who are medically overweight and people who just don't care about losing weight, why is it that some of us lose weight and others don't?

I think it all comes down to one word: responsibility.

The only person responsible for weight loss is you. No matter what's happened in your life, you, and only you, have the power to lose weight if you really want to.

Blaming the inability to lose weight on other factors is nothing more than a way that you deny that losing weight is your sole responsibility.

What to do about it: take responsibility! Part of the new mind-set that you must adopt by constantly thinking about what you eat is that weight loss, like any other changes you make, is solely your responsibility. If you have to say "Only I'm responsible for my weight loss!" out loud 1,000 times in order to convince yourself, then do that. It's time to stop blaming others or outside forces and take the bull by the horns – it's your show...get on with it!

Think about it. This is your life we're talking about here!

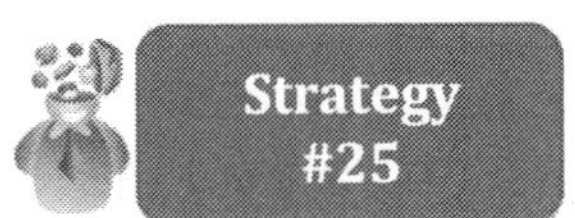

Think About Cheating

It is understandable why people cheat. They want to reward themselves after being "good" for a certain period of time. Perhaps they go off their diet for a meal or more after a week or two of staying on it. On the surface, you wouldn't think that's such a bad idea. But it **is** a bad idea on two counts.

First, why would you reward yourself by doing something that you **know** is no good for you? Would you reward yourself for driving without getting into an accident by deliberately hitting a telephone pole? Would you reward yourself for working out diligently by being a couch potato for a week, thereby undoing all the good you've done? Of course not. From a purely logical sense, it makes no sense to cheat.

Second, for some people, one cheat may be the beginning of a reversal of all the good work you've done. Eating fat after being on a low-fat diet may trigger something that results in a backward slide.

And think about it from another point of view. Let's say you're on your program religiously for two weeks – 14 days – 336 hours. Is it worth jeopardizing those 20,160 minutes by eating the wrong foods for 5 or 10 minutes? Wrong foods that might only deliver a couple of moments of "taste pleasure" to your brain?

What to do about it: simple – reward yourself in some other way. Make an agreement with yourself that for every week or month or "X" number of pounds lost, you'll buy

yourself something special: jewelry, clothing, music, concert tickets – whatever. Cheating never works!

Think about it. This is your life we're talking about here!

A reader commented: "This section was helpful. I have trouble stopping the cheating."

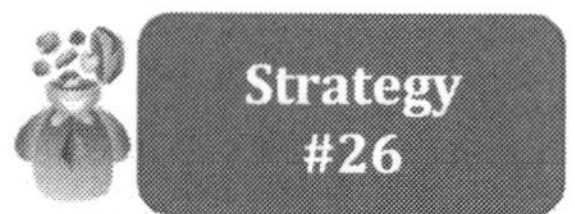

Think About How Much Weight You Want To Lose

Let's suppose you want to lose 35 pounds, and based on what you've read and discussed with your doctor, you want to do this within 6 months.
Thinking that "I want to lose 35 pounds" may seem like a large amount, and you may get frustrated when a week goes by and you only lose one pound. In fact, many people give up because the amount they lose in any given week is a fraction of the total, and they wind up saying "I'll never lose that much!"

What to do about it: you must set goals that break down the weight in bite-size pieces (excuse the pun!). One way is that your goal, using the above example, is 1.5 pounds per week (which equals 6 pounds per month or 36 pounds over 6 months). 1.5 per week is very reasonable and doable!

Set goals that are reasonable, and then concentrate on meeting each individual goal. Plan to reward yourself (not with food!) after each month's goal is met. Another way is to set 10-pound drops as a goal, and reward yourself after each 10 pound drop.

Think about it. This is your life we're talking about here!

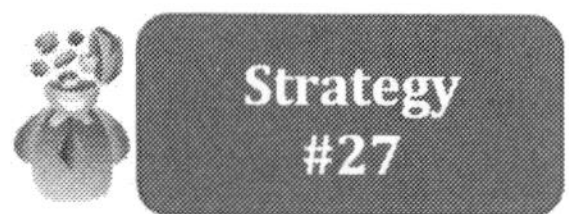

Think About The Scale

During the weight loss process, the scale can be your friend or your enemy, or at least it feels that way. Do you find yourself dreading getting on the scale, thinking that if you lost any weight, it might only be a miniscule amount…or worse, that you gained after dieting for a week?

When you weigh yourself, you step off the scale either happy or not. When you've worked hard dieting and it's not reflected on the scale, it can lead to an immediate reaction: "This just isn't working. I give up."

If you weigh yourself every day, daily fluctuations can account for short-term gains or staying even, despite following a strict diet regimen. Also, many people weigh more at night than in the morning.

I strongly believe in weighing yourself every day, without fail. I also think you should get a digital scale, and they are not expensive. It tells your weight loss in tenths of a pound. While it may take a week to lose 1.5 pounds (see previous "think about") you might lose 2/10 one day, 3/10 another, etc. It all adds up! iVillage.com reports that "people who step on the scale daily lost twice as much as those who weigh-in on a weekly basis. For your truest weight, hop on the scale early in the morning."

If you only weigh in once a week, that gives you a strong tendency to cheat for 3, 4, 5 or even more days, and starve yourself 1 or 2 days before you weigh in just to avoid gaining. That's not the way, obviously.

Dr. Lazarus correctly points out that the scale is NOT the only measure of your progress, and that's important. In addition to patting yourself on the back when you lose ounces and pounds, you should also feel good:

- Every time you make a food and drink substitution from something bad to something good.
- Every time you make time for a brisk walk, bike riding or other fun exercise.
- Every time you look at a nutrition facts label to better evaluate a food or drink.
- Every time you drop a clothing size.
- Every time someone says that you look thinner.
- Every time you notice positive changes in your body, both inside and out.

In short, every time you take a positive step to lose weight and eat healthy.

What to do about it: make up your mind to weigh yourself every morning and to be thrilled when you lost 2/10 of a pound!

Think about it. This is your life we're talking about here!

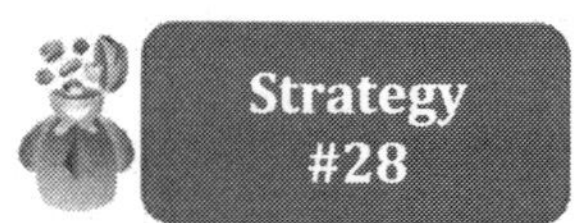

Think About Hunger

I'm convinced that so much of what we eat occurs when we are **not** hungry. Some of us have been conditioned to eat three square meals a day; others have been brought up on a big, hearty dinner, always at dinner time.

To be hungry is to have a strong desire for food, usually accompanied by some degree of discomfort, weakness or pain from going too long without food. Be honest with yourself: how often does your stomach really growl from hunger pains? Probably not very often.

So if we eat when we're not hungry, we're really adding food to our bodies that we don't need. Hunger pangs are the body's way of telling us that it needs more nourishment. When you don't feel hungry, in most cases, your body is not calling out for food.

There are many cases where you have to eat when you're not hungry. In today's hurry-up society, just getting everyone together for dinner isn't always the easiest thing, so you may end up eating when you're not hungry.

If you must eat when you're not hungry, follow your diet program religiously.

But what about the times when you genuinely are hungry? When you get those "hunger pangs?" The sensation we feel and call hunger pangs occurs when there are contractions in the stomach wall because it is not as full as it usually is.

Eating when truly hungry is among the most dangerous of times, because the gut reaction (excuse the pun please!) is to eat food fast in order to stop the hunger pangs. The faster you eat food in this state, the more food you are likely to eat, because you want to feel full, because feeling full is the opposite of feeling hunger pangs.

There is another class of hunger as Dr. Ethan Lazarus points out: "Our satiety center (controls feelings of hunger) is located in the same region of the brain in which we experience depression, anxiety and reward. Our satiety center drives our eating behavior. Many of my heaviest patients are constantly hungry, because their satiety centers have malfunctioned." If you *really* are constantly hungry, seeking a medical opinion is warranted.

What to do about it: when you're hungry, eat as slow as possible. The hunger pangs will go away. Just give them a short time. Follow the same eating routine that you do when you're not feeling hungry. Don't do anything differently simply because you feel hunger pangs.

Think about it. This is your life we're talking about here!

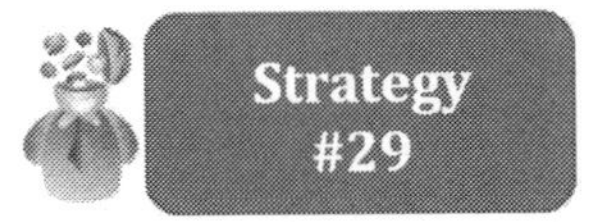

Think About What Your Body Needs

Doctors and nutrition specialists (accredited professionals like registered Dietitians or Certified Nutrition Specialists), all agree that the body needs six major food groups, liquids and nutrients:

- Protein
- Fat
- Carbohydrates
- Vitamins
- Minerals
- Water

Eliminating any of these six key building blocks can not only cause problems, but can retard weight loss. That's why most proven and sensible diet programs have a balance. Even low-carb diets still require that you have some carbs – and some carbs are much more beneficial than others.

Many of us don't get enough vitamins that occur naturally in food. And while one-a-day vitamin pills can easily make up the difference, many people don't even take vitamins.

Many of us don't drink enough water. While soda, coffee and other drinks contain water, they also contain other stuff, like sugar, that is not good for us. We all need to drink much more water.

It is critical to get the right balance with these six building blocks so you don't omit any of them.

What to do about it: with your doctor's or nutrition specialist's help, determine the optimal amount of each of the six you need, and then learn what foods contain them naturally. If you're on a low-fat diet program, make sure you still get enough fat, and the <u>right</u> fat. Spend time to learn about the various diet programs and how much of the six groups listed above they recommend.

Think about it. This is your life we're talking about here!

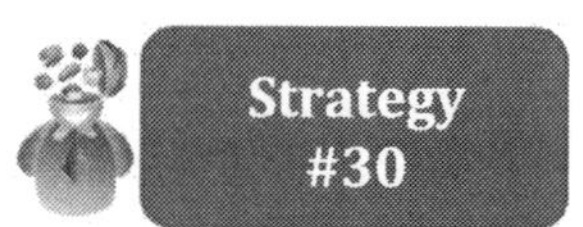

Think About Diet Programs and Your Profile

The ultimate diet you choose to follow needs to be based on many factors. Taking the time to sort them out and discuss them with your doctor and nutrition specialist is critical. Some or all of these factors could affect the diet you go with:

- Current ailments (i.e. salt intake must be restricted if you have high blood pressure)
- Genetics (i.e. parents who have had heart problems may be an indicator that you will, and that can affect your dietary choices)
- Medications you're taking (some drugs should not be taken with certain foods)
- Ease of following the diet (i.e. some people find counting points is easier than the ways other programs are set up) – you want a diet that's easy to follow and not frustrating
- Metabolism (i.e. how fast you digest food)
- Age, weight, height
- Muscle tone, bone structure
- Food allergies (i.e. you may be allergic to certain foods)
- Food addictions (i.e. you may be addicted to certain foods)
- Food tolerances (i.e. some people have digestive problems with dairy products)
- Taste – if you love fruits and vegetables, a fruit and vegetable-rich diet may be better for you

The ideal program is one where you enjoy most or all the foods on the diet, and none of them interfere with medication, allergies, addictions and tolerances.

And yes, dieting is somewhat complex given all the above factors. That's why all of the "lose weight fast" miracle pills just don't work. You really need to clearly understand the relationship between foods and how they affect your body. Spend the time to learn and make the right decisions.

What to do about it: start making a list of all of the foods that you cannot have based on the factors listed above. Then, consult with your doctor and nutrition specialist to nail down a specific program that is easy to follow and that one you can live with.

Think about it. This is your life we're talking about here!

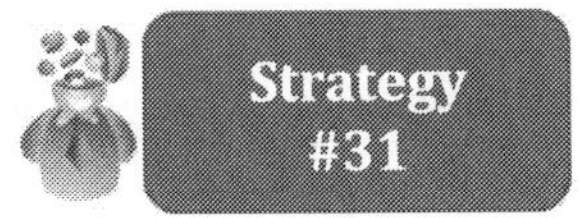

Think About the Value of Food Studies

It seems like every day there's a new study out that tells us that some specific food is good or bad for us. With this "information overload" – what are we supposed to do? Should we be altering our diets every time we read about a new development?

Recently I read that dark chocolate is better for you than milk chocolate in terms of having more anti-oxidants, which are good for you. And we all know about the studies that show red wine is better than white wine in helping to lower cholesterol.

Should we all be running out and adding dark chocolate and red wine to our diets?
The basic answer is probably not. Here's how I look at it.

These studies can be divided into two groups: those showing **major** changes vs. those showing **minor** changes.

If a study shows that a dietary change resulted in 30% or more people being helped, I consider that major and worthy of consideration. But if the change is less than 30% as most studies are, I consider those minor, and I would not rush out to make those changes. And if the sample sizes are small, I question the validity in the first place. Plus, you may have to drink so much red wine or eat so much dark chocolate to even see the benefits.

You see, losing weight is a major, major factor in your short- and long-term health – so you don't want to risk that under any circumstances. Unless it is a major study with thousands of participants, and the change experienced is dramatic, and the results have been replicated elsewhere, I would not change your diet based on any single study.

What do to about it: only consider changing your diet – with your doctor's and nutrition specialist's approval -- when the benefits of adding, changing or removing a food from your diet are 30% or more in published studies from reputable sources.

Think about it. This is your life we're talking about here!

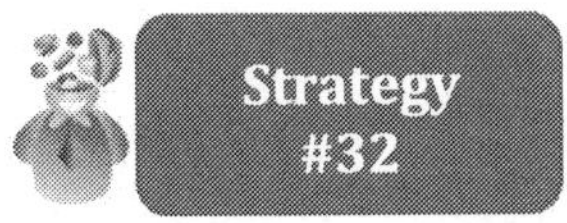

Think About How Fast to Lose Weight

The ads proclaim "Lose 30 pounds in 30 days!" and "Burn a pound a day while you sleep!" Yet you ask most doctors and nutrition specialists how fast you should lose weight, they typically respond with "no more than a couple of pounds a week." Even on some medically sound diets, you can lose 5 to 10 pounds the first week, but after that, you should be at the 1-2 pounds per week level. So who is right?

The professionals, for sure. Some of these copywriters (I consider some of them to be irresponsible) are appealing to everyone who responds to fast weight loss via a "magic pill." People that try the latest fads, pills, patches mostly jump from one unsuccessful program to another. Because of the ads, their expectations are ridiculously high and are rarely met.

Medically, it's dangerous to lose too much weight too fast. The only way to lose 30 pounds in 30 days is by starvation and/or food intake that is incredibly unhealthy and could lead to medical complications.

Since most of us who need to lose weight need to lose anywhere from 10 to 50 pounds, losing one or two pounds a week is still very good. So if you need to drop 20, we're talking only 10 to 20 weeks at a healthy, steady pace to do so!

Also, when people lose weight fast, they tend to put it back on fast. When people lose weight slowly, they tend to keep it off much longer, because the body has adapted over a period of time.

You should be prepared that you won't lose weight every day, even small amounts like 1/10th or 2/10th of a pound. Staying the same or even gaining a little is normal and can't be avoided. Pat yourself on the back if you lose a little each day during the week, and on one day you stay even and on another day (maybe a hot day when you drank more water than usual) you even gain a tad. Losing a little, staying even or gaining a smidge are all things to pat yourself on the back about – because they are all signs of progress. Gaining a pound or two is not!

What to do about it: forget about losing weight fast. Figure out how long it should take you to lose the weight you need to, and then enjoy the process.

Think about it. This is your life we're talking about here!

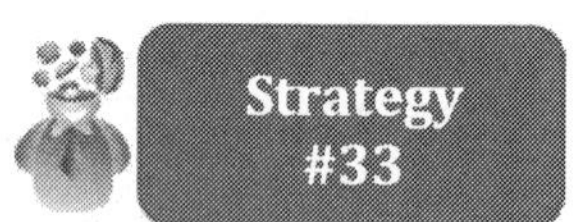

Think About Those Silly Dieting Quotes

You hear people say things that on the surface sound good, but in reality they are really quite silly. Examples:

- "You can eat everything in moderation."
- "No one should deny him or herself anything."
- "Cheating once in a while is OK."

Of course, these, and most others like them, are bogus and don't help your weight loss efforts. Assuming that at some point you've designed a diet program for yourself, there will be some foods that you can have and some that you can't. You just won't be able to eat everything. The only quote you need to embrace is: "You can do anything you set your mind to!"

That's why the first quote is wrong. You **cannot** eat anything or everything in moderation. You can only eat what your particular plan proscribes.

The second quote is simply something people say as a rationalization to have something they shouldn't. People who say this are not serious about losing weight.

As for the third one, cheating makes absolutely no sense.

What to do about it: don't listen to what people say about dieting that sounds like these sayings. Once your mind is made up and you're on a good track for weight loss success, nothing anyone says can be allowed to affect you.

Think about it. This is your life we're talking about here!

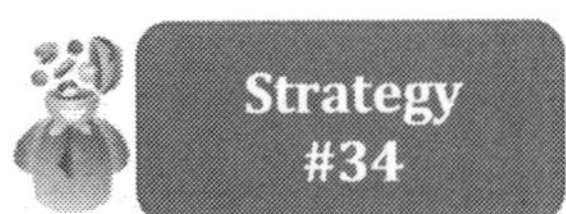

Think About the Power of Substitution

The basis for all sound diets is that you can eat certain foods and stay away from others. That's a given. At the core of successful weight loss is your ability to substitute good foods and drinks for bad ones.

Whether it's a point system or you're counting calories or carbs, the bottom line is that you need to understand substitutions.

In this day and age, there are some substitutions that are so easy to make or buy and easy to get used to:

- Replace cookies and cake with fruit. Fruit, containing natural sugar, tastes very sweet and is much better for you than foods where sugar is added. However, some people who have sugar problems should not load up on fruit.
- Replace regular ice cream with no-sugar-added varieties.

- Replace "bad" nuts with "good" nuts. Depending on which diet program you're on, stop eating nuts that are unhealthy and replace them with nuts that are good for you.
- Use natural peanut butter instead of processed peanut butter that contains salt, sweeteners and fatty oils. I'll bet you can't tell the difference!
- Replace instant oatmeal with the natural one. Though it takes longer to cook, it isn't highly processed like the instant kind.
- Replace white rice and especially instant white rice with brown rice.
- Replace white bread with whole grain breads.
- Replace French fries with a sweet potato.
- Replace **creamed** corn or spinach with **steamed** corn or spinach salad.
- Replace apple pie with baked apples.
- Replace fried chicken with broiled chicken.
- Replace processed foods with fresh foods.

Most of the substitutions you make should be painless. You should be able to get to the point very quickly where you don't miss the unhealthy foods you've replaced with foods that are not unhealthy.

What to do about it: make substitutions a top priority! They will be the easiest and fastest things you can do to jump start your diet.

Think about it. This is your life we're talking about here!

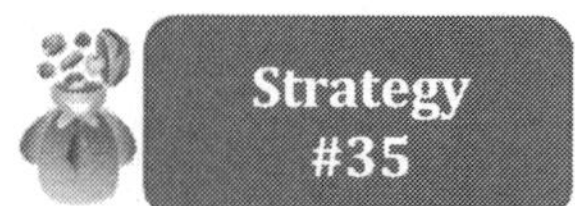

Think About the Holidays and Dieting Resolutions

Unless today, the day you're reading this page, happens to be December 31st, making a resolution to start dieting on January 1st is another one of those rationalizations we use to justify eating poorly prior to the first of the year.

Picking a point in the future to start dieting is simply putting it off, and in the time between now and that date, you're going to be putting on the pounds faster as your "last fling" before you start a diet that is probably not going to last. So what have you accomplished with a New Year's resolution? Not much.

If you make this resolution anytime between Thanksgiving and the third week in December, you're going to have lots of occasions to overeat:

- Thanksgiving
- Christmas, Hanukkah, Kawanza and other holidays

- Family get-togethers, most common at this time of year
- Breaks from school
- New Year's Eve parties
- New Year's Day parties

This four-week period is probably one of the worst in terms of people overeating and putting on the weight. That's undoubtedly why people started making resolutions in the first place.

What to do about it: the time to start eating healthy is today. Don't delay another day!

Think about it. This is your life we're talking about here!

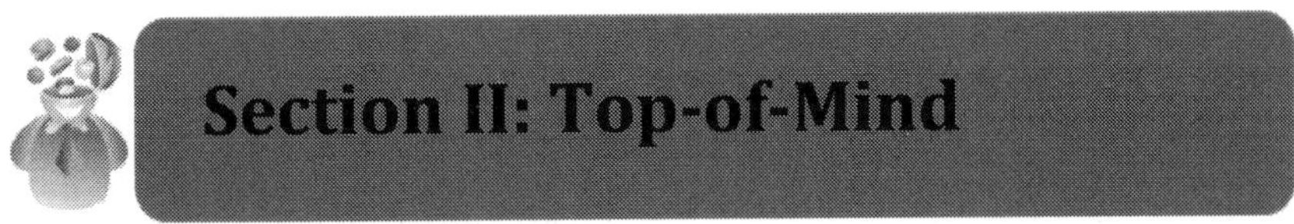

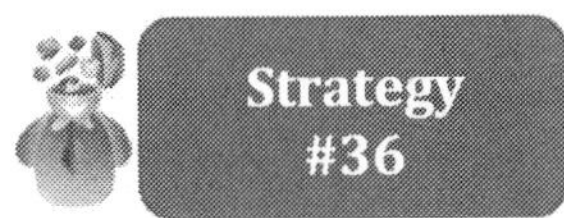

Think About Working with Your Doctor And Nutrition Specialist

I cannot overemphasize the importance of working with your doctor and nutrition specialist – your weight loss team – to design a program of diet and exercise that's right for you.

Your doctor will combine results of recent blood tests, knowledge of what medicines you take, an understanding of what kinds of food you eat, how overweight you are, EKG results and other information to make specific recommendations.

Your nutrition specialist will take the doctor's recommendations and fine tune them into a diet, combining that with your personality and other information. He or she will educate you about specific foods and food groups, and explain how they will help you lose weight. You will learn which foods to eat, in what quantity and which foods to avoid.

Co-author Marilyn Diamond (*Young For Life*), with Dr. Donald Schnell, points out that with the abundance of food in the U.S., so many people are deficient in key nutrients, especially overweightt people. How can that be? She says, in an interview in *Life Extension* Magazine, "food is plentiful, but most of it is processed, laden with cellular and neurotoxic chemicals, dyes, preservatives and additives; it is irradiated, fractionated, microwaved, sprayed with pesticides, fungicides and herbicides; it is stored for long periods or shipped in hot weather; it is contaminated and genetically modified." Take this into account when working with your MD and nutrition specialist in formulating your food intake game plan, so that you get the greatest nutritional value from the calories you consume.

Dr. Mark Hyman, in a *Huffington Post article*, concludes that 40 years of nutritional research shows that **despite the abundance of food, 80% of Americans are Vitamin-D deficient and 90% don't get enough Omega-3 fats**, "which are crucial for staving off inflammation and controlling blood sugar levels." Much of this nutritional deficiency stems from the fact that "foods are stripped of their nutrients during the refining process." Example: refining whole wheat flour into white reduces fiber by 80%! Game plans are different for all people and should be customized to your personal decision.

What to do about it: when you've made up your mind that you will take weight loss seriously and do everything in your power to succeed, the first step is to visit with your doctor. Your doctor should write a Rx for a nutrition specialist consult, and bring your current blood test results to the nutrition specialist.

Think about it. This is your life we're talking about here!

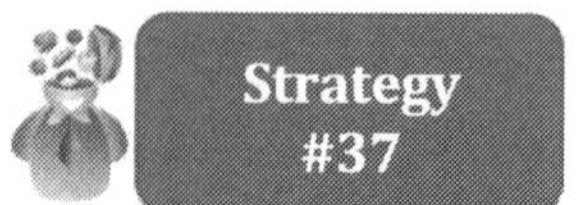

Think About Talking to Yourself

One of the most useful tricks I've found in the dieting process is to talk to myself. My conversations with myself typically are:

- "OK, am I really hungry? Do I need to really eat now?"
- "Should I eat this, or is there a good substitute?"
- "C'mon Irv, chew slower!"
- "Don't take so much food."
- "Talk more, eat less."
- "This doesn't taste that good. No need to finish it."
- "Why am I doing this?"
- "This has way too many carbs. Don't eat it."

Talking to yourself is one good way to keep reminding yourself of what you need to do. Talking to yourself makes it easier for you to remember the key points of your diet program. And the best place to talk to yourself when you're eating out is before you take food from the buffet or before you choose your selections from the menu.

When you start to see results, you'll find yourself uttering these statements to yourself:

- "Wow, four straight weeks of losing weight!"
- "That workout sure felt great."
- "I'm getting my stamina back."
- "Three more pounds. Awesome!"
- "I can't believe I used to drink regular soda."
- "I lost another size...now I can wear some favorites I haven't been able to wear in a while."

What to do about it: start talking to yourself! Remind yourself what to eat and what not to eat, and congratulate yourself on your successes.

Think about it. This is your life we're talking about here!

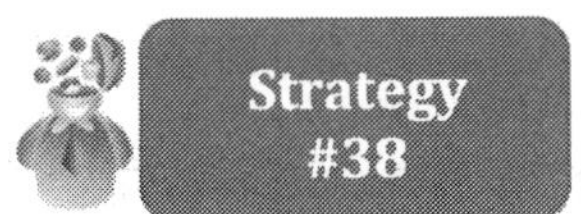

Think About the Cost of Food

Dieting can save you money! A lot of money!

How about that for an added bonus over and above your weight loss?

There are many ways you will save money once you're on a steady weight-loss program:

- When you eat out, you'll be ordering less food and spending less as a result. Not only will you save on the cost of the food, but the tax and tip will be lower also!
- Because you'll be eating less food, when you food shop every week, you'll be buying less food and saving money.
- If you can wean yourself off soda and fruit drinks and drink water instead, you'll save a bundle!
- If you eat out less frequently because you've made up your mind that eating is not as important as it used to be, big savings there too!

You never hear diet ads talk about how much money you can save...they just **want** your money.

Blogger and scientist Darya Rose (www.summertomato.com) offers 7 ways to save money while eating healthy:

- Eat at home as often as possible. If you cut out dining out and taking out by 3 meals, you'll save a bundle.
- Shop on weekends when you have more time to make better food choices.
- Shop for foods that are in season at local farmers markets. Cut out the middleman!

- Combine leafy greens with beans, grains and herbs to make meals that cost a couple of bucks.
- Buy in bulk. But choose wisely in terms of foods that are good for you.
- Eat less meat, one of the easiest ways to save money. Even if you love meat, substitute burgers for that $35 steak.
- Eat canned fish that, in many cases, is as good for you as fresh.

Author and blogger Scott Christ, writing in www.lifehack.org suggests eating beans, as they are one of the most affordable, nutrient-dense sources of protein and fiber. Plus, they are "super cheap."

Here is a list of "20 Budget-Friendly Superfoods," courtesy of Cleveland Clinic Wellness written by Jill Provost, with cost per typical serving. Read the entire article here: http://tinyurl.com/mdpwwdv.

- Bananas — 24 cents for a small banana
- Pears — 33 cents for a medium size pear
- Watermelon — 26 cents for one cup
- Prunes — 19 cents for ¼ cup
- Broccoli — 36 cents for one cup
- Collard Greens — 27 cents for one cup
- Romaine Lettuce — 27 cents for one cup
- Carrots — 29 cents for one cup
- Potatoes — 11 cents for one baked potato
- Onions — 18 cents for one cup
- Cabbage — 8 cents for one cup
- Parsley — 11 cents for one cup
- Barley — 7 cents for ½ cup
- Salmon — 72 cents for 3 ounces
- Turkey — 36 cents for 3 ounces
- Beans — 4 to 14 cents for ½ cup (depends on bean type)
- Lentils — 6 cents for ½ cup
- Sunflower Seeds — 16 cents for ¼ cup
- Canola Oil — 2 cents for 1 tbsp.
- Yogurt — 62 cents for one cup

What to do about it: the sooner you start dieting seriously, the faster you'll start saving money. Could be hundreds of dollars a year!

Think about it. This is your life we're talking about here!

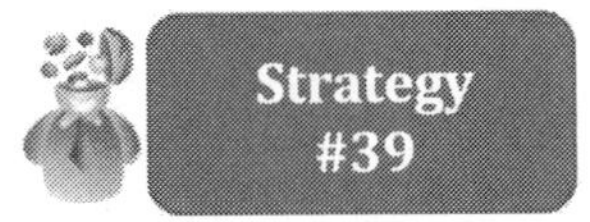

Think About Weight and Your Career

While not hiring a heavy person or giving a thin person an advantage is discrimination and illegal in the U.S., it happens every day. And it's so hard to prove as well. Surely you have heard of lawsuits stemming from firings of overweight people and airlines attempting to penalize consumers who can't squeeze into one seat, or even charging based on how much they weigh.

Publicly, employers will say that a person's looks, his/her weight, appearance, etc., are not taken into account in the hiring process.

But for many employers, the opposite is true, and least "off the record." It's hard to blame them, for they have some pretty good arguments as to why they should be allowed to base hiring decisions based on weight:

- Heavier people tend to have more medical problems, resulting in more sick days, higher insurance costs, and lower productivity.
- Many customers and clients don't like working with overweight people, especially in certain industries.
- Many jobs require people to not be overweight, simply by the nature of those jobs: dancers, athletes, etc.

Studies summarized at www.dietsinreview.com bear this out:

- Only 5% of CEOs in the U.S. were obese in 2009.
- 45% to 61% of top male CEOs were overweight.
- Only 5% of overweight CEOs are women.
- 95% of Americans feel obesity will lead to discrimination.

I give my sincerest apologies to those of you that are heavy and have experienced employment discrimination. It's wrong, but it does exist, and always will. It's extremely difficult to change human nature and the added costs that go along with hiring overweight people.

You have zero control over a prospective employer's feelings about hiring an overweight person, nor about a current employer's disposition to keep you employed. **What you do have control over is the ability to lose weight and remove the obstacle of not getting hired and advancing due to your weight.**

This is not a knock against the capabilities of heavy people. I know many that are superb workers. It's simply a statement of what tends to happen in the real world: given two equally qualified candidates for either employment or advancement, the thinner ones will have an advantage. Sad, but usually true.

What to do about it: getting a good job and advancing without the hindrance of weight is a great motivator to lose weight.

Think about it. This is your life we're talking about here!

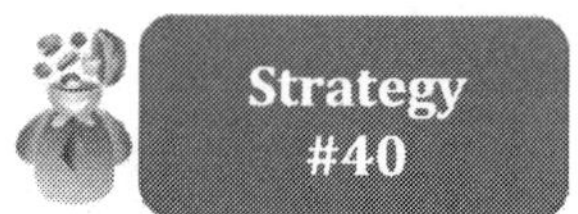

Think About the Short-Term Effects of Weight Loss

Within a very short time (usually a week or so) of starting a serious diet program coupled with regular exercise, you will see a lot of immediate benefits and changes:

- You will start to see the pounds come off.
- You'll feel healthier overall.
- Clothes that were tight will start to feel more comfortable.
- Some medical problems such as headaches may start to subside.
- People will notice and start commenting.
- If you're between clothing sizes, you may actually drop a size in the short-term.
- You won't feel sleepy after meals.
- You'll have more energy.
- You may even be more productive at work or in school.
- You'll start enjoying food more because you're getting the taste sensations to last longer.
- You'll start to save money!

And most importantly, you'll have made the first steps on a weight-loss journey that has a long list of benefits in the long-term.

What to do about it: enjoy every benefit of weight loss as it happens. Congratulate yourself on how smart you were to get serious in the first place.

Think about it. This is your life we're talking about here!

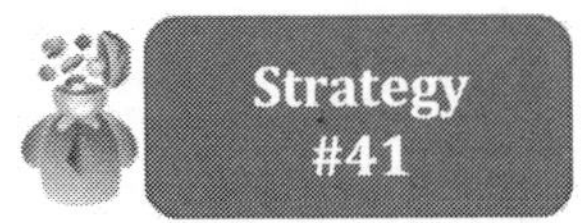

Think About the Long-Term Effects of Weight Loss

As you stay on your diet for more and more time, you will start to see dramatic benefits and enjoy tremendous results of your weight loss:

- You will start dropping sizes in clothing, leading to a better selection of clothes that look good on you.
- More and more people will comment on your weight loss.
- There's a very good chance you will be able to stop taking certain medications that were necessary when you were overweight.
- You'll be able to participate in sports and other physical activities such as dancing, hiking and swimming – activities that you probably couldn't partake in previously.
- You will have eliminated weight discrimination as a possible hindrance to finding a job and advancing.
- If you're married, your love life will improve because your partner will be more attracted to you, and because lovemaking will be easier.
- If you're not married or dating someone, you'll be more attractive to others.
- Chances are good that you won't contract certain illnesses that you may have when you were overweight, such as adult-onset diabetes.
- You'll greatly reduce the chances of getting a heart attack or other major illnesses that are associated with obesity.
- You'll stop huffing and puffing and shortness of breath will be a thing of the past.
- You'll start enjoying life because so many of the inconveniences that have plagued you will disappear.
- You'll find that you enjoy many new activities that replace your focus on eating.

And most important of all, you'll really feel great – physically and mentally.

What to do about it: just do it! I could fill this book with a thousand short- and long-term benefits of weight loss, but that's not necessary.

Think about it. This is your life we're talking about here!

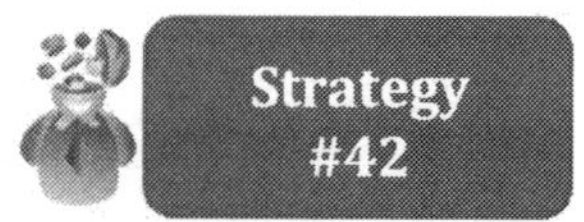

Think About Food Labels

Years ago legislation was passed requiring food manufacturers to label their foods with the mounts and percentages of ingredients. Coupled with the proactive desire by some of them to let people know what's in their foods, it has never been easier to determine just how good or bad certain foods are for you. Many restaurants publish calorie and ingredient counts on their menus.

You need to become familiar with these labels, and look at them while you're shopping for food. The reason is simple: you will almost always be surprised, perhaps stunned, at what goes into food. You will find that foods that you think are healthy or those with healthy sounding names contain ingredients that are not right for whatever diet program you're following. There are a couple of key areas on food labels:

- **Serving size**. This tells you the recommended serving – how much you should eat or drink. Look at how many servings there are in the entire package of food. So if it's a candy bar or a bag of potato chips, the serving size is listed, such as ½ of the bar or approximately 30 chips. Keep this in mind as you read the rest of this section. And keep in mind serving sizes when it comes to liquids as well. For example, many coffee creamers list "one level teaspoon" as the serving size, and therefore can claim that it is fat and sugar free. Well, not quite, for two reasons. The FDA's rule allows sugar and fat to be "rounded down" to zero when there is less than half a gram involved. So that's misleading. Second, most people don't use one level teaspoon; they turn over the container and pour, using far more, and getting far more fat and sugar than they imagined!

- **Servings per container**. Since all the numbers and percentages relate to a single serving, the servings per container can be critical. If there are **two** servings per container for a candy bar, then you would **double** the numbers if you end up eating the entire bar or container. So a candy bar with 2 servings per container showing 24 grams of fat and 36% of the recommended daily value (I'll explain that in a moment) means that if you eat the entire bar, you're actually eating 48 grams of fat accounting for 72% of your daily recommendation! Conversely, if you eat just ¼ of that bar, you're only getting 12 grams and 18%. I'm not encouraging you to eat more than one serving, just to be aware that you need to understand that servings per container is not as simple as you might think!

- **Calories and calories from fat**. This is the number of calories per serving. If you're counting calories, this is an important number. Be sure to multiply or divide by the servings per container only if you eat more or less than a single serving.

- **% Daily Value**. This column represents the percentage of the daily recommended amount of specific components of food that the government has established as appropriate. Your doctor may or may not agree with these, which you should discuss. These percentages are usually based on a 2,000 calorie diet, but some packages have two columns, one for 2,000 calories and the other for 2,500 calories. So if the label shows that a 4-serving size bag of chips has 10% of the daily recommended amount of sodium (salt), then eating the entire bag delivers a whopping 40%. Same multiplication and division applies.

- **Grams and milligrams**. Next to each item (fat, saturated fat, cholesterol, sodium, potassium, carbohydrates, dietary fiber, sugar and protein) you'll see the number of grams (g) or milligrams (mg). If you're counting these numbers as part of your diet program, it's easy to see how much you're getting. Same multiplication/division rules.

- **Vitamins**. Certain vitamins are listed and like the other components, they relate to the serving size and servings per container.

- **Ingredients**. Here is the listing of what goes into your food. By reading this, you may be very surprised to find that certain foods that you would never suspect of having sugar actually do. Or you may find that foods you thought had no saturated fat do.

Getting to know food labels is essential to successful dieting because it helps you avoid foods that contain ingredients you should not have. These labels are really very easy to understand – they are all set up the same way so whether you're looking at the label for cream cheese or popcorn or natural peanut butter, you only have to learn how to read the labels once.

What to do about it: simple, learn how to read food labels if you don't how already. And then pay attention to them when shopping. It's critical for your diet program. One of the bonus guidebooks explains food labels in greater detail!

Think about it. This is your life we're talking about here!

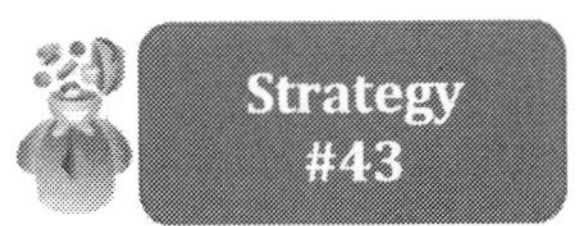

Think About Two Questions to Ask Yourself Before You Eat

We are all so tempted by food, whether it's at home, in the restaurant, at a party, in the office or while driving.

What's worse, we tend to eat foods that we know ahead of time aren't that tasty, simply because they are all that's available, or because they come with the entrée in a restaurant.

Does this sound familiar? You order a steak and it comes with vegetables and mashed potatoes. You take a forkful of the potatoes, and they aren't very good. In many cases, you'll eat them anyway, simply because they are **there**.

Or you'll look for a snack at home, and because there's nothing healthy around, you'll eat something that you know you shouldn't have. Or because you're lazy and don't feel like preparing something that's on your diet, you'll resort to gobbling down cold cuts or heating up a TV dinner.

Or you'll be at a party and while you're at the smorgasbord table, you take much more food than you should, because *it looks so good!*

What to do about it: before taking or eating any food, ask yourself two important questions, and get in the habit of asking them every time:

- ***Will I enjoy this food -- will it really taste good?***
- ***Is this food bad for me -- is it something I should stay away from?***

If you're serious about your diet, these questions represent another barrier between you and unhealthy foods.

Think about it. This is your life we're talking about here!

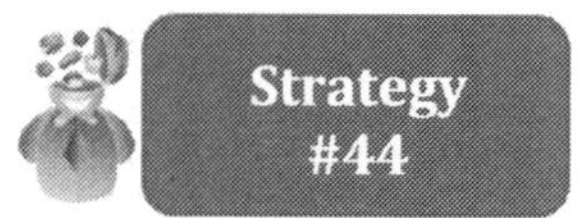

Think One at a Time

What do all of these common foods have in common?

- M&M's
- French fries
- Onion rings
- Nuts
- Potato chips
- Chunks of cheese

They are all foods where we tend to eat a handful or forkful at a time. When you grab for M&M's at a party, you always take a handful and many of us tend to take that entire handful and pop it into our mouths in one fell swoop. That was me!

Let's say you're at a restaurant, and you take a forkful of French fries. And let's say you pick up four fries and eat them all at once. Whatever taste sensation you get probably doesn't last for more than 5 seconds.

And let's say that you got 24 fries. At 4 fries per forkful, you get 6 forkfuls and 6 instances of getting some taste pleasure (assuming the fries taste good in the first place). At 5 seconds per taste sensation, that's 30 seconds of enjoyment.

Now let's suppose you eat just one at a time and as I recommended earlier, you chew each one and enjoy each one for 10 seconds. And let's say that you're real smart about this and you only eat 12 of the 24 fries. Because you're eating one at a time and chewing longer, you're getting a whopping 120 seconds of taste enjoyment from **half** of the fries. That means ½ the fat, ½ the carbs and ½ the sodium than you would have gotten by eating all 24 fries.

Bottom line, by training yourself to eat one fry, one M&M, one chunk of cheese at a time and chew it longer, you can easily cut down on the total amount of food you eat and get much more enjoyment. When you find yourself wanting to eat a lot of food, ask yourself why? Are you really, truly hungry, or are you eating for another reason. When you're totally honest with yourself, you'll start making better decisions.

What to do about it: think of "one" as the friendliest number there is. You may think I'm nuts for suggesting this, but it works. And since losing weight is the goal here, anything you can to do reach that goal makes sense.

Think about it. This is your life we're talking about here!

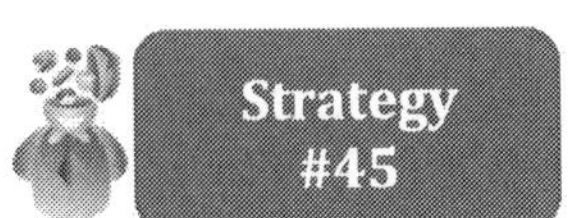

Think About Eating When You're Not Hungry

I'm convinced, beyond any shadow of a doubt that we all eat when we're not hungry, and as a result, that contributes to weight gain.

Of course, it's not possible to eat **only** when we are hungry. If your family has breakfast every day at 8am because that's the optimal time due to schedules, you may be hungry at that time on Monday but not hungry at the same time on Tuesday. The same holds true for your other meals.

If we all ate **only** when we're hungry, we'd all probably be thin. But because we eat both when we're hungry and when we're not, we tend to eat a lot more than we need to.

Logically, the thing to do would be to wait until you're hungry, and eat then. But that might result in eating breakfast at noon, lunch at 4pm and dinner at 10pm. Clearly that doesn't make sense.

What to do about it: spread out the food you eat so you can eat whenever you're hungry. If you're on a 2,000-calorie a day diet, and you find that you eat a total of five times during the day, just make sure you don't go over 2,000 calories. Yes, this takes effort, but if you've read this far in this book, you know that effort is required to lose and keep the weight off.

On some days, you may be able to eat only when hungry, so on those days you might only eat 3 times. It all comes down to a little advance planning and keeping track of points, calories, grams or whatever measuring stick you use.

Think about it. This is your life we're talking about here!

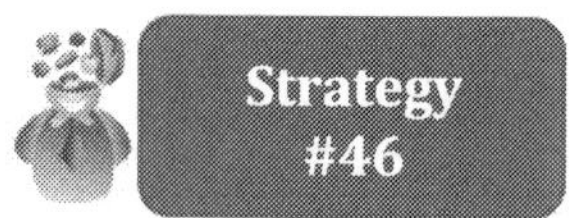

Think About Grazing

No, you're not a cow or a sheep. And no, you don't eat grass or hay. But many people are finding that grazing is a good way to satisfy your eating desires and lose weight. So what is grazing?

Grazing is a buzzword that has become popular to describe eating 6-10 times per day. Rather than eat three set meals per day, you eat constantly. By eating this often, theoretically you never get hungry. The key is to spread out your food intake across the entire 6 to 10 eating sessions. So if it's calories that you're counting, you could consume no more than 200 calories at a time (on average) and you could eat 10 times per day (if you're on a 2,000 calorie diet).

200 calories may not go far, but because you're eating often, you may only be an hour or so away from the next 200 calories. Your grazing schedule may allow you to eat small portions at these times:

- 7am
- 8:30am
- 10am
- 11am
- 12:30pm
- 2pm
- 4pm

- 6pm
- 7:30pm
- 8:30pm

Depending on the diet you're following, this might mean just two eggs at 7am, an orange at 8:30, a chunk of cheese at 10am and so forth. **What's great about this kind of eating – as long as you stick to it – is that you get to eat often!** The downside, and it is a big one, is that you have to be meticulous in dividing up your daily intake into 6 or 8 or 10 sessions. But hey, if it works for you, it's well worth the time and effort, right?

What to do about it: for the first couple of weeks on the grazing plan, keep a written journal of what you eat until it becomes second nature. Remember that one mistake – eating 1,000 extra calories because you forgot to keep track – can ruin the entire day.

Think about it. This is your life we're talking about here!

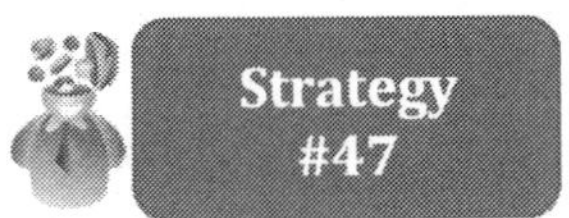

Think About Breakfast

There are lots of reasons why breakfast is an important meal. The two most important, in my mind, are:

- Eating a healthy breakfast jump-starts your metabolism after you've been asleep all night.

- If you skip breakfast, you probably will become over-hungry for lunch and eat a lot more than you should. If you skip both breakfast and lunch, you will almost certainly overeat for dinner.

Let's look at each of these reasons for eating breakfast in greater detail.

When you wake up in the morning, your body has not had any food (think of food as fuel, like gas in a car) since dinner or an evening snack the night before. That may be as many as 12 hours or more. Like a car, your body needs energy to run.

Many people aren't hungry in the morning, claim they get sick from eating breakfast or don't have the time because they are in a rush. In this case, eating a small meal is OK even if you're not hungry, because you need to get your body going. In terms of people that might get sick from breakfast, it may be a matter of trying out different foods or drinks. Surely you won't get sick from every possible breakfast food! And an excuse like "I don't have time" is rubbish. Everyone has 5 minutes to grab some fruit or oatmeal. The time excuse is just baloney. You need to spend a few minutes to figure out how to change your schedule so you do have time for breakfast.

The second reason is as important as the first: skip breakfast and you throw your body off-kilter, many times resulting in overeating when your body starts begging for food. Mother Nature Network (www.mnn.com) says that skipping breakfast increases your insulin response, so going without breakfast can actually increase your risk of obesity.

One of the most commonly recommended foods for breakfast is oatmeal. While instant oatmeal in packets is convenient, they are loaded with sugar. The best oatmeal are called "steel cut" and they take 20 minutes to make, but well worth the time because they are much healthier for you. We make oatmeal on the weekend and it lasts all week long.

I eat one form of protein for breakfast every day because I've read in many sources that the protein gives you a sense of feeling full for a longer period of time. When I do that, I'm rarely hungry before 1 or 2 in the afternoon.

Registered dietician and author Bonnie Taub-Dix (*Read It Before You Eat It)*, talks about five reasons why you need to eat breakfast:

- Breakfast is necessary to fill our minds and bodies after going without food during the evening and nighttime.
- Without morning food, your blood sugar levels could resemble a roller coaster, leading to fatigue and irritability.
- Skipping breakfast often leads to a high-calorie, mid-morning snack or a heavy lunch.
- Studies show that breakfast can aid in keeping disease away.
- Good habits are contagious. Start off right in the morning to ensure that you'll continue eating well during the day.

Another registered dietician and author Keri Gans (*The Small Change Diet*), writing in www.Health.USNews.com, identifies five typical breakfast mistakes:

- **Not eating enough protein**. Most people do not get nearly enough protein for breakfast.
- **Too little fiber**. Fiber keeps you fuller longer, while sugar does the opposite. Yeah, that iced donut tastes great, but it does you no good.
- **No fat**. A meal with no fat can make you hungry again within an hour. You need a little good fat for breakfast.
- **Not enough food**. If you don't eat enough food to satisfy you, you'll be hungry mid-morning, and likely to snack on junk.
- **Eating breakfast too late**. The longer you wait to eat breakfast, the hungrier you will be, and more likely to overeat.

Plus, eating breakfast leads to smarter kids. A University of Pennsylvania School of Nursing report in *Bottom Line Personal* that kids who did not eat breakfast daily scored 4.6 points lower on verbal and performance IQ tests. Breakfast provides fuel to the brain, something kids need every day. On the other hand, underperforming kids in inner-city Boston who participated in a free school breakfast program had higher math scores, behavior marks and better attendance.

What to do about it: make the short time it takes to find a breakfast that works for you, and then eat breakfast every day. It's just that simple.

Think about it. This is your life we're talking about here!

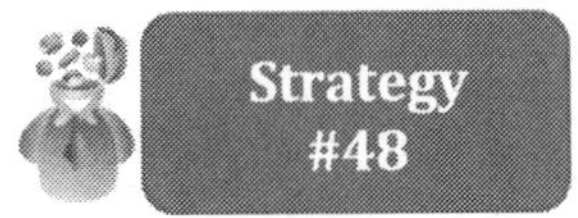

Think About Lunch

Lunch is a little different than breakfast. You may find yourself in any of these situations, all of which can disrupt the way you want to eat:

- You're asked to lunch by the boss or a client or your co-workers.
- The food served in your company cafeteria leaves a lot to be desired.
- A meeting runs late and you have just a few minutes to grab lunch.
- It's someone's birthday, and there's a cake and cookies.
- The company orders lunch for everyone, but there's nothing you like, or it's all fattening foods.
- The food truck at the factory doesn't have any healthy foods.

These are all situations in which you might end up eating foods you don't even like, eating too much or eating when you're not hungry or even when you're over-hungry. In any of these situations, you tend to eat the wrong thing and put on weight.

What to do about it: whenever you're in a situation like these, have a plan so you know ahead of time how to react:

- ***When you're asked out to lunch, in most cases you can't decline. Treat this as any dining out experience and follow your plan of eating the right foods. No one cares what you eat, and there's no need to be embarrassed if you don't finish everything on your plate.***
- ***If you can't find something acceptable in the company cafeteria, start bringing your own lunch. It will be healthier, and will cost a lot less.***

- ***Make the assumption that <u>all</u> meetings will run late. Knowing this, perhaps you eat a little before the meeting and a little after (like a mini grazing plan), so you're not rushed.***
- ***It's hard to say 'no' to birthday cake, so take a very small piece and nibble at it. Take it back to your office so you don't have to throw away the rest of it in front of everyone, and throw it out in the privacy of your office or cubicle.***
- ***When the company orders lunch, stay on the phone so you can avoid eating something you don't like or something that is not healthy for you. No one is going to criticize you for working!***

Think about it. This is your life we're talking about here!

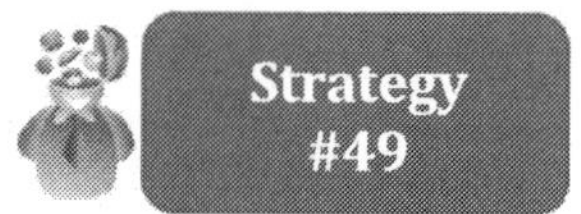

Think About Dinner

For most of us, dinner has become the "big" meal of the day. Our mind-set, whether we eat home or dine out, is that it is a big meal. We don't have that same mindset for breakfast or lunch. Perhaps it's a celebration of the completion of a hard day at work, or gathering the family together for the first time during the day. Whatever the reason, the concept of dinner being a big meal needs to change.

For one thing, it's the closest meal to bedtime, and the last thing you want is a load of food in your stomach while you're sleeping. Unless you work out after dinner and burn it all off, having a big meal for dinner makes absolutely no sense.

We also tend to eat out for dinner more often than any other meal. And when we eat out, we tend to eat more food, and we eat food that other people have prepared. We don't know what ingredients have been used. When we eat at home, we know what we're putting into each dish. When we eat out, we usually don't.

What to do about it: on a top-level, start thinking of dinner as the "healthy smaller" meal, where an extra effort is made to eat healthy and cut down the volume of food. I have a salad for dinner with a small portion of protein, almost every day! Create a visual picture in your mind of a pile of food settling into your stomach as you sleep, and how bad that is for you. If you're counting calories, carbs or fat, shift some of the allocation to other meals and/or snacks. Go to restaurants that have calorie counts on the menus.

Think about it. This is your life we're talking about here!

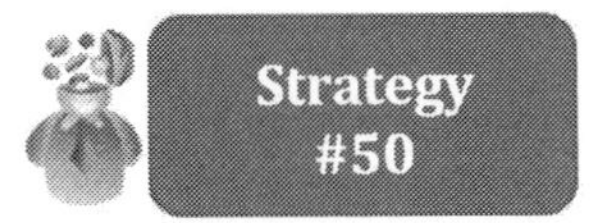

Think About Eating Out Less

I'll be the first to tell you that I enjoy eating out...and who doesn't? And so do most Americans: almost half of all the money we spend on food is spent on eating outside the home. That's a huge number. It's bad for our wallets and bad for our health.

As I mentioned in the last section, when we eat out we usually eat more food and eat food that has ingredients that are not good for us. Let's look at this in greater detail.

Most restaurants embrace the "oversized portions" philosophy and serve plates that are overflowing with food. One of the exceptions to this general rule is expensive restaurants that serve smaller portions and put time and effort into "food decoration" and display. But for the big chains and most restaurants, big portions and salad/buffet/dessert bars with unlimited food is the order of the day. Obviously, that results in us eating a lot more than we should.

Another key factor is the ingredients used in preparing the food. Unless you ask your server what is in each dish, you'll never know. Chances are high that ingredients you shouldn't have are used in dishes where you wouldn't think they would show up.

One good example is sauces. Many sauces have sugar and salt added. If you're watching either or both, you could be eating far too much salt and/or sugar without knowing it. It's the same with soups.

Since I believe so strongly in the dangers of added sugar, I ask what ingredients are in sauces and other food preparations when I eat out. I also look for sugar-free desserts (some of which taste pretty darn good) when dining out. Don't be afraid to speak up and ask.

Finally, eating out is expensive. If you were to cut down the amount of times you eat out per month by just one time that would save you as much as $1,000 or more, depending on how many people are in your family.

What to do about it: eat out less. If you eat out four times or less per month, eliminate one dining out trip. If you eat out five to ten times, eliminate two. More than ten, eliminate 25% of the number of times you eat out.

Ask servers what goes into sauces etc., and get in the habit of eating less food and leave over more, especially foods that are not good for you. Eat only half your meal, take home the rest, and you now have lunch or dinner for the next day.

Here's a novel idea from my friend Linda Pretyka: using the money you've saved by not eating out, buy a meal for a needy family!

Think about it. This is your life we're talking about here!

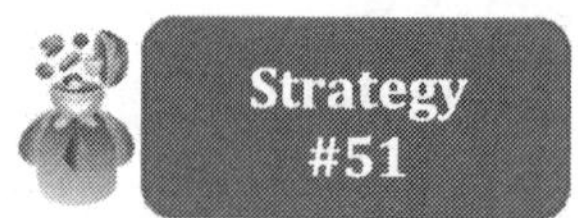

Think About Food and Dieting Information Overload

We're all bombarded by ads, news and information about food, dieting and illnesses relating to food. On the one hand are ads with mouthwatering pictures that are designed to entice you to run out and buy whatever is being advertised or go to the restaurant or fast-food joint.

On the other end of the spectrum are news stories, studies, research and "factoids" that talk about what foods are bad for you. To further complicate things, newspapers, magazines and the web are loaded with pitches for all kinds of weight-loss products, and most of them take the "magic bullet" approach.

How are we supposed to absorb all of this and make sense out of it? How are we supposed to remember every single study that comes out while we shop or eat out? And, in fact, are all of those studies valid? Should we believe the ads that claim you can burn off weight while you sleep (see next section) or dismiss them all?

I hear people talk about how confusing this all is, and how it's so easy to simply throw up your hands and say "This is too much to deal with." I used to feel the same way until I made up my mind and got serious about weight loss.

What to do about it: it's actually quite simple. When you make up your mind to lose weight the right way, and you choose a program that's medically sound and easy for you to follow, just be true to your program.

Once you make up your mind that you're not going to have fries or onion rings, ads for them will not sway you. Once you make up your mind that you will lose weight slowly and steadily, ads proclaiming fast weight loss will have no impact on you. And when you read studies in the news, you'll know which ones to pay attention to, and which to ignore.

Think about it. This is your life we're talking about here!

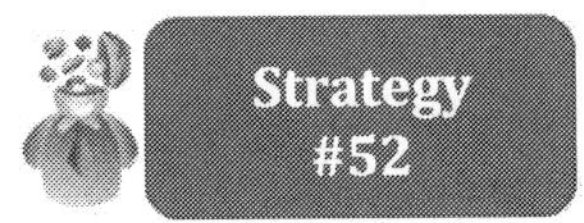

Think About Weight Loss Advertising

Aside from "get rich quick" schemes, I don't think any other category of advertising has attracted more charlatans, con artists and ads with outrageous claims than the dieting/weight loss category.

I'm not talking about the Jenny Craigs or Weight Watchers of the world or bona-fide products that are medically sound. I'm talking about ads that boldly claim you can:

- Lose 15 pounds while you sleep!
- Eat anything you want, as much as you want!
- Lose pounds and inches like crazy!
- Burn fat without exercising!
- Melt away 22.5 lbs with Apple Cider Vinegar!
- Lose your appetite and feel satisfied!
- Eat anything and reduce cholesterol levels!
- Eliminate cellulite and excess fat pockets before your eyes!
- Stimulate your body's natural fat-burning ability!

While some of these claims are **technically** true, the context in which they are presented leads people to believe that anyone can basically eat a ton of food, never exercise, pop a pill once a day, and wake up the next morning pounds lighter. And sadly, some people, perhaps millions, fall for these ads, spend their hard-earned money on them, and then fail, wondering where they went wrong.

But what about the testimonials shown in these ads, you ask? The woman who dropped 35 pounds in 22 days, or the guy who went down 8 sizes in 6 weeks? These testimonials fall into two categories: actors who say these things because it's a new product and testimonials don't exist; and valid testimonials that are not representative of everyone who buys the product. In fact, the FTC reports that 55% of 300 weight-loss ads reviewed included at least one unsubstantiated claim for weight loss!

If you look closely at the next diet commercial you see, you'll see the disclaimer that is typically worded like this: **results like this are not typical**. Or, **do not expect dramatic weight loss**. Having these disclaimers allows for certain claims to be made, and while they made be legally acceptable, they hide the full story.

But what about their guarantee, you ask. These companies know that most people won't ask for their money back, so they have no problem or risk in putting in guarantees. In this case, these guarantees are worthless.

What to do about it: 99.99% of people who try "lose weight fast" products will fail. If you want to waste your money, time and effort, go right ahead. Instead, since you've made up your mind to do it right, ignore these ads no matter how enticing they are.

Think about it. This is your life we're talking about here!

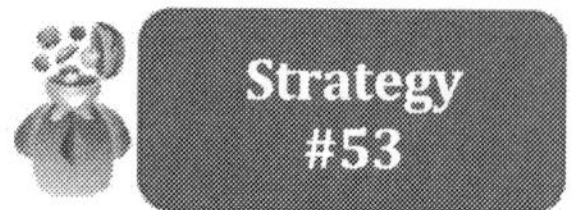

Think About Your Weight and Clothing

Personally, clothing that doesn't fit well as a result of weight gain is one of the most constant and annoying reminders that one is heavy. Despite fashion designers' attempts to create good-looking clothes for plus sized people, clothing that overweight people end up wearing are often uncomfortable, not terribly stylish, often don't look good on and can't possibly accentuate a figure that is, well, not a good figure. While there are clothes that are stylish, they tend to be expensive.

When you wear clothes, no matter how well they look, they tend to get soaked from perspiration under the arms, on the back and other places. Not only is this uncomfortable, it is embarrassing. One result of this is your clothes need to be washed or dry-cleaned more often.

What to do about it: get the weight off so you can enjoy the clothes you've not been able to wear since before you gained weight. Pull out some photos from times when you were thinner, and imagine yourself getting back to that point. Then, just do it!

Think about it. This is your life we're talking about here!

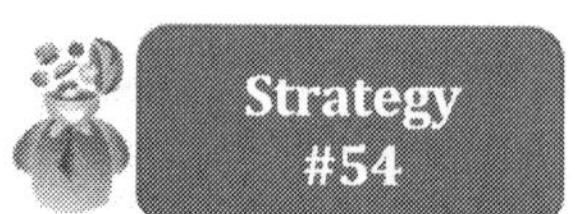

Think About Snacking While Watching TV

I think the common phrase "couch potato" needs to be changed to more accurately reflect what we all do while watching TV: couch eaters.

For a whole host of reasons, we've made it a tradition to snack while watching TV, in the same way we do at movie theaters. It seems that we just can't sit still and watch the big screen or the small screen without eating. For many, it has become a habit that we just can't seem to break – you grab a snack even if you're not hungry – simply because you're so used to eating while watching TV.

For some of us, we need to sit down in front of the TV with food that we eat during the show and during the commercials. For others, commercial breaks result in the mad dash to the refrigerator or cookie jar. In fact, iVillage.com found that 71% of women polled admitted to reaching for a snack **simply because "it's there."** Whether at work or home, remove unhealthy snacks so that they are out of eyesight. Since most of our TV watching is a night, the worst time of the day to eat, we're hurting ourselves by being couch eaters.

What to do about it: there are three things you can do to get out of this habit:

- ***Watch TV less. If you cut TV watching down from 3 hours to 2 hours, you'll snack 33% less!***
- ***Make a rule that the only place your family is allowed to eat is in the kitchen or dining area...and stick to it!***
- ***To keep your hands and mind busy during slow parts of a program and during commercials, start doing other activities instead of eating: go online and surf or answer emails, write a letter, read the newspaper or magazine, do a crossword or other puzzle, knit, sew, exercise, fold laundry, organize photos, etc. Anything but eat!***

Think about it. This is your life we're talking about here!

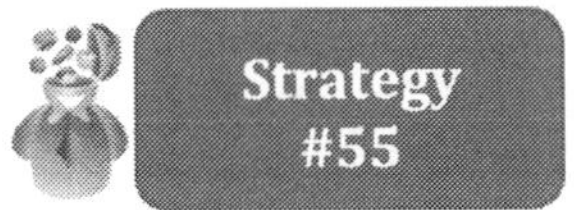

Think About Food and Stress

One of the often-used excuses that we use to justify eating is that we're under stress. I'm sure you recognize when these situations occur, and that if you're heavy, this might be one of those times when you eat when you shouldn't.

Chances are you don't think about this, but stress is a leading cause of medical problems, resulting in the fact that 9 of 10 doctor visits by men can be attributed to stress (American Institute of Stress). Stress can be directly responsible for heart disease, high blood pressure, stroke, cancer and more. Getting rid of stress should be a major goal for you.

What to do about it: there are many ways to relieve stress:

- ***Do something physical: go for a run, hit a punching bag, yell and scream (where no one can hear you), lift weights, etc.***
- ***Talk it out: get with your partner or best friend and talk about the problem and how to deal with it.***
- ***Learn to relax: when stress occurs, use meditation, yoga or other types of relaxation techniques to dissipate the stress.***

- ***Get more stuff going on in your life: boredom is a direct cause of stress in addition to other sources of stress; the fuller your life, the better off you are.***
- ***Lose weight: being heavy in itself is stressful, so the more you lose, the better you'll feel.***

If you must snack when stress hits, certain foods are better than others. According to Elizabeth Sommer, author of "Food & Mood," designate certain foods as "stress snacks" (Reader's Digest):

- ***Whole-grain crackers can enhance the release of serotonin, a chemical when released in the brain induces a sense of calm.***
- ***Milk's calcium, magnesium and potassium may help keep blood pressure down, and drinking warm milk often relaxes people.***
- ***Cereal seems to be associated with lower levels of the stress hormone corsitol.***

Think about it. This is your life we're talking about here!

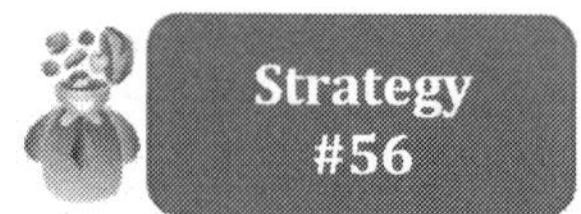

Think About Genetics and Weight Loss

There are plenty of people who believe that weight gain is "in the genes" and if your parents or siblings are fat, you too will be destined for a life of being overweight. There's nothing you can do about it, because you're "stuck" with fat genes.

The World Health Organization concluded "while it is possible that single or multiple gene effects may cause overweight and obesity directly, and indeed do so in some individuals, this does not appear to be the case in the majority of people."

Our genes may make it harder for us to lose weight, but certainly not impossible. Some genes may give us a slower metabolism rate than other people; genes can affect the amount of muscle and fat in our bodies; and people whose parents had "love handles" might be more inclined to develop love handles too. Dr. Lazarus says that genetics can play an important role, and environment "pulls the trigger" on weight gain.

But none of the experts say that genetics determines whether or not you can lose weight. The net of this is that if you have a slow metabolism gene from your dad and/or a love handle gene from mom, you're going to have to work a little harder and smarter to overcome them. It's just like in basketball: if you're not born 6'6 and have average ball-playing skills, you'll have to work harder than someone who is blessed with that height and talent.

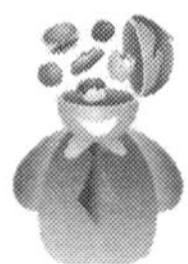

What to do about it: if you honestly (and that's the key word here) believe some of your genes might be contributing to your weight problem, discuss this with your doctor and nutrition specialist when planning which diet program you're going to follow. This is one additional factor to take into account.

Think about it. This is your life we're talking about here!

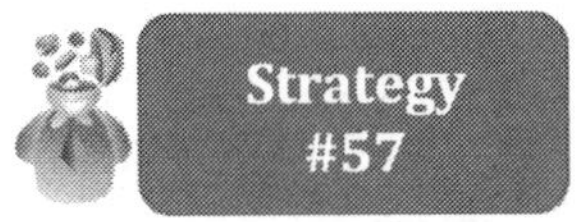

Think About Smoking and Weight Gain/Loss

If you smoke, you may have concluded two important things:

- The nicotine found in cigarettes acts as an appetite suppressant and alleviates the need for snacking that non-smokers or people quitting smoking experience.
- You may be very reluctant to quit smoking because you fear you'll immediately gain a lot of weight. When you stop smoking, your blood sugar will most likely drop, giving you the urge to snack on sweets in response.

If you're overweight and smoke, I hope you know you're combining two of the worst risk factors and taking a major chance with your life.

What to do about it: you need to stop smoking <u>and</u> lose weight if you want to live...plain and simple. The experts advise:

- ***Upon quitting smoking, drink lots of fruit juices for the first three days, which will stabilize your blood sugar levels. Also, the acidity of the juices should help your body get rid of the nicotine, thus shortening the withdrawal symptoms.***
- ***Turn three meals into six or more. Spread out your daily food allotment throughout the day so you can snack more often, when urges occur.***
- ***Exercise. While every day is recommended, working out for just 20-30 minutes every other day is going to help you.***

Of course, talk with your doctor and nutrition professional before quitting and making dietary changes or starting to exercise. They may recommend certain prescription drugs that can help you quit smoking and prevent weight gain after.

Think about it. This is your life we're talking about here!

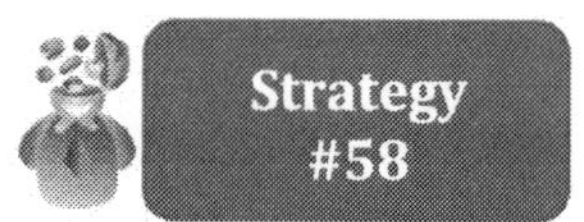

Think About Generalizations about Food and Weight Loss

When I listen to people talk about weight loss, dieting, being overweight, diets, and related matters, I hear a lot of generalizations and hearsay that just makes no sense.

One of my pet peeves in general, and one I hear over and over again with regard to weight loss, goes something like this: "They say it's a good idea to fast once a week to get rid of the toxins in your body." You might hear this from a friend, family member or someone at work. Chances are you trust the person who said it, and you may even accept it as fact.

But here's the peeve, worth repeating: who is the "they" referred to? Did the person who told you this hear it from a doctor? See it on TV? Read it in a book? Or more likely, hear it from someone else that may or may not have heard it from the original source.

The key point for this strategy: generalizations don't always apply to you and your unique circumstances. Figure out which ones will work for you.

What to do about it: whenever someone recommends that you do anything involving your body, check it out. Ask who the "they" is? Go to your favorite search engine online and enter "fasting and weight loss" or whatever the "advice" is and read up on it. Talk to your doctor and nutrition specialist if necessary. No matter how much you trust someone, they may be unknowingly passing on bad information, or at least, information that is not right for you.

Think about it. This is your life we're talking about here!

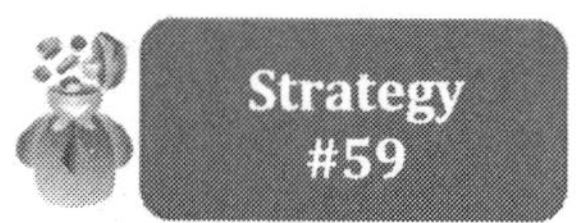

Think About Some Unusual Measures

The more research I did for this book, the more ideas kept coming in – ways that people have been thinking about and implementing in order to lose weight and keep the weight off. Some of those are:

- **Food visualization**. Several people convince themselves that certain foods are actually poisoning their bodies. They associate these foods with the skull and crossbones or with the word "poison" and they find that whenever they see that food, the association is so strong that they have no desire to eat that food.

- **Eat salads, fruits and or vegetables at night.** Eating a dark green salad every night as a main course, with a little of protein is one of the most important changes I made to my eating routine. I dress up my salad with toasted almond slivers, small amounts of cranberries, a sensible amount of dressing and turn it into a meal that leaves me full and satisfied. Why? Because the body slows down at night, the last thing you want to feed it is carbs and sugar. And many salad ingredients are mostly water! Many times I eat fruit and nuts.

- **Evening/midnight snacks that might be OK.** If you absolutely, positively must have a snack after dinner, replace the bad stuff (you know exactly what I mean!) with these suggestions that are healthy and should keep you tied over until breakfast:

    - A handful of peanuts and a few chunks of fresh cantaloupe
    - A ¼ cup of low-fat cottage cheese
    - One slice of whole wheat bread with no-sugar-added peanut butter
    - A handful of carrots or other veggies
    - A cold glass of water or seltzer

What to do about it: just like you plan out the rest of the day, plan what you're going to eat if you must at night.

Think about it. This is your life we're talking about here!

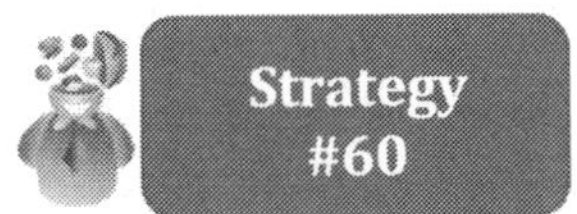

Think About Keeping a Journal

I think by now you realize that you must make a real commitment to losing weight vs. simply trying the latest fad diet or product.

Part of this promise to yourself is keeping written records of what you've achieved. This "journal" should include your food plan, your medical information, your nutrition specialist's recommendations, and a simple daily chart of your weight.

We talked earlier about losing weight steadily and slowly, perhaps one to two pounds a week. Two pounds a week equals about 3/10th of a pound per day. If you can lose 3/10th of a pound every day, you will lose about eight pounds a month and almost 50 pounds in 6 months. See how it adds up?

Because you eat every day, and because I recommend that you weigh yourself every morning, completely naked, you will see results on a daily basis for every day that you comply with the food plan you've created for yourself.

Some days you might lose 2/10th or 4/10th. Other days you might lose only 1/10th or half a pound. Don't be discouraged if it's not 3/10th every day. In addition to your weight losses, your journal should include what foods you eat, substitutions you made that day and when you ate.

What to do about it: make the commitment to yourself to put results in writing. After a little up-front work, I'm talking about a minute or two a day to write down your weight. But don't stop there!

Wellness writer Jennifer Cohen reports that a Kaiser Permanente study found that people who wrote down what they ate doubled their weight loss!

And make sure to get a digital scale that shows your weight in tenths of a pound.

Think about it. This is your life we're talking about here!

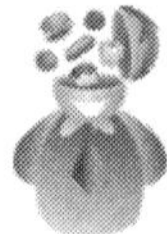

Section III: Your Relationships

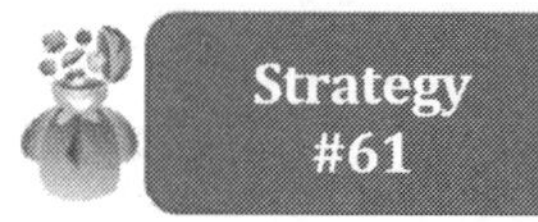

Think About How Weight Affects Your Partner

Whenever I see a couple where one person is thin and the other very heavy, I always wonder if they can be **truly** happy. Yes, they may love each other. And yes, they may enjoy being with each other.

One reader writes: "my husband has always been thin and in control of his eating. My being heavy has hurt our relationship."

But I always reach the same conclusion: for most people in this situation, there must be many times when the thin one wishes the heavy one wasn't heavy. It's only human nature. Things are more difficult when one is heavy and one isn't – a few examples – in many relationships:

- Lovemaking is not likely to be as enjoyable.
- Deep down inside, you are embarrassed the way the heavy one looks. Perhaps more embarrassed with certain people than others, but almost always embarrassed.
- The heavy one can't look good in clothes and certainly can't look sexy for his/her partner.

And I'm sure you can think about many more problems, some big and some small, that come with a partner who is heavy.

But the biggie is that the heavy one might die prematurely, become disabled, require extensive medical care, and the thinner one is left holding the bag. All the love in the world that the thinner one has for the other one is fine and dandy, but you can be sure the heavy one, in effect, is depriving the thinner one of a lot of quality time, simply by being heavy.

For an interesting take on relationships and weight, read this short but powerful article by emotional eating expert Dr. Roger Gould:
http://tinyurl.com/kr57ovm.

What to do about it: if you're the heavy one, think about how your weight is affecting your partner. Surely you'll agree that it is, or will, deprive your partner of what life has to offer in so many ways. Your partner is, or certainly should be, the most important person in your life – think about making the right decision for him or her.

On a practical basis, author and registered dietitian Cynthia Sass offers five ways to work with your partner to ensure you both eat healthy:

- ***Eat different foods, together. You don't need to eat the same thing, because we're all different. Author's note: my wife is on Weight Watchers and my diet was created with my doctor and nutrition specialist. While we sometimes end up eating the same food, most of the time we don't. And that works!***
- ***Personalize your portions. Chances are you and your partner don't need the same amount of food.***
- ***You don't always have to eat together. If he's coming home late, it's not necessary to wait for him for dinner because that might not be good for you.***
- ***Break out of a rut centered around food – i.e. popcorn while watching TV together. Do things together that are not centered around food.***
- ***Focus on your love life – instead of food.***

Think about it. This is your life we're talking about here!

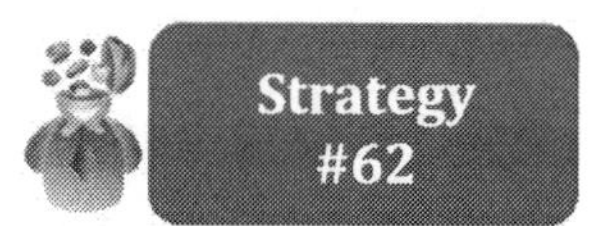

Think About How Eating Habits Affect Your Kids

Recently I saw something that made me cringe. Though I've seen this many times before, as I'm sure you have, I get sick to my stomach whenever I see this.

There was a family of three waiting in the airport. Mom and dad were at least 300 pounds each if not more. The little boy looked like he was about 8 years old, and at least 150 if not 200 pounds. As they interacted, they seemed like nice people, and in most respects, they may be very good parents, but with one huge exception.

It's one thing to let yourself go and bloat up to obesity and threaten your own life, but it's quite another thing to bring a child into this world and raise him or her in the same fashion. This couple obviously has given up on themselves, but how can they saddle a young child with all that weight? That's just not right; in fact it's downright awful. That boy will be behind the 8-ball for his whole life:

- He'll be taunted throughout his school years.
- He won't have many friends, and if he does, they'll all be fat like him.
- The only dates he'll get are with overweight girls.
- He won't be able to play sports; if he tries to play sports, he'll be picked last or not at all. And it might be dangerous to play sports.
- He'll wear baggy and loose fitting clothes to hide his weight.
- He'll be shy and introverted because he'll wrap himself up in TV and videogames, losing out on the normal socialization process.
- He may be discriminated against when he applies for jobs.
- If he gets married, chances are it will be to a fat girl, and chances are the entire cycle will be repeated with their children.

But most of all children who are overweight or obese are coming down with "adult" diseases and conditions at extremely young ages (review the statistics in *Truth* to refresh your memory of how dire this can be). Your child may also resent you for your habits that he/she mimicked. This is really a very major issue, and you have the power to make positive changes!

Kids at school will react to the fat child by laughing, giggling, smirking, staring, turning away, making faces, making jokes, taunting and worse – bullying.

Even family members, perhaps more subtly, will make an overweight child feel hurt, embarrassed, worthless and more. And they might criticize your parenting skills.

The child will be called names like chubby, fatso, porker, big boy, earthquake, fat ass, big butt, and a lot worse.

Do you really want this to happen?

If you think "it can't happen to my kid," take a look at some of these extremely sobering stats, all from "Your Kids Are Getting So Big" (*NY Post, 9/5/2010)*:

- Most American kids eat three snacks a day, up from one or two in the 1980's and 1990's.
- The average teenager gets 37% of their calories outside of the home, including 17% from fast food.
- Most kids drink 2-3 cans of sugar-sweetened soda per day, and each can has 15 teaspoons of sugar.
- Most teen boys drink enough soda to get 34 teaspoons of sugar a day, far more than the recommended amount of 5-8 tsp.
- Pizza consumption has increased 425% since the 1970's.

A researcher at Johns Hopkins University School of Medicine believes that children born after 2000 have a 30% chance of developing diabetes over their lifetime. We can't let our kids start life this way!

Dr. Manny Alvarez, senior managing health editor of FoxNews.com, says that "Being overweight can cause an imbalance in your reproductive hormones, which affects your menstrual cycles and may prevent ovulation. Hypertensive disorders, like preeclampsia, during pregnancy are the leading cause of maternal and fetal death and illness." Bottom line: lose all the weight before you get pregnant to give your child-to-be the best opportunity for health and fitness from the second he/she is born.

Dr. Michael Goran, director of the Childhood Obesity Research Center at the University of Southern California, says that his research shows that High Fructose Corn Syrup, a very prevalent sweetener, promotes the development of obesity in infants.

In "7 Surprising Effects of Obesity" by Liz Neporent (*abcnews.go.com*), "overweight women have a harder time getting pregnant." Over 90% developed a condition associated with infertility. She adds, "obesity increases a woman's chance of having a preterm baby, especially when her BMI is 35 or higher." Premature birth is the leading cause of infant death and long-term disabilities.

That's not all. Senior News Editor Rick Nauert, PhD reports in www.psychcentral.com that a BYU study of 8,000+ families found that babies predominantly fed formula were 2½ times more likely to become obese toddlers than babies breastfed for the first six months. Plus, putting babies to bed with a bottle increased the risk of childhood obesity by 36% (*Pediatric Obesity*). And, introducing solid foods too soon (before 4 months of age), increased childhood obesity risk by 40%. Are we unknowingly doing things that will result in obese kids?

Eating Disorders as a Result of Dieting

Recent research published in *Pediatrics* by Mayo Clinic researchers concludes that obese children and teenagers who lose weight in an unhealthy manner are more likely to develop eating disorders. According to the report, at least six percent of children suffer from eating disorders, and over 55% are females in high school. Parents need to be aware of this because when a child loses a lot of weight, the development of eating disorders may be overshadowed by the celebration of the weight loss.

Leigh Garfield, LCSW, BCD is a private practice psychotherapist specializing in the treatment of eating disorders, disordered eating and body image issues. Based on her years of experience, she commented on the diet/eating disorder phenomenon: "Dieting emphasizes body weight and size, rather than health and wellness. The diet mentality is constructed with eating disordered beliefs and thinking patterns. The dieting messages create fears of fatness and emphasize restrictive eating and excessive exercise.
These are underlying symptoms of eating disorders that often go undetected in a dieting teen. In fact, dieters are often rewarded for behaviors and attitudes that are actually warning signs. The key to successful treatment of an eating disorder is early identification. This cannot happen when dieting reinforces what are often symptoms of a deadly disorder."

Leigh (theredinc@aol.com in Central NJ) has served on the Board of the New Jersey Chapter of the American Anorexia/Bulimia Association, and is past President of the Eating Disorders Association of New Jersey and has lectured extensively on issues regarding food and eating and other mental health topics.

Adds Leslie Sim, clinical director of the Mayo Clinic's eating disorders program, "When formerly overweight or obese adolescents come into our clinic, they look like the average kid, but their hair's falling out and they're not menstruating and they're very, very sick kids – and they're not being identified because of their weight."

What to do about it: this is the most important decision you will ever have to make. If you have obese children, or if you are obese and are planning to have children, you MUST make up your mind to break this tragic cycle. Do not raise a kid or bring one into this world if you can't give that child a chance to grow up happy and healthy, and not as a fat kid whose life will hold little value. Make sure you feed yourself well during pregnancy and remember what you just read in the paragraph before this one!

Plus, don't get your kids in the habit of expecting a "junk food reward" when they do their homework or chores. Saying "take out the garbage and you get a candy bar" is essentially programming your kid that food is a reward for doing something good, or for not doing something bad.

If you are having trouble getting your child to eat healthier, or if he or she is being resistive to your efforts, take your child to the doctor, and have your doctor talk frankly and openly about weight and how it will affect the rest of his or her life. Getting through to your child is critical.

Your child needs your help and nurturing through this most difficult time. They don't know how to handle ridicule at school and if it occurs, snide comments at home. If you have any doubt about how to help your kid lose weight, get into therapy now, or contact an organization like Shapedown (shapedown.com) that combines sensible weight loss with family-based treatment.

Special Videos to Show Your Children

These are all "must views" for your family:

- ***The Scarecrow: https://www.youtube.com/watch?v=lUtnas5ScSE***
- ***Polar Bears Drinking Soda: http://www.theRealBears.org***
- ***Sugar is Killing Us: www.youtube.com/watch?v=Yda8RtOcVFU***

Think about it. This is your kids' life we're talking about here! Think long and hard about it. Make the right decision. Do it now.

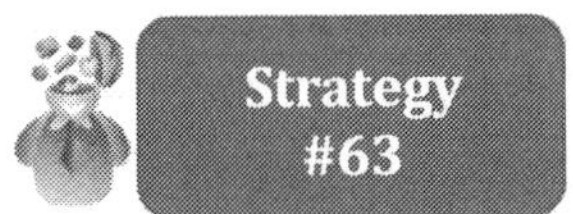

Think About Hugging, Kissing and Holding Hands

The Beatles sang about holding hands...countless other songs talk about hugging and kissing. These are among the most natural things we do with the people we love.

For those who are thin, there's no second thought – you just hug, kiss and hold hands. But for heavier people, these can be uncomfortable and not very romantic. I recall that when I was heavier, simple things like these were not nearly as enjoyable as they are now!

I've seen heavy people trying to hold hands, but because the way their arms are "bowed out" to follow the contour of their bodies, holding hands is just not that simple. For overweight couples I've seen, it looks very awkward and it just doesn't look like much fun. Hugging can also be a problem if you can't get your arms around the person you want to hug. Getting into the right position to kiss someone is also problematical.

As a result, many heavier people don't hug, kiss and hold hands or show affection to each other as often as they want to. And they have the same problem hugging their kids; everyone agrees this is very important.

What to do about it: there's no easy answer, no trick, but to lose the weight so these and other romantic activities become enjoyable, natural and fun. Envision how much more enjoyable your love lives will be if you are both thinner. Keep hugging, kissing and holding hands while you lose weight.

Think about it. This is your life we're talking about here!

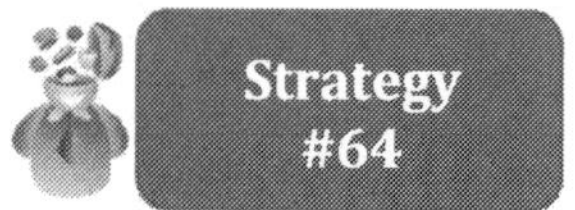

Think About Weight and Sex

I came across a statistic that I had to read a couple of times to make sure it was not a misprint. The May/June 2003 issue of *AARP Magazine* (for 50+ consumers) reported that 50% of women would choose chocolate over making love. Is that a sad commentary or what?

Let's look at this a little closer. There could be lots of reasons why women would prefer chocolate and I'm not going to attempt to explain any of them. They would include not having a partner, a partner who is not a good lover, medical issues, hormonal changes, just not enjoyable, etc.

My personal conclusion is that the only reason of importance here is that some portion of those tens of millions of women who chose chocolate over making love is because they and/or their partners are overweight and sex is just no fun or is actually annoying or even painful. So for the women in this group, you're basically replacing something that's immensely pleasurable and calorie-free with something that lasts for a few seconds and puts on even more weight. Yikes, what's going on here?

Of course, I understand that it's difficult to have a good love life when you're overweight or obese. I don't have to describe the problems because they should be evident to anyone reading this book.

What's important is that amongst everything we do in life, lovemaking is one of the most special, precious, passionate and downright pleasurable things you can do. To miss out on it is just a travesty.

What to do about it: think long and hard about how much better your life would be if you and your partner could make love without your weight(s) interfering. It's time to decide once and for all that you don't want to miss out on sex.

Think about it. This is your sex life we're talking about here!

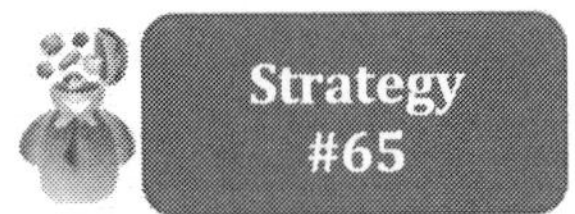

Think About Getting Family and Friends to Help & Support You

This weight loss program that I'm recommending is one that should be supported by family, friends and co-workers.

It is not something to be done in secret.

The more people that know what you're doing, the more support and encouragement you'll get, and the more positive feedback you'll receive when your weight loss becomes noticeable.

Take the time to explain in detail what you're doing, so that others will provide support in the way that's good for you. Perhaps they will prepare something special for you when getting together for a family dinner.

Even better, try to get your partner and/or other family members and friends to read *The Mind Diet* with you. By doing this, you'll be supporting others and they will be supporting you. You'll also share what you've learned so that everyone in your "group" gets the benefit of what's working.

What to do about it: make this a big deal with your friends and family. Make it out to be (and it is), one of the most important things you've ever done, and ask for their support and help. Reader suggestion: "Don't be afraid to ask or even TELL them what kind of support you need – stand up for yourself! I had to ask my family to put junk food out of sight."

Think about it. This is your life we're talking about here!

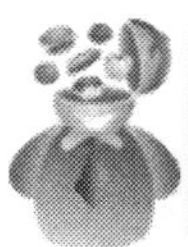

Section IV: Weight Loss Products

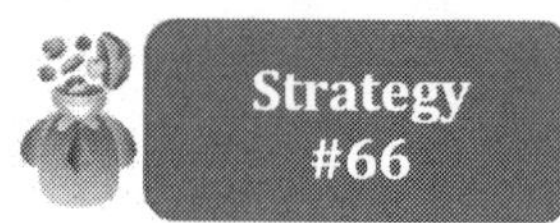

Think About Which Weight Loss Program is Right for You

You're faced with literally hundreds of choices of ways you can lose weight – in person programs, online programs, food provider programs, energy and candy bars, and on and on and on.

How do you absorb all of these and choose one? The most effective diet program you can choose will take into account all of these factors, so it's a good idea to make a comprehensive list, including:

- Foods you can't stand to eat
- Foods you enjoy eating
- Your personal medical history
- Your family medical history
- Medications that you're taking
- Food allergies you might have
- How much exercise you get
- Your ability to deal with stress
- How much weight you need to lose
- Your age
- Your gender
- Programs you tried that didn't work

In addition to all of these, perhaps the most important one is your personality and your ability to follow and stick with any given program. Some of us are good at, and don't mind, keeping track of points or calories or what you've eaten during the day, so those people may gravitate towards programs that require you to keep track (something which is good as it reinforces the thought processes in this book).

Others don't have the patience to keep track, so if you're in this group, look for a program that's still easy to follow. One of the things I like about some programs is that they are simple to follow and I don't have to remember a whole lot. Of course, as I recommend in this book, I spent time learning about the program and what I can and can't eat.

So with all those choices out there, it's not as difficult as you might think to choose the program that's right for you.

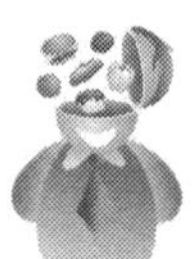

What to do about it: talk over all the above points with your doctor and nutrition specialist, and make an informed decision after you've read about what's involved in each diet program. If you get inspiration from weekly meetings, support groups and speakers, that's great. Choose the one that medically makes the most sense and that you can follow and that is OK with your healthcare professionals.

Think about it. This is your life we're talking about here!

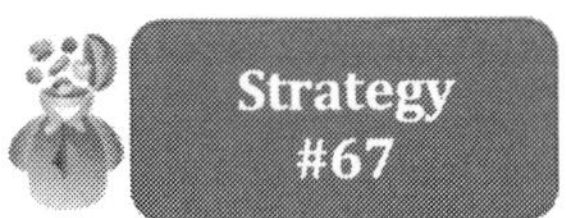

Think About Understanding the Program You Choose

Years ago, I first learned about The Atkins Diet from a friend, who had lost 25 pounds on that diet. Since eating more fat and not many carbs was a foreign concept to me, I bought the book and read it thoroughly. I understood the program and why it was so successful.

Learning and understanding the program helped me become a real believer in this kind of diet and more importantly, a real believer in that I would be successful with it. Not only did I come to understand the how's and why's, but reading the book quickly ingrained in me what kinds of foods were OK and what kinds were not. While there are variations on Atkins and other fine programs, I just happened to latch onto that one. I have since switched to a different diet recommended by my doctor and nutrition specialist.

Regardless of the program you ultimately end up with, you will find the same thing once you take the time to learn and understand it.

What to do about it: before you consult with your doctor and nutrition specialist, think about which program to choose, read up on those you think might work, so that you can have a very intelligent conversation with your health care professionals.

Think about it. This is your life we're talking about here!

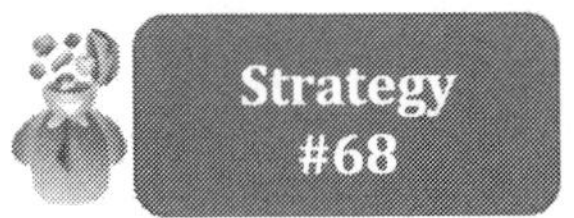

Think About Weight Loss Products

As a rule, I never eat anything unless I have a pretty good idea of what it is and the effects it can have. Just because a friend pops diet pills or an ad proclaims that the latest "fat burner"

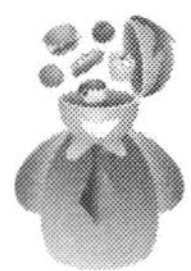

will burn fat when I sleep, there are just too many potential disasters out there, so I don't take any chances.

If you do a search at your favorite search engine for "weight loss products," you'll see thousands, including:

- Books
- Videos
- Customized diet plans
- Supplements
- Nutrition calculator
- Drugs, supplements and pills
- Herbal products
- Shakes and drinks
- Healthy TV dinners
- Weight loss programs
- Patches
- Many others, including wacky things like electronic muscle stimulators, appetite suppressing eyeglasses and magic weight-loss earrings!

Just because a product is sold or advertised doesn't mean it's any good. In this country, anyone can sell anything, and products are not banned until the FTC or other agencies get involved. The primary exception is prescription drugs. So when you see products in your supermarket, health-food store or in mail order ads, don't assume they are OK.

What to do about it: don't buy any products that you have not discussed with your doctor or nutrition specialist. Many of them can bring on nasty side effects, and others may interfere with medication you're taking. No matter how slick the ads or that your best friend is taking it, check it out with your doctor. The Food and Drug Administration (FDA) has banned 111 ingredients once found in non-prescription diet products -- they are potentially harmful and none of them have proved effective in weight-loss.

Think about it. This is your life we're talking about here!

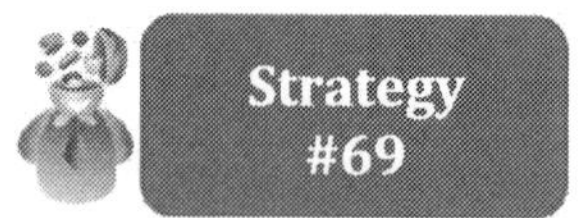

Think About Weight Loss Operations

Surgery is a very big decision, one not to be taken lightly.

As Dr. Ethan Lazarus points out, "Obesity is a deadly disease. For the right patient, surgery may be the only acceptable option." For the morbidly obese, surgery is the only proven strategy shown to reduce morbidity and mortality.

In 2013 there are three common surgical procedures:

- Gastric bypass (http://tinyurl.com/lx5o8ew)
- Adjustable gastric band (http://tinyurl.com/z4l8p)
- Sleeve gastrectomy (http://tinyurl.com/l77ejbp)

This book is not the forum to discuss these. I've provided Wikipedia links to get you started on learning about these procedures. The same is true of weight-loss drugs. They must be discussed with your healthcare professionals, and are actually recommended in some cases.

What to do about it: if you think you might be the right kind of candidate for surgery, the first step is find a surgeon with deep experience in obesity-related procedures and have an open and frank discussion with him/her about your situation.

Think about it. This is **really** your life we're talking about here!

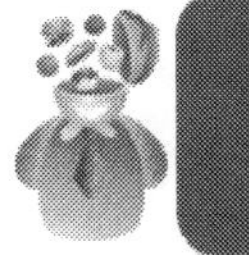

Section V: The Art of Eating

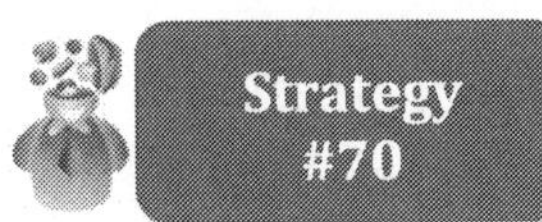

Think About How You Chew Food

I touched on the "art of chewing" earlier, but now I'll spend some more time on it, because chewing correctly is the easiest thing you can do to enjoy food and lose weight. And you can start immediately!

Believe it or not, there is a group of about 60,000 people who belong to "Slow Food" a group that embodies what I'm talking about. Take the speed out of eating and enjoy the taste is what they're all about. So what I'm preaching is something that they, and millions of others, embrace.

It's OK to **think** that you need to eat slower and chew more. But let's go one step further. I've developed the "Rule of 14" when it comes to chewing. From now on, chew every piece

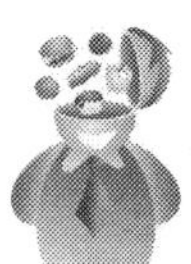

of food for 14 seconds or 14 chews, whichever you prefer. That's right. Count seconds or chews and you'll start seeing results instantly:

- You'll enjoy the food more, because you'll get a lot more taste sensations.
- You'll take a lot longer to eat, which is good.
- You'll eat less food, because you'll get hungry before you finish.
- You'll lose weight because you won't be eating everything.

"I'm not going to bother to count how many times I chew" is the response I hear to this technique. Some people think I'm nuts. Here's my response: it works! While you don't have to do everything I recommend in this book, you need to do a lot of them to succeed. It just so happens that this is one of the easiest things I recommend. And no one has to know you're doing it. You don't count out loud, so what's the big deal?

What to do about it: just do it. Period. End of story.

Think about it. This is your life we're talking about here!

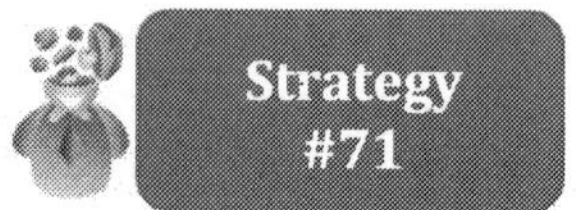

Think About Volume

The fact of the matter is, we don't need to eat much food to live healthy lives. Tens of millions of people around the world eat a lot less than we do, and have fewer medical problems than we do.

The trouble is that food has become such a part of our lives and it is in so much abundance here in America. It's cheap, it's available 24 hours a day and it tastes so good. And most restaurants serve giant-sized portions. Hey, if our entire food supply tasted like airline food, we'd all be as thin as rails.

The simplest way to look at any diet or weight loss program is that we need to eat less, to cut down on our volume.

If you're counting calories, and you eat 25% less food, you'll ingest 25% fewer calories. If you count fat or carbs, eating 25% less means you'll get 25% less carbs or fat. It really is that simple.

What to do about it: concentrate on taste, not volume. What's better -- to get 25 mouthfuls of an entrée where you hardly appreciate the taste, or 15 mouthfuls where you enjoy every single one? And 40% fewer calories, carbs, fat and salt to boot!

Think about it. This is your life we're talking about here!

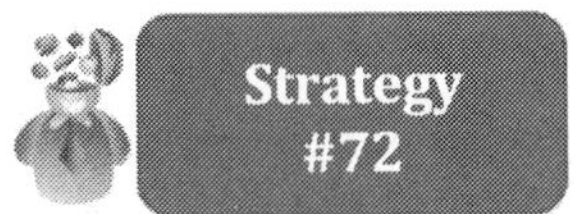

Think About Piece Size

I've come to the conclusion that most people eat pieces of food that are way too big, and can't possibly enjoy them as a result. In watching people in restaurants and eating at parties, I can't help but wonder why. Why are they eating a forkful of cake that is so big that it is practically falling off the fork? Why are they eating half a dozen French fries at once? Why are they eating ¼ of their cheeseburger in one bite?

Since I couldn't understand this behavior, I actually asked people why they eat such large pieces of food. Most of time I got one of two responses:

- This is the way I've always eaten.
- I have no idea. I never thought about it.

Well, now is the time to think about it. If you eat big pieces because you always have, it's time to change, for several reasons:

- Eating big chunks of food is not healthy and it makes it much harder for the body to swallow and digest it.
- You can't possibly enjoy the taste of food when your jaws are working overtime to make sure the food can be swallowed.

What to do about it: think small. Eat one French fry or onion ring at a time, or even half (see next section) of one. Cut steak into pieces no larger than ½" square and ½" thick. Whether a soda, water, shake or juice, sip your drinks instead of chugging.

Think about it. This is your life we're talking about here!

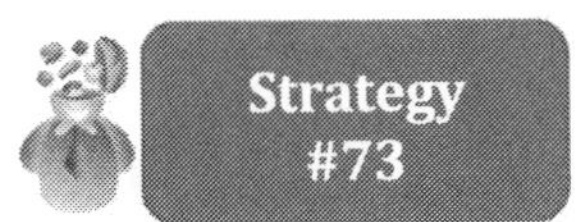

Think ½

The fraction one-half is a very important one in the grand scheme of weight loss according to *The Mind Diet.* It has three main purposes, and you need to remember one-half whenever you eat:

- **½ sized portions**. Whenever you eat out, plan on eating only ½ of your meal, and bringing home the rest for another day. Restaurant portions are way oversized anyhow, so eating half is approximately what you should be served in the first place.

- **½ of a piece**. Get in the habit of eating half a piece instead of the whole piece. If you take a chunk of pineapple from a buffet plate, cut it in half instead of swallowing the entire piece. Eat half of a French fry or onion ring. While you don't have to eat ½ of an M&M, certainly eat half of a cookie.

- **½ inch bite sizes**. When cutting any kind of food, like meat, poultry, fish, pork, etc., aim for ½" square pieces. I've seen too many people eat pieces of steak that look like they're 2 to 3 inches square.

What to do about it: think ½.

Think about it. This is your life we're talking about here!

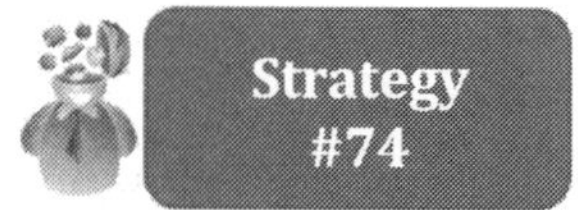

Think About The Eating Experience

When I watched people eating in restaurants, I noticed there were two types: those that had their focus solely on the food; and those where the food was not the main focus, but conversation and enjoyment of the people they were with was.

Most of the time when we eat with others, it's an enjoyable experience. We talk about the game we're watching or the latest developments at work or family matters, but the eating experience is just a part of a bigger experience – enjoying the people we're breaking bread with.

And here's the key: when food is not the focus, and you're talking a lot and having a good time, you tend to eat slower and eat less. When the food is the focus, you tend to eat faster and eat more.

What to do about it: if your focus is on the food, change it to focus on the people you're with. Talk more, eat less and have a great time. Weight loss will follow.

Think about it. This is your life we're talking about here!

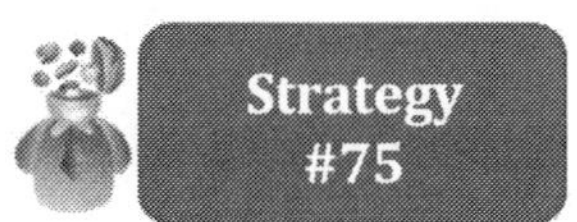

Think About Being Tired From Food

I don't know about you, but I find that I get tired from food – when I eat too much and from specific foods. For me, sugar and carbs make me sleepy. Protein doesn't have that effect. That was one of the reasons (among many) that I chose a low-carb diet over other programs. I can't afford to be tired during the workday, and I don't want to be tired on weekends!

According to *Redbook*, fats, because they stay in your stomach longer than non-fats, can divert blood away from your brain, muscles and other tissues. This can leave you tired for as long as 6 hours! Protein, as I discovered, primes your brain to produce a chemical called dopamine, which keeps you alert. Carbs are responsible for the production of serotonin in your body – it's a calming brain chemical.

One of the surprising aspects of coffee is that while it can wake you up in the short term, it can knock you out hours later. Same with alcohol. For every glass of alcohol or coffee, drink a glass of water to counteract the long-term effect.

What to do about it: using the knowledge of what foods and drinks make you tired, eliminate them or reduce the amount you have so that food and drink will not cause you to be tired. This is where a diary or journal comes in handy.

Think about it. This is your life we're talking about here!

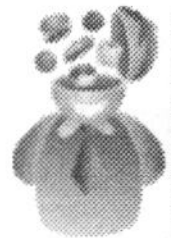

Section VI: Eating Situations

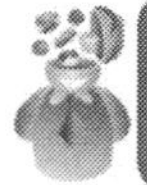

Strategy
#76

Think About Eating Out

It's no secret that the more you eat out, the more weight you'll gain. Why is that? There are three main reasons:

- You'll eat more because most restaurants serve a lot of food. Because food is so cheap to produce, restaurants serve more of it in order to leave you with the feeling that you're getting great value for your money. In fact, at many restaurants, the portions **are two to eight times** larger than the recommended serving. Because portions have been increasing steadily over time, many of us don't recognize the difference between 8 ounces and 16 ounces, or if we do, we ignore it.
- You don't know what's in the foods when you eat out. This is particularly true of sauces, dressings, and other ingredients used in food preparation. A lot of sugar is used in food preparations that would surprise you.
- With few exceptions, the food you eat when you dine out is not as healthy as what you eat at home. Eating out puts you in the frame of mind to order whatever you want and not pay attention to whether or not what you order is right for you.

Does this mean that you shouldn't eat out? Of course not. But like everything else you think about, you need to think about the entire dining out process, and make changes that will work for you.

What to do about it: make up your mind that you're going to take half of your meal home in a doggie bag, for starters. Now you have two meals for the price of one. Start your meals with non-creamy soup (not canned!) and salads, which will fill you up without too many calories. Go easy on salad dressings – get them "on the side" so you control the amount. Ask what's in the BBQ sauce, and if it's loaded with sugar, brush most of it off – you'll still get plenty of BBQ sauce flavor as long as a little of the sauce remains.

Think about it. This is your life we're talking about here!

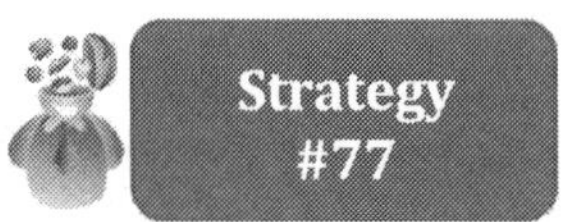

Think About Eating At Parties

Parties are another difficult time for us. Your family or friends work hard to prepare, and for most parties that are small, it's easy to stand out if you don't eat. Very few party hosts serve only healthy food – there always seems to be chips and dips, candies, nuts, etc. Yes, there are fruit platters and cheese trays as well.

To make matters worse, we've all experienced going to parties where the host or hostess is intent on making sure everyone eats, and in some cases, eats a lot. The more dishes that are made from scratch, the higher the desire it is for guests to eat.

Parties and other gatherings where the emphasis is on food doesn't mean that you have to be "bad" and have no choices. We **always** have choices, whether we're at a restaurant, party or at home.

What to do about it: seek out the foods that are good for you, and enjoy them. Circulate more, talk more and get involved in the non-food aspects of the party. If your host pushes food on you, pull him or her aside and explain that you're making a major effort to lose weight, and that while you've had a taste of his/her dishes, you've reached your limit. Be polite, and firm. They'll understand.

Think about it. This is your life we're talking about here!

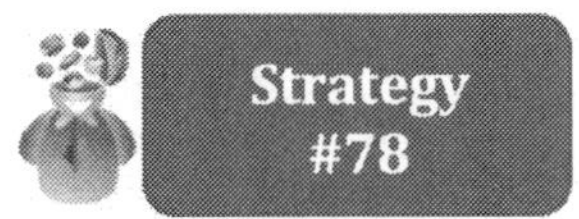

Think About Buffets

They're everywhere. Buffets are one of the most difficult eating environments to deal with. Not only is there so much food, but there's such a big selection. There are all-buffet restaurants, and Sunday buffets/brunches are traditions at many eating establishments around the country.

If you go on a cruise, buffets at all hours are one of the main attractions. And at many resorts, buffets are part of the fare.

Clearly if we had to pay for food from buffets by the ounce, we'd all take a lot less food, right? Of course. Since it's all included in one price, we tend to think of it as "free." And when we're an invited guest to a wedding or company party, the buffet is indeed free.

We've been so conditioned to taking food and filling up our plates that we don't even think about it anymore: fill up the plate until it can't hold any more, eat it all and then go back for more. That's the drill.

One uncontrollable binge at a buffet can undo a week's worth of dieting, and that becomes very frustrating when it happens.

What to do about it: planning and raising your consciousness. Hopefully everything in this book is teaching you to think about every situation involving food. This is no different. Plan ahead of time what your buffet strategy will be. Go heavy on salad, fruit and other filling foods that are healthy for you. Fill only half of your plate each trip. Eat very slowly. Drink a lot of water or other liquids. Set a goal in your mind that you won't eat more at a buffet than you would eat at home. Pick a table farthest from the buffet so it's a long walk back. Take a lap around the buffet before you pick up your plate – so

you know where the good foods are. Don't take seconds. Alcohol has calories too – so go easy and have more water and other non-alcoholic drinks. Check out a great article on this topic, quoting University of Cornell Food & Brand Lab director Brian Wansink with more ideas: http://consumer.healthday.com/Article.asp?AID=675526

Think about it. This is your life we're talking about here!

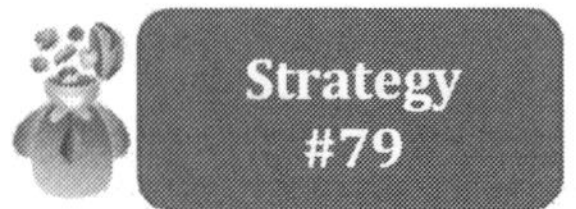

Think About Serving Sizes

Do you know what the recommended serving sizes are for the foods you eat?

Most people don't.

And for those that do know that a portion of chicken is 4 ounces, many of them don't know what 4 ounces looks like. Many people are served a chicken breast and assume it's a portion, that it's about 4 ounces. Well, as I'm sure you know, chicken breasts come in different sizes and many weigh a lot more than 4 ounces.

What about cereal? You pour some into a bowl, but do you know if you've poured out one portion, two portions or even more? If a portion is supposed to be ¼ of a cup, how much cereal is that?

One of the primary reasons we eat too much is because we ignore serving sizes and we don't know what recommended servings look like.

What to do about it: take the time to learn about serving sizes and how to accurately estimate them. Whether you're eating at home or in a restaurant, eating twice as much as you should because you can't estimate serving sizes accurately is a wasted opportunity to lose weight and keep it off. Sure it's one more thing to worry about, but you're serious about losing weight, right?

Think about it. This is your life we're talking about here!

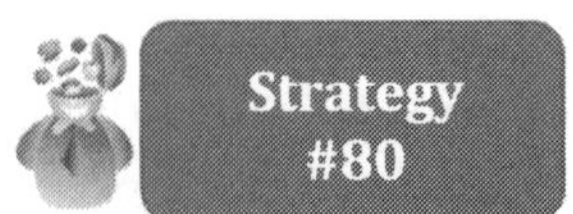

Think About Supermarket/Delicatessen Prepared Foods

Here are a couple of questions to test your prepared foods IQ:

- Do you have any idea how much mayonnaise is used in their potato and macaroni salads? Or their tuna and chicken salads?
- What's really in their "health salads?"
- What's in the sauce on their BBQ ribs?

The plain fact is, you really don't know what's in prepared foods unless you ask. But you can be sure, for example, that there is probably more mayonnaise in their salads than you would use at home.

Let's face it, prepared foods often taste great, and when you're in a hurry, they are an easy way to prepare lunch or dinner. And they are cheaper than a restaurant, but more expensive than making the same dish at home. But unless you watch out for what ingredients they use, you'll be retarding your weight loss program every time you eat prepared foods.

What to do about it: in two words – read and ask. Read signs that tell you what's in prepared foods and labels on prepared foods that are in packages or containers. If you can't find signs or labels, ask the person behind the counter what's in the foods you're considering. Unless they're very busy, they should be happy to tell you – assuming they know the answers to your questions. Sometimes you can simply look at some foods and know they're overloaded with mayo and other stuff that's not good for you!

Think about it. This is your life we're talking about here!

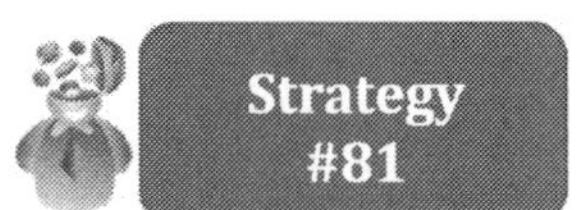

Think About Fast Foods

Just about every health care professional will tell you there's absolutely nothing good with fast foods (perhaps with some exceptions like salads that have been introduced in recent years). Yet so many of us ignore this advice, and keep on gobbling down everything that the fast food chains offer. Despite this, 75% of us consume fast food at least once a week, and of that group, 20% eat fast food three or more times a week! That's a whole lotta bad stuff going into our bellies!

The bigger problem is that fast food joints are everywhere; they spend a ton of money on ads that motivate you, especially kids; and the food really does taste pretty darn good. For people on the run, drive through windows make it easy to pull in, order, get your food and be on your way in minutes – and so many of us eat while we're driving or as passengers.

In the logical side of our brain, we all know that eating fast food isn't going to help us lose weight. But in the emotional side, fast food is easy and tastes great, and when you see those ads or get within 100 feet of one, you can practically taste those Big Macs, fries, onion rings, fried chicken and everything else they offer. It's truly hard to resist.

To give you a sense how just how bad some of the popular fast food items are, check out this infographic from LifeHack.com of fast food items each with over 1,000 calories – you'll be astounded: http://tinyurl.com/kwqvr3t. Examples:

- Outback Steakhouse Aussie Cheese Fries: 2,140 calories
- Quiznos Large Tuna Melt: 2,090 "
- Nathan's Fish N Chips: 1,537 "

In a depressing article "The Chicken Which Should be Banned" on mercola.com, we read that only 50% of a Chicken McNugget is actually chicken, and the other 50% contains corn derivatives, sugars, leavening agents and a long litany of synthetic ingredients, most of which are not good for you. Back in 2003, Federal Judge Robert Sweet said, "Chicken McNuggets…are a McFrankenstein creation of various elements not utilized by the home cook."

Part of the problem is that fast-food places are everywhere. Of all restaurant visits in the U.S., a whopping 78% were at fast-food outlets, according to the National Restaurant Association. If we all cut down visits by 10%, that would help!

For more scary stuff like this, check out www.EatDrinkPolitics.com. Michele Simon is a public health lawyer specializing in legal strategies to counter corporate tactics that harm the public's health. Simon has been researching and writing about the food industry and food politics since 1996. Well worth the visit.

But resist you must if you want to lose weight and keep it off. I'm not saying that you can never eat fast food, but (a) you've got to make it an infrequent stop; and (b) when you eat there, you've got to choose wisely.

What to do about it: when you get the urge to go to any of the fast food chains, think about just how bad fast food is for you. Think about how one meal can set you back a week or more. And if you must eat there, stay away from the fries and the onion rings and other dishes that you know are loaded with fat and salt. And if you have kids, make sure you don't reward them by going to a fast food place – if you do that, you'll actually be reinforcing that fast food is OK, something that you don't want to do.

Think about it. This is your life we're talking about here!

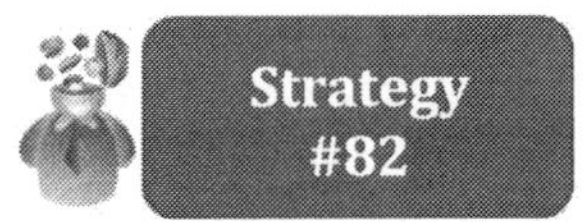

Think About Eating Alone

There are times when we eat alone. Most of us don't like to eat alone. It's generally no fun, there's no one to talk to, and as a result, the focus is on the food. As I've said earlier, you never want to focus on the food during a meal.

When you eat alone, you tend to eat more food than when someone else is present. If you're married or living with someone, and you're eating alone, there's no one around to watch what you're eating, so you tend to eat more for that very reason.

What to do about it: you need to decrease the importance of food when you eat alone. If you know you'll be eating by yourself, plan activities before and after dinner so that you're busy, and as a result the meal becomes something you need to do. The other activities are what you get pleasure from, and they need to be what you focus on. Also, while you're eating, do another activity: surf the web, watch TV, read, etc. Keep your mind off the food and on whatever else you're doing. Finally, prior to the meal, drink a lot of water so that you're not terribly hungry when you eat.

Think about it. This is your life we're talking about here!

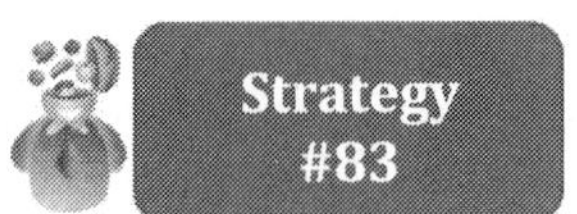

Think About Snacking

Picture the scene: you get an interoffice email that freshly baked chocolate chip cookies are in the snack room, compliments of one of your co-workers, vendors or clients. Or you go to your buddy's house to watch the game and he's got every snack known to mankind right there for the asking. Or you just have this urge to eat after your favorite TV shows are over.

And as I'm sure you already know, most snack foods are high in carbohydrates, and what you may not know is that carbs are a leading saboteur of weight loss. When you snack on carbs, the feeling of being full (when you don't feel like eating) doesn't last very long. You get hungry relatively soon after snacking on carbs. If you snack on protein, for example, the feeling of being full will last a lot longer. Here's why. It takes longer for protein to break down and become digested, and because of that, you have the feeling of being "full" for longer than carbs and sugar.

What to do about it: eat protein, not carbs or sugar when you need to snack. Second, snack only when you feel physically hungry, and you know when that is! And take small

portions – take a small plate and fill it halfway. Drink a lot, and focus on the people you're with and the activity that's going on. Drink water or seltzer before snacking.

Think about it. This is your life we're talking about here!

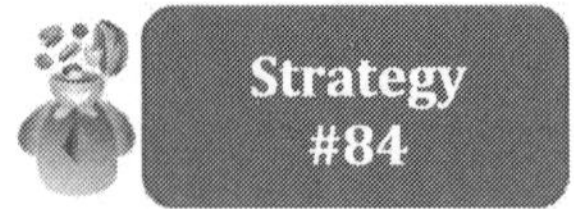

Think About Eating in Uncomfortable Situations

We've all been in situations where people try to heap as much food upon us as possible.

For many of us, it's difficult to say "no" to your host or hostess.

In these cases you're caught between a rock and a hard place: you don't want to say no but you also realize that the last thing you want to eat is another plateful. Plus, the more people around the table, the more embarrassing this is.

What to do about it: simple – eat as slowly as possible! You're not going to hear "c'mon, have some more" if you're not finished with your first portion. By the time you get done eating, everyone else will have finished, and the "food pusher" will no longer feel the need to get you to eat more.

Think about it. This is your life we're talking about here!

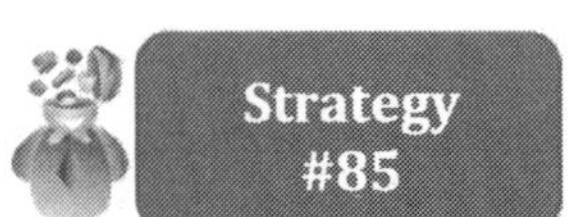

Think About Food Shopping

When you're in the supermarket, you're often tempted to buy certain foods based on promotional displays, coupons and price reductions. Today's modern grocery stores employ a wide array of tactics in order to get you to buy. Most of them are fine, such as price reductions.

Chances are that once you buy something, you're going to eat it. It's not human nature to spend money on food and then throw it away. So in terms of your weight-loss philosophy, don't buy any foods that are not right for you.

If there is a promotional display or a reduced price or a "buy one, get one free" promotion for a food that is not on your plan, don't buy it. If you're on a low carb diet and see an incredible special for potato chips, don't buy them.

What to do about it: remind yourself on the way into the store that you're here only to buy the foods that are on your diet program, and nothing else, no matter how appealing or cheap. Prepare a list prior to shopping and focus on it. Move quickly from location to location where the foods on your list are, bypassing everything else!

Think about it. This is your life we're talking about here!

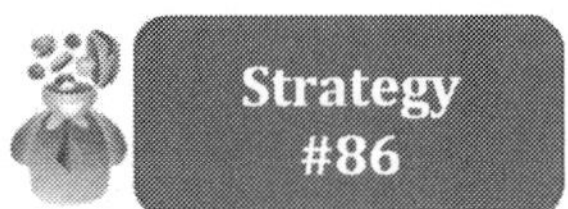

Think About Eating While You're On An Airplane

On many flights these days, you either get or can purchase sandwiches, snacks and other food items. In this environment, unless you're busy reading or working, you're a captive audience to food. Because it's there, right in front of you the temptation is to go ahead and eat it, especially when everyone around you is.

While airline food has improved over the years, it's still nothing to write home about. Before you're offered the food, think about whether or not you really want it. If you're not hungry, why even take the food.

What to do about it: think about cutting out food on airplanes and other places where the quality is average, especially if you're not even hungry in the first place. Bring your own snacks that you know are healthy for you. At the very least, cut down the amount of food you eat in these situations. In this day and age where airlines charge for everything, skip the airline food and bring your own snacks!

Think about it. This is your life we're talking about here!

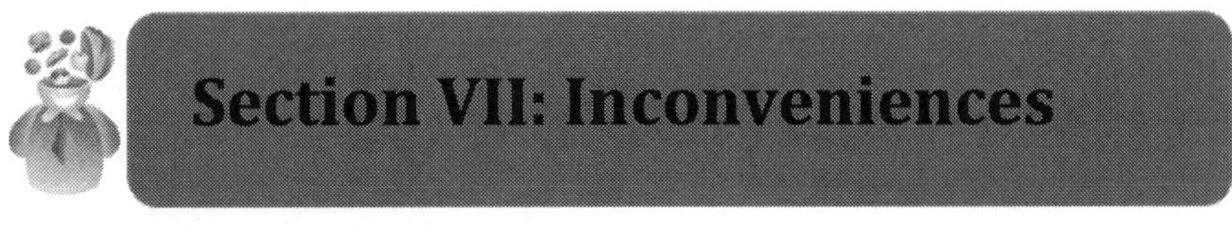

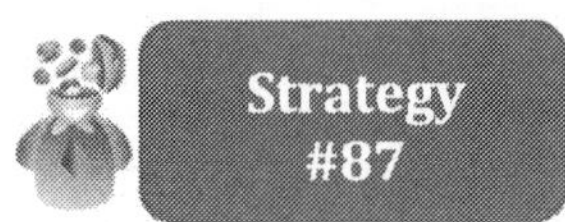

Think About Driving

Driving when you're overweight can be downright annoying and uncomfortable, especially if you have a smaller car and don't have air conditioning.

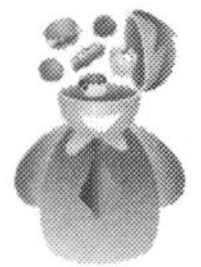

There's the difficulty of getting in and out of the car or truck, particularly if it's a small vehicle and a tight fit. Once you're in the driver's seat, you may have to move it back so driving is actually uncomfortable and maybe even dangerous, if your arms are too far away from the steering wheel.

And if it's a hot, humid day and you don't have air conditioning, it can get really hot and sticky, much more so than if you were not heavy.

On average, people drive 30 minutes to an hour to work and the same or more back, depending on rush-hour traffic. That adds up to a lot of hours –about 250 to 500 hours per year. That's a tremendous amount of time to be uncomfortable.

What to do about it: next time you're ready to eat foods that are not on your diet, think of how uncomfortable you are when driving, and then put the food down. Think of the days when you're thinner and driving will be fun and enjoyable.

Think about it. This is your life we're talking about here!

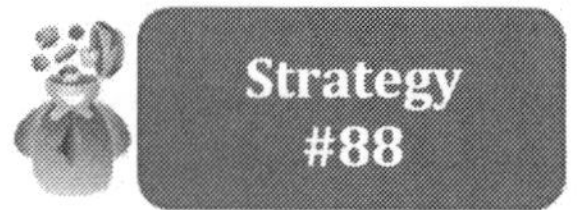

Think About Going to the Bathroom

OK, it's not the most pleasant topic in the word, but remembering just how inconvenient going to the bathroom can be when you're overweight, especially for those who are obese or even morbidly obese, is worth considering as another reason to eat healthy.

For starters, there are lots of occasions when stalls are very small and you have to squeeze in, such as on airplanes, restaurants and other public places. Even for thinner people, it's sometimes a tight fit. Those times are certainly an annoyance.

When I was heavier, I didn't like going to the bathroom. Now that I'm much thinner, it doesn't bother me. For reasons that I have no intention of going into here, the smells and everything else associated with doing your business is 100 times worse when you're heavy. It isn't a pretty picture.

What to do about it: add this annoyance to a growing list of inconveniences and annoyances that you endure when you're overweight. Use them as motivation when you're tempted by food.

Think about it. This is your life we're talking about here!

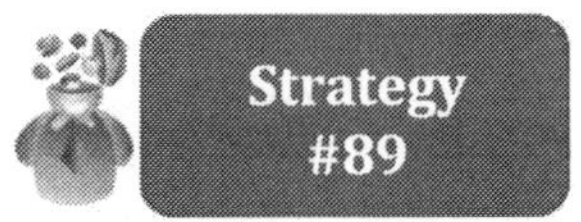

Think About Traveling by Plane, Bus or Train

Some of the airlines have tried charging extra for overweight people who could not fit into one standard seat. While that's a potentially a discriminatory situation, it does highlight yet another problem overweight people face.

Putting that issue aside, unless you fly first class, coach seats are cramped with very little leg room, even for thinner people. I can't begin to imagine not only the annoyance but the potential pain and discomfort felt by overweight people in coach seats. And how heavier people impact the people they sit next to.

Also, while planes are air conditioned, there are times when the air is off or lowered, and those can be uncomfortable as well. I know I sweat during those times, so I can imagine the discomfort of heavier people.

The same problems can occur on crowded buses and trains. Add in the fact that you might have to stand for an hour or more if there are no seats, and you have a recipe for a nightmarish trip.

What to do about it: the more often you fly or travel by bus or train, the greater the number of times you're going to be annoyed. Think about this inconvenience and add it to other inconveniences while you're away from home.

Think about it. This is your life we're talking about here!

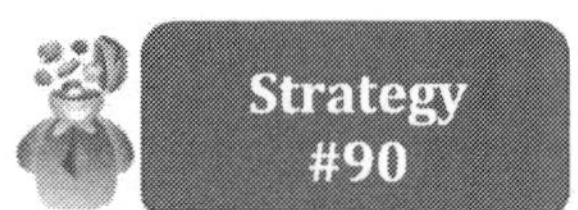

Think About Walking

Part of my research for this book involved watching overweight people walk. I've classified heavy people's "walking styles" into three categories:

- **Semi-Normal**. Those who are 10-20 pounds overweight almost walk like thin people – one foot directly in front of the other. While walking doesn't appear to be an issue, there are other walking-related issues I'll discuss that in a minute.
- **Altered Steppers**. This group of people clearly has altered their gait and manner of walking because of their weight. They don't walk in a straight line very well,

sometimes veering right or left, and in many cases, cut off the person they are walking with. They appear to be off balance in some cases.

- **Waddlers**. These severely overweight people walk with their feet pointed outwards and with every step, they shift a lot of weight back and forth between their feet. It almost looks like they are walking from side to side at the same time they are moving forward.

In all of these groups, I also saw that they had trouble with inclines and declines, steps and uneven surfaces. Their ability to walk in these situations was clearly hampered by their weight.

In addition to all these walking problems, being overweight affects walking in a medical sense also. The more weight you have, especially around your gut and butt, the more strain there is on your back and leg muscles when you are walking.

Being overweight for too long can lead to severe medical problems and result in you walking less and less, and when you do walk, it is with increasing pain and discomfort.

Walking has numerous benefits in addition to aiding in weight loss. Rich Weil, Director of the New York Obesity Research Center Weight Loss Program at St. Luke's Roosevelt Hospital in New York City, offers 10 really good reasons to walk:

- Helps prevent type 2 diabetes.
- Strengthens your heart if you're male.
- Strengthens your heart if you're female.
- It's good for your brain.
- Walking is good for your bones.
- Helps alleviate symptoms of depression.
- Reduces the risk of breast and colon cancer.
- Improves overall cardiorespiratory fitness.
- Short burst of walking improves fitness, especially in sedentary people.
- Improves physical function and helps prevent physical disability

What to do about it: because walking is so integral to our lives, walking should be a major motivator for you to lose weight. With every step you take, think about how much easier and pain-free walking would be if you were not carrying around all this excess weight. Plus, think about how life would be if your weight led to a condition where you had to severely restrict your walking.

Think about it. This is your life we're talking about here!

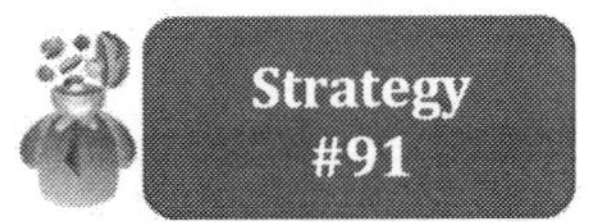

Think About Sleeping

There's no question that overweight people have more trouble sleeping that thin people. Since getting a good night's sleep is critical to how we function during the day, those that don't sleep well are immediately behind the eight ball during the day. The average American now sleeps 1-2 hours less than we did some 40-50 years ago. Women who sleep less than 5 hours a night are 32% more likely to gain weight than those who sleep at least 7 hours (University of Chicago study).

Overweight people have trouble sleeping for two reasons: breathing and position. When you're heavy, breathing is harder, because you need a lot more oxygen to keep your body operating, even while sleeping. And because of the excess weight, your heart works harder and requires more oxygen as well. And you tend to snore more often, which can wake you up periodically (or often) throughout the night.

Secondly, when you're overweight, it's hard to find a comfortable position for any length of time. You're always tossing and turning. Just about every position is not good for your back and other parts of your body.

A University of Chicago study in 2010 found that people who slept well lost much more fat than those who did not sleep well. During this study, researchers found that the level of a hormone called Ghrelin rose in those that did not sleep well. Higher Ghrelin levels have been shown to reduce energy expenditure, stimulate the desire to eat, increase feelings of hunger and promote the retention of fat. Other studies, including one involving children, found that those kids who got the least sleep had a 4.2 times higher risk of becoming obese, and the heaviest children had the unhealthiest blood profiles.

What to do about it: since sleep is, or should, be roughly 1/3 of your 24-hour day, it's critical to sleep well. There's no easy solution to this problem until you lose weight. So remind yourself at least three times a day how important losing weight is so you can sleep well: when you go to bed, say to yourself "If I were thinner, I could look forward to a great night's sleep."

When you wake up, say to yourself "If I were thinner, I would wake up refreshed and not have aches and pains." And whenever you get tired during the day, say to yourself "If I were thinner and had slept well last night, I wouldn't get tired during the day."

Think about it. This is your life we're talking about here!

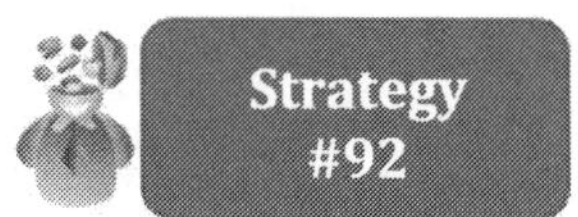

Think About Sweating

No one likes to sweat. Sweating is both annoying and usually embarrassing. For people who are not overweight, it's not a big problem. A little powder or deodorant spray and you're set for the day.

For overweight people, it's a different story. The heavier you are, the more sweat you produce, and it almost always becomes a nuisance and embarrassment. I won't go into an explanation as to why heavier people sweat more, but I can tell you that losing weight will go a long way to resolving this problem.

What to do about it: like sleeping, use sweating as a motivator to help you lose weight. Every time you sweat and it's uncomfortable and/or embarrassing, say to yourself, "When I'm thin, this won't happen!"

Think about it. This is your life we're talking about here!

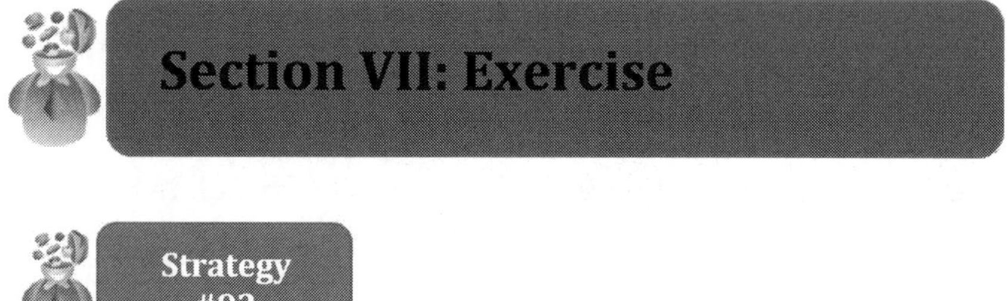

Strategy
#93

Think About Energy

One of the most significant benefits you'll see when you start to lose weight is an increase in your energy level. You'll feel tired less and you'll start to enjoy doing things because of your increased energy.

When you have more energy, you become a different person!

If you've sat by, watching people playing sports, dancing, walking on the beach or simply taking a stroll around town, and you couldn't participate because you are overweight, you can start doing those activities once you have more energy.

Energy goes way beyond giving you the ability to partake in activities that you can't when you are heavy.

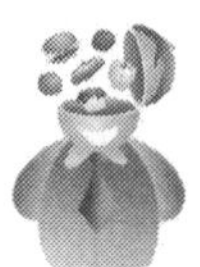

You will reach a state where your entire body, and most importantly your mind, is energized. With this new found sense of energy, vitality and zest, you will enjoy life more!

What to do about it: in a word, exercise. Read the rest of this section carefully, because exercise is the key to energy and one of the three components of successful weight loss.

Think about it. This is your life we're talking about here!

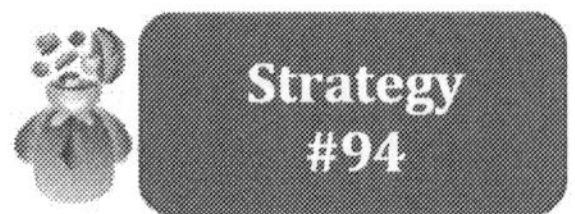

Think About Exercise

As you know from the beginning of this book, exercise is one of the three cornerstones of successful weight loss. The other two are a sound medical diet program and a change in your mindset, which is the purpose of this book.

If you're not prepared to exercise, then you won't lose as much weight, plain and simple. And I don't mean intense or lengthy workouts. More on that in a moment, but first, here's my story as it relates to exercise.

I love playing basketball. And when I got out of shape, I couldn't do more than just shoot around. When I got serious about weight loss and started exercising, I built up my stamina to the point where I could participate in basketball games. First, I had enough steam for half court. And then I found that I could play several full court games in an evening and not wear down!

Most people, myself included, look at exercise as boring and tedious. After all, how much fun can walking on a treadmill and lifting weights be? When I made up my mind to lose weight the right way -- that included making up my mind to exercise – working out wasn't as boring.

I've since taken up bike riding. The great thing about bike riding is it gets you outdoors into the sunlight and fresh air, and easier on your body than running. A half hour ride a day burns about 200 to 300 calories and is very refreshing and invigorating.

Now, it's very important to discuss exercise with your doctor. Depending on how much you're overweight, the amount and type of exercise will vary. In fact, many gyms require a doctor's prescription in order for you to work out. So as part of the overall planning with your doc, include exercise planning as well.

What to do about it: once you've made up your mind that you can't lose weight unless you exercise, get right to it. Not tomorrow, next week or next month. Meet with your physician ASAP and start a program.

Think about it. This is your life we're talking about here!

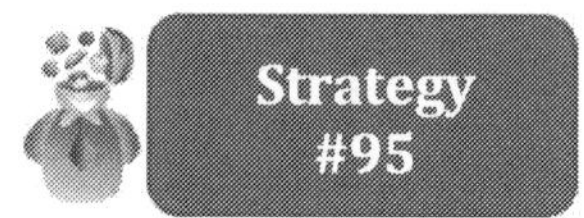

Think About The Type and Quantity of Exercise You Need

Most people think you need lots of strenuous exercise for it to have any benefit, you know, "no pain, no gain." Nothing is further from the truth. Yes, walking slowly for 10 minutes isn't going to help you, but you don't need to kill yourself either.

Most experts agree that if you can do 30-60 minutes a day for 3 to 5 days a week, you'll see some benefit. Of course, those numbers depend a lot on how much weight you have to lose, how sedentary you've been, and other factors.

Once you're on a diet program coupled with exercise, your body will get better and better at burning off fat and calories. They go hand in hand. Plus, you'll be able to steadily increase the amount of time you spend exercising and/or the number of days a week you exercise as your body adjusts to improved nutrition and your exercise regimen.

Typically, exercises that are good for dieters include walking at a brisk pace, jogging, swimming, jumping rope, aerobics exercises, bike riding, hiking, and playing games like basketball, soccer, football, etc., where running is involved.

Don't make the biggest mistake that people often do when starting to exercise, especially after being sedentary for a while. They try to do too much too fast, and wind up pulling muscles or worse. I've done that.

What to do about it: your doctor and professional staff at a reputable gym can craft a training program for you, one that takes into account your medical history and other factors. Get your exercise program going now. There are plenty of things you can do outside of a gym, including walking around the neighborhood, playing fun workouts on a Wii or similar system and parking far away from the entrance to work or the mall, so you walk more.

Think about it. This is your life we're talking about here!

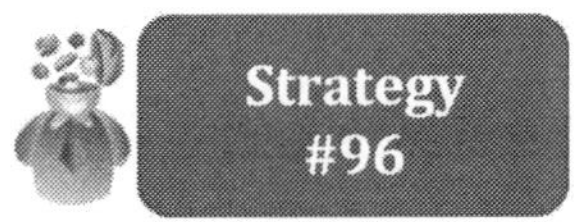

Think About Getting Motivated For Exercising

Yep, it sure does take an effort to get off your butt and start exercising. And it's so easy to put it off until tomorrow, next week or next month.

But a really exciting thing happens when you start to exercise, in concert with a proper diet and what you're learning in this book. It becomes enjoyable. You look forward to it. You come out of it feeling relaxed, juiced up and mentally more alert.

Here's a "slice of life" story that, for me, sums up one of the many values of getting exercise. In 2011, my six-year old niece was a non-stop blur of activity. At a party, we would take turns playing with her. Playing consisted of chasing her around the house and vice-versa. "Come run with me" was the request/command, and it was fun.

But while I wasn't running fast, it wasn't walking either, and she kept each of us running for a good half-hour. In my heavy days, I would have never lasted that long, but because I walk and ride constantly, I had no problem keeping up, and with no huffing or puffing.

The rewards of exercise are physical and mental, and they translate into being able to participate in activities you once could not, and enjoying people a whole lot more. So how exactly do you get motivated to start exercising?

What to do about it: focus on what you will be able to do once you've started exercising. Picture yourself running a mini-marathon, playing a full set of tennis, keeping up with your nieces and nephews, or whatever sounds like fun.

Think about it. This is your life we're talking about here!

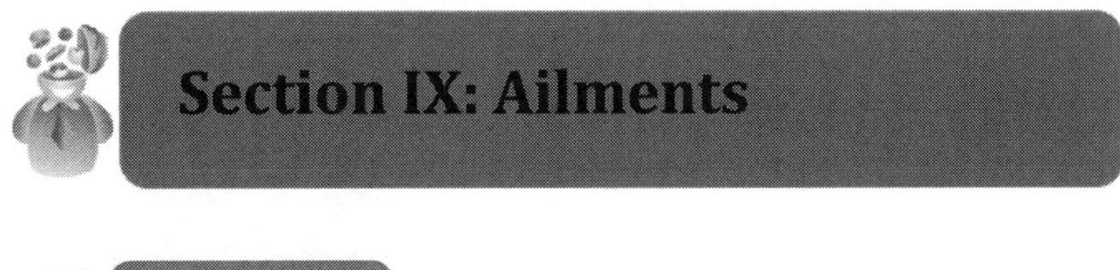

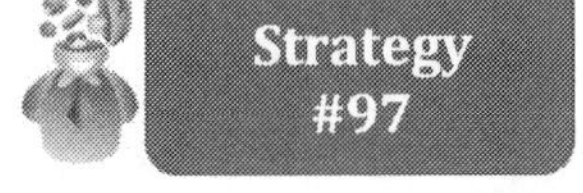

Think About High Blood Pressure

Before we talk about the relationship between weight and high blood pressure, let's define blood pressure and hypertension so we're on the same page. Blood pressure is the force of blood against the walls of arteries. During the day, your blood pressure rises and falls. When your blood pressure stays elevated over time, it is called high blood pressure.

The medical term for high blood pressure is *hypertension*. High blood pressure is dangerous because it makes the heart work too hard and contributes to atherosclerosis (hardening of the arteries). A blood pressure level of 140/90 mmHg or higher is considered high. More than 50 million American adults have high blood pressure.

Middle-aged Americans – those who are the most sedentary -- face a 90% chance of developing high blood pressure during their lives. That's where the relationship between weight, exercise and high blood pressure comes in.

The heavier you are, and the more inactive you are, the greater the chance you have, or will develop, hypertension. And in most cases, you'll need to be on medication for potentially your entire life. But with weight loss and increased exercise, you can turn back the effects of high blood pressure and even get off the medication you're taking (or may take in the future).

What to do about it: lose weight and exercise, two of the three pillars of successful weight loss according to countless experts in all health-related professions. No one needs high blood pressure. There's no benefit to having it. And the medication isn't cheap.

Think about it. This is your life we're talking about here!

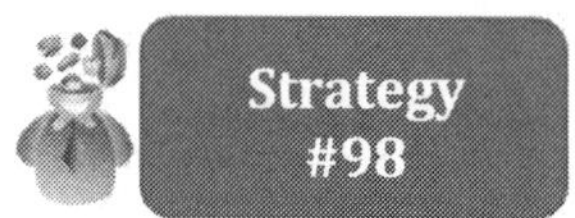

Think About Diabetes

Diabetes is a disorder of the way our bodies use the food we digest for growth and energy. Most of the food that we eat is broken down by digestive juices into a simple sugar called glucose. Glucose is the main source of fuel for the body. After the digestion process, the glucose passes into our bloodstream where it is available for body cells to use for growth and energy.

Insulin must be present in order for the glucose to get into the cells. Insulin is a hormone produced by the pancreas. When we eat, the pancreas automatically produces the correct amount of insulin that is needed to move the glucose from our blood into the cells. When you have diabetes, the pancreas produces little or no insulin, or the body cells do not respond to the insulin that is produced.

What happens next is that the glucose builds up in the blood, overflows into the urine, and passes out of the body. Even though the blood contains large amounts of glucose, it passes out of the body. That's why diabetics need to inject insulin into their bodies. Diabetics fight a daily battle of preventing their blood sugar levels from being too high or too low.

There is a direct link between the type of food you eat and the probability that you will get diabetes. Also, African-Americans, Native Americans and Hispanics are more prone to diabetes than other groups. What's significant is that if you are in any of these three groups AND you eat a lot of foods that are not good for you, you dramatically increase your chances for diabetes.

Many people are "pre-diabetic," which means they are dangerously close to diabetes. Most people in this situation don't even know it!

Eating too much refined sugar (the kind that comes in a box that we use to prepare cakes and cookies and lots of other foods) moves you closer to a diabetic condition. So does eating too many carbohydrates, such as bread, pretzels, candy and others.

What to do about it: you don't want to get diabetes, that's for sure. Get with your doctor and nutrition specialist and learn about what foods are good for you and what foods are not, depending on your genetics and medical history.

Think about it. This is your life we're talking about here!

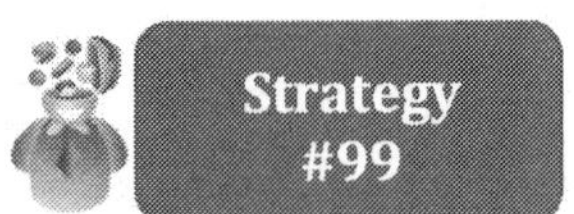

Think About Cancer

The World Health Organization's International Agency for Research on Cancer estimates that being overweight and inactive accounts for one-quarter to one-third of worldwide cases of breast cancer, colon cancer, endometrial cancer, kidney cancer and esophageal cancer. Most people have no clue that being fat can increase your risk for cancer.

Researchers have concluded that being overweight and inactive produces basic hormonal and metabolic changes that make it easier for cancer to gain a foothold. The link centers around the role of body fat. Most people think of fat as an inert substance that merely collects and results in us wearing larger sized clothes. But it's more than that: fat cells behave like endocrine cells, constantly producing and secreting a wide variety of hormones into the bloodstream. These substances send signals to other parts of the body that, under certain conditions, seem to make it easier for certain cancers to grow. So in addition to diabetes and hypertension, being fat could be a cause of cancer.

According to Dr. Steven Mittelman of the Children's Hospital (Los Angeles), "Obesity seems to increase the risk of developing cancer, but also from dying from cancer. We found that obesity actually directly accelerates leukemia cells' growth and progression and also makes it so that the leukemia cells are harder to treat."

What to do about it: how much more bad news do you need before you start dieting and exercising?

Think about it. This is your life we're talking about here!

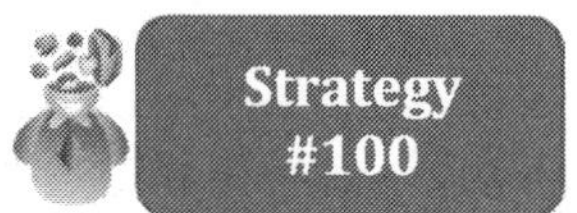

Think About Problems With Your Legs

This is real simple. Your legs support the rest of your body. The more weight they have to carry around, the more wear and tear there is on your legs.

Your legs are made up of bones, muscles, veins, arteries and tissue, and all of those can be negatively impacted by a big belly. For example, the veins in your lower legs carry blood back to the heart. The pressure of a large love handle may upset the system that carries blood "uphill" to your heart, eventually causing damage or destruction. This results in higher blood pressure in the lower legs, which can cause swelling, thickening of the skin, and sometimes ulceration of the skin.

Varicose veins can be the result of being overweight for a long period of time, and if you're on your feet a lot and are overweight, that's a double whammy. Anyway you look at it, nothing positive happens to your legs when you're fat.

There's new evidence that indicates lymphodema in legs – pain and swelling due to a blockage of the lymph nodes in the groin area – is linked to obesity.

What to do about it: think about how important your legs are to the enjoyment of life. So many activities require your legs to be in tip-top shape, and if your legs start to deteriorate, you can say "good-bye" to a lot of fun stuff.

Think about it. This is your life we're talking about here!

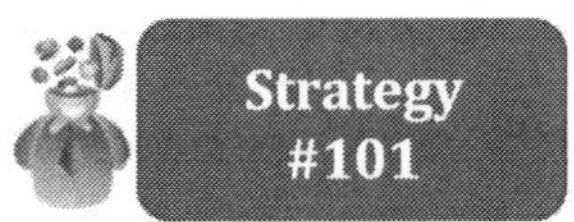

Think About Back Issues

Something like 80% of us will experience back pain at some point in our lives. It's inevitable, but if you're overweight, your chances of getting back pain (if you don't already have it) increase significantly.

Obesity causes back pain because the excess weight puts pressure on the spine and discs. When you're fat, your stomach muscles weaken, and as a result, there is more strain on the back and the muscles in your back.

Back pain of all types can be extremely painful. Back pain is one of the most common causes for missed time at work that costs the American economy billions of dollars per year. Plus, it can take a long time to recover from back pain – I know, I've been there.

What to do about it: some effects of excess weight you may be able to tolerate, but not back pain. If you've had it, you know. If you haven't, lose weight before your back becomes a real problem.

Think about it. This is your life we're talking about here!

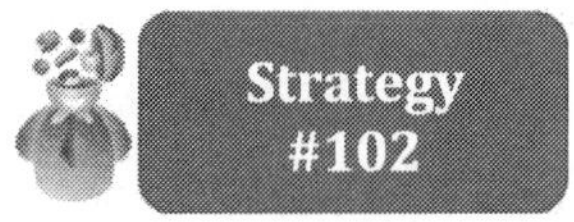

Think About Heart Problems

Clearly your heart is the most important organ in your body. Without it functioning properly, you just don't live. There's no doubt in most people's minds that the heavier you are, the greater your chance for heart disease, including heart attacks. And the more fat you have around your belly, the worse it is. The American Heart Association lists obesity as one of the primary risk factors for heart disease. A few stats to scare you:

- A weight gain of only 20 pounds **doubles** your risk of heart disease.
- Coronary heart disease is more than twice as common in obese men under 45, than in men of normal weight.
- Strokes are twice as common in obese people.
- Nearly 70% of the diagnosed cases of heart disease in America are related to obesity.

I could go on and on about how excess weight affects your heart, but I won't. I'm sure you have read and heard countless times how obesity puts a strain on your heart. While doctors, nutritionists and other health professionals may differ on various diets, they all agree that you've got to lose weight to prevent major heart disease.

What to do about it: clearly this is the top reason to lose weight – to make sure you stay alive. Remember the stats above when you're tempted by foods that you know you shouldn't have.

Think about it. This is your life we're talking about here!

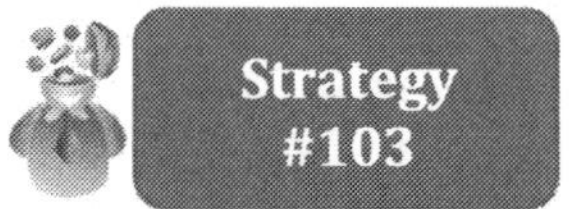

Think About Problems With Your Lungs

One doesn't ordinarily think about the effect being overweight has on your lungs, but it's another issue you've got to face. Our lungs purify the blood that is sent back to your heart. Thus, the lungs and heart are closely intertwined with each other.

The bottom line here is that any problems with your heart can negatively impact your lungs and vice-versa. Overworked hearts mean overworked lungs. Smoke-filled lungs mean potential problems for your heart.

What to do about it: if you smoke, better stop pronto, because all you're doing is adding more fuel to the fire, dramatically increasing your chances for an early death, and making it more difficult for the heart and lungs to work together. If you don't smoke, thinking about how being overweight can impact your lungs is another reason to lose weight.

Think about it. This is your life we're talking about here!

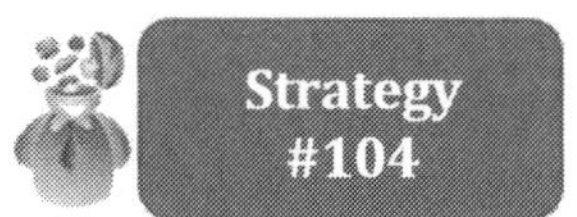

Think About Breathing Concerns

When I was overweight and didn't get any exercise, I remember huffing and puffing when doing the simplest things, like walking up a flight of 6 or 7 steps, or lifting something. I remember it was such an annoyance, and it scared me because I knew it was not normal.

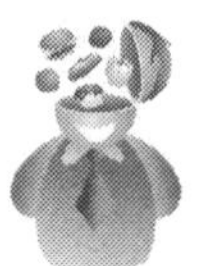

My breathing was one of the first things I thought about, because unlike other ailments that may not have obvious symptoms, I couldn't ignore difficulty breathing simply because you breathe several times every single minute!

In the famous Framingham study, researchers concluded that how well you breathe directly affects how long you'll live, and is a good predictor of your general health and vigor. So if you huff and puff, sometimes gasp for air, or worse, think about breathing in the same way you think about your heart and lungs – all are critical to your health and well-being.

What to do about it: every single time breathing is difficult, remind yourself that you, and only you, can lose weight and get rid of this problem, once and for all. Whenever you huff and puff, visualize in your mind that every piece of junk food you eat makes every breath you take harder.

Think about it. This is your life we're talking about here!

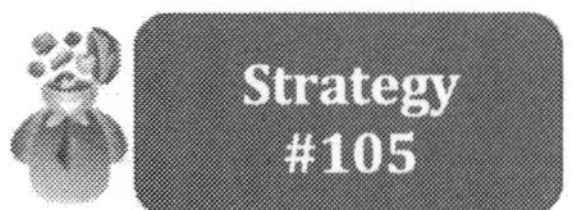

Think About Kidney Problems

Kidney disease is another one of those things that most people never think about until it happens to them or someone they know. And as you may know, passing kidney stones is one of the most painful things you can experience.

Your kidneys function to filter your blood constantly. Essential glucose, amino acids, hormones and other vitamins are returned to the blood stream after this filtering process occurs. The excess waste is discarded through the urine. The more fat tissues the body contains, the harder the kidneys have to work to complete this filtering and elimination task. Bottom line, the more you weigh, the greater your risk of kidney disease.

When your kidneys fail, you have several treatment choices, none of them being pleasant or fun. You can go for hemodialysis, where a machine cleans and filters your blood to rid your body of harmful wastes, extra salt, and extra water. These treatments last 3 to 5 hours each, and you need to do them three times a week.

Peritoneal dialysis is another procedure that removes extra water, wastes, and chemicals from your body, via a catheter (small tube) that is inserted into your abdomen. This catheter stays there permanently to help transport the dialysis solution to and from your abdomen. You can get a serious abdominal infection from this procedure.

Finally, you could opt for a kidney transplant. Another alternative that you can't possibly want. So there it is: kidney failure, often a result or by-product of obesity, is something you never want to happen to you.

What to do about it: from time to time, envision what life would be like if your kidneys failed. Imagine having a transplant operation or having to deal with all the issues surrounding the other two procedures. Then think about the fact that you can avoid this whole mess by losing weight!

Think about it. This is your life we're talking about here!

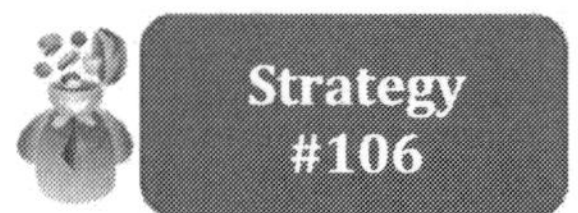

Think About Issues With Your Muscles, Joints And Bones

Being overweight can and usually does have a significant impact on bones, joints and muscles in addition to your major organs. That's because bones, joints and muscles all are strained by the added pressures resulting from being fat.

Let' say you're 50 pounds overweight. Imagine if you had to carry around a breadbox weighing 50 pounds 16 hours a day (except while sleeping). How would that feel? Could you even do it for more than a couple of minutes?

Of course not, but that's **exactly** what your muscles, joints and bones are doing…day after day, month after month, year after year. They are supporting weight and becoming weaker and weaker as time goes by. That's why overweight people typically get a whole range of problems involving muscles, joints and bones.

Muscles are affected because they directly hold up the excess flab around your belly, and the more weight you have, the more stretched and tense they become. Have lower back pain? In many cases, that's a direct result from too much belly fat.

Joints and bones are affected because they are not designed to carry excessive weight. If you're heavy, don't you have aches and pains in your knees and/or ankles? Those pains, and others, occur because of the weight placed on them. If we assume that about 2/3 of your total weight is concentrated on and above your hips, then your legs have to carry 2/3 of whatever you weigh.

In many people, legs are fairly thin, even if they are 50 or 100 pounds overweight. How many times have you seen obese people with thin legs? Imagine 200, 300 or 400 pounds all being supported by thin legs? It's no wonder that people in those situations have leg, foot, muscle, joint and bone problems.

What to do about it: while you're losing weight, you must get with your doctor and exercise professionals to start strengthening your muscles.

Also, discuss with your doctor if you need any calcium supplements or others in order to help your body support your weight during the time you're losing weight. This is critical – don't put it off!

Think about it. This is your life we're talking about here!

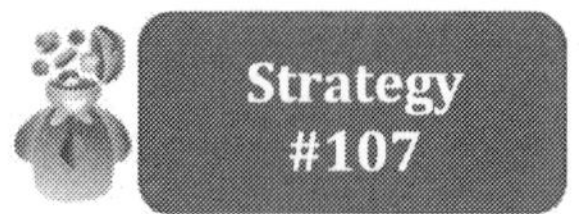

Think About Headaches That Obesity Causes

Certain foods may be the culprit behind a variety of headaches, so if you get headaches regularly, you may need to isolate which foods may be causing them, and then eliminate them from your diet. These foods and drinks are known triggers that can set off migraine and other headaches:

Drinks

- Red or white wine
- Other alcoholic drinks
- Coffee, tea
- Cola soft drinks
- Aspartame (in food or drinks)
- Caffeine (in food or drinks)

Foods

- Chocolate
- Cheese, particularly ripened cheeses such as cheddar, Gruyere, Brie
- Pickled foods
- Nuts
- Bananas
- Citrus fruits
- MSG
- Freshly baked bread
- Sour cream, yogurt
- Lima beans, navy beans, pea pods
- Figs

- Pork
- Pizza (sorry about that!)
- Fermented sausages, bologna, hot dogs, pepperoni
- Sauerkraut

And here's a more general statistic, from the New England Center for Headache: obese people have double the risk for chronic daily headaches than people who are not obese. So in addition to specific foods, just being overweight can cause a lot more headaches.

What to do about it: next time you get a headache, make a note of what you ate prior to the headache in your journal. Eliminate those foods that may be responsible and see if the headaches recur. If they do, ask your doctor about more sophisticated testing procedures.

Think about it. This is your life we're talking about here!

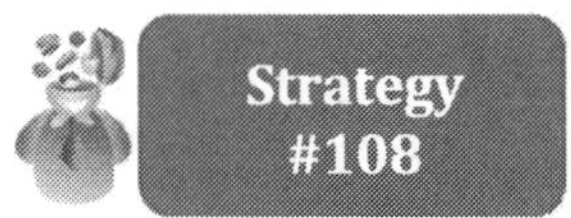

Think About Acid Reflux

Acid reflux is the most common stomach disorder in the U.S., affecting tens of millions of us; about ¾ of those are women. The technical name is gastroesophageal reflux (GERD) and it occurs when acid from your stomach backs up into the esophagus, which is the pipeline that transports food from your mouth to your stomach. When you have acid reflux, you have heart burn, chest pain, difficulty swallowing, food regurgitation, and/or chronic hoarseness.

If you have acid reflux, then you know how annoying it can be. Doctors and nutrition specialists recommend the following dietary changes in order to reduce or eliminate acid reflux. Starting with weight loss, they also suggest avoiding:

- Fatty foods
- Large meals
- Eating or drinking late at night
- Potentially irritating foods and beverages:
    - Citrus fruits and juices
    - Caffeine
    - Carbonated drinks
    - Spicy foods
    - Tomatoes
    - Mints
    - Chocolate

For the vast majority of acid reflux sufferers, weight loss and avoiding these foods does the trick. Hopefully you won't need medication or worse, surgery.

What to do about it: let your doctor and nutrition specialist know that you have acid reflux, so that they can take that into account when planning your eating plan.

Think about it. This is your life we're talking about here!

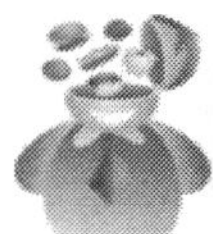

Section X: What's in the Foods You Eat

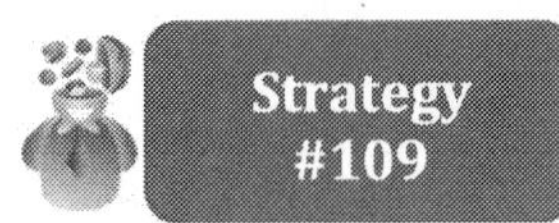

Think About Calories

It's a simple fact of life: when you boil down every single diet there is, you wind up with the same conclusion: losing weight is all about the calories. But it's not simply the fewer calories you eat, the more weight you lose. It's also about the foods you consume.

Where the diets differ is in **which** foods are recommended in order to limit your caloric intake. 2,000 calories is still 2,000 calories whether it's high in fat or low in fat. But the purpose here is not to compare specific diets, but to get across the importance of calories in your quest to lose weight.

In my observations, most people overestimate the amount of calories burned by any specific activity, and they underestimate the amount of calories in portions of food. I hear statements like, "I rode my bike for a half hour; I must have burned 500 calories." Or, "It's only one donut, how many calories could it be?"

Well, if you check out one of many calorie burning calculators online (one I like is: www.calorie-count.com), you'll find that riding a bike for 30 minutes burns about 200 calories (of course, that depends on how fast you rode and what you weigh). And one donut is about 200 calories as well.

So in this example, you need to work for 30 minutes just to counter the calories in a single donut, which may take you all of a couple of minutes to eat! And if you take the time to identify the "worst offenders" you'll really be amazed. A few examples:

- One chocolate chip muffin can have close to 600 calories.
- Bagels have 300 calories and up.
- The fast-food burgers can also have close to 600 calories.
- A mocha coconut Frappucino with whipped cream has over 700 calories!

Let's look at the simple fact that not all calories are equal – which is what a lot of people think. Two examples:

- The effect of protein in reducing appetite is much more beneficial than the same number of calories consumed from fat and carbs.
- Even with sugar: fructose can stimulate your appetite, causing you to eat more, compared to the same number of calories from glucose.

Once you understand how calories work and get a sense for how to burn them off, you'll be better able to plan your diet program and exercises that much better.

What to do about it: discuss calories with your doctor and nutrition specialist in the general framework of the diet plan you're putting together. Become aware of which foods are very high in calories, particularly those where you get a lot of calories for a very small portion.

Think about it. This is your life we're talking about here!

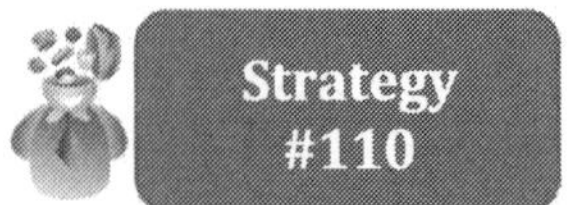

Think About Caffeine

Millions of people drink coffee and colas with caffeine, as well as foods that contain caffeine, for two reasons: the "kick" it provides and to increase the body's metabolism in order to lose weight faster. The fact is, it's not a good idea to consume caffeine for either of those reasons.

Caffeine occurs in the leaves, seeds and/or fruit of plants, including cocoa-beans, tea, coffee, cola and guarana. When entering your blood stream, caffeine is rapidly absorbed, reaching peak levels 45 to 60 minutes after being taken. Here are the effects that caffeine causes:

- It can trigger a rise in your blood sugar, followed by a sharp fall, which will have the effect of making you hungrier.
- It can raise your blood sugar and insulin levels, leading to "insulin resistance," which in turn can increase your risk for heart disease and Type II diabetes.
- It increases your heart rate.

- Since caffeine is a diuretic, it increases water loss, and while water loss decreases your overall weight, it's not fat loss, and it's temporary.

Studies also show that ingesting large amounts of caffeine have no significant impact on weight loss. Dr. Atkins once said "Excessive caffeine may cause unstable blood sugar and should be avoided by those who suspect they are caffeine dependent. Everyone should try to avoid caffeine."

What to do about it: start drinking water, seltzer, decaffeinated coffee, tea and other healthy drinks.

Think about it. This is your life we're talking about here!

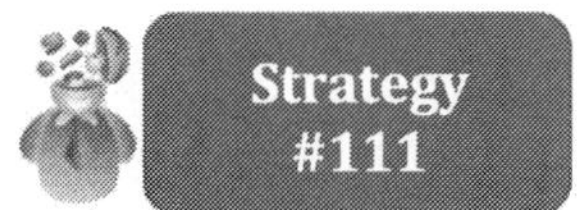

Think About Protein

Proteins are extremely important to the proper functioning of your body. They are composed of amino acids and are required for the structure, function and regulation of the cells in your body, including your tissues and organs. Every living cell and all body fluids (except bile and urine) contain protein. The cells of muscles, tendons, and ligaments are maintained with protein. Children and adolescents require protein for growth and development.

Protein helps reduce two main risk factors for kidney disease, help build muscles, reduce body fat and lowers risks of various diseases.

How much protein should you consume? It all depends on a wide range of factors, and the ones best suited to answer it are your medical doctor, obesity specialist and nutrition specialist. Based on your blood test results as recommended in the next guidebook, your intake of protein needs to be adjusted to the optimal amount. Protein prevents muscle tissue from breaking down and it repairs all body tissues such as your skin and teeth. Two to three portions of protein generally gives you the grams you need.

If you feel hungry frequently, it could be a sign you're not getting enough protein, so you can satisfy your hunger and help your body by snacking on protein.

If you fail to get enough protein, it could lead to weakened bones, especially in the thighs, hip and spine. Research at Harvard and Tufts proves the lower your intake of protein, the weaker your bones.

What to do about it: this is easy! Eat more protein – which is found in meat, eggs, cheese and other dairy products. Eat protein with every meal, and considering eating it before other parts of the meal because it's healthier. And, start snacking on protein instead of fats and carbs. Of course, plan your protein intake with your doctor and nutrition specialist.

Think about it. This is your life we're talking about here!

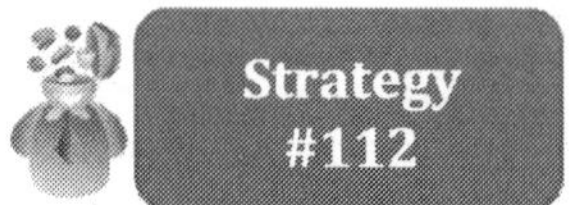

Think About Sugar

You know, if we didn't have a sweet tooth (actually a sweet tongue), we'd all be a lot better off. While sugar and everything that sugar is in tastes good, it is at the root of a lot of medical problems resulting from obesity. Quite simply, the more sugar in your bloodstream, the closer you are to getting diabetes and other maladies. But, not all sugar is bad. Basically, there are three types.

- **Natural**. This sugar occurs naturally in the foods you eat – pineapple, bananas, blueberries – and is the most beneficial kind of sugar, but you can't eat an unlimited amount of it. And dried fruit often contains a lot of sugar that is not good for you.
- **Added**. These foods may or may not contain sugar naturally, and for taste, sugar of various types is added: cookies/cakes, fruit juices, sodas, BBQ sauce and many, many more.
- **Substitutes**. Products like saccharin, aspartame and others provide a sweet taste without the harmful effects of added sugar, but they have chemicals that many think are just as bad. Sucralose (known as Splenda), is 600 times sweeter than sugar, and "sugar alcohols" (sorbitol, xylitol, lactitol, mannitol, and maltitol) are found in many of today's sugar-free candies, cookies, and chewing gums. By the way, sugar alcohols are a lot like laxatives – they can and often do, cause diarrhea – so be warned.

Your best bet is Stevia, an all natural sweetener that tastes good (I get Zevia brand soda sweetened with Stevia). Along with naturally flavored seltzer, I've found two great replacements for soda and diet soda.

The average American eats about 20 teaspoons of sugar a day, and over half (about 60%) comes from corn sweeteners used in sodas and other sweetened drinks (high fructose corn syrup or HFCS). Most of the balance (about 40%) is from sucrose (table sugar). So, most of our sugar intake is from added sugar – the worst kind! And we've increased our sugar intake by 30% in just four years (1996 to 2000). It's getting out of hand! The USDA recommends we eat no more than 10 teaspoons a day. Here are some foods where a single portion gives you more than you entire day's worth of sugar:

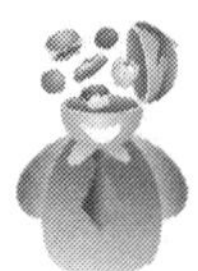

- Low fat, fruit flavored yogurt 7.00 tsp
- Pancake syrup, ¼ cup 10.25
- Hostess Lemon Fruit Pie 11.50
- McDonald's Vanilla Shake 12.00
- Sunkist Orange Soda 13.00
- Fruitopia Strawberry Passion Awareness 17.75
- Dairy Queen Mr. Misty Slush 28.00

In an interesting study among juveniles in prison, they found that a group of these kids who had most sugar eliminated from what they were fed had a 50% drop in serious misbehaviors, and an 80% drop in kids who continually got in trouble. So sugar consumption may be responsible for negative behaviors as well.

What to do about it: cut out 90% or more of added sugar and switch to foods with Stevia. At a party, reach for fresh fruit instead of cookies and cakes – sweet but much better for you that empty calories in cookies and cakes.

Think about it. This is your life we're talking about here!

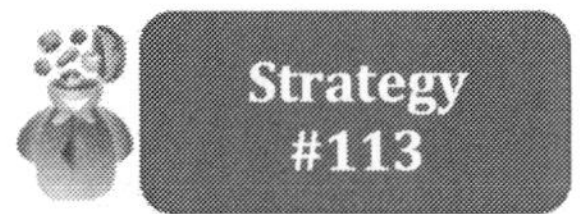

Think About Cholesterol

Much has been written about cholesterol, and while miracle drugs lower your bad cholesterol levels, millions of Americans still have cholesterol counts that are way too high. Cholesterol is a soft, waxy substance found in your bloodstream as well as your cells. It has beneficial uses: it helps form cell membranes, some hormones and serves other important bodily functions. But too much of it is a major risk for heart disease and ultimately, heart attacks and strokes.

Your body manufactures cholesterol, and the rest of it comes from animal products, such as meat, poultry, fish, eggs, butter, cheese and whole milk. You won't find cholesterol in food grown on plants like fruits and vegetables. Cholesterol cannot dissolve in your bloodstream, so it has to be transported to and from cells by special carriers called lipoproteins. In addition to your overall cholesterol count, which should be 200 or less according to most experts, you need to watch two types of cholesterol as well:

- LDL (low-density lipoprotein), commonly known as "bad" cholesterol. Too much of it clogs your arteries. You want this count to be 100 or less.
- HDL (high-density lipoprotein), commonly known as "good" cholesterol. You want this count to be 40 or higher.

This is a fairly simplistic discussion of cholesterol; you need to talk to your doctor and nutrition specialist about optimal levels for you. The bottom line here is that the more foods you eat that raise your overall cholesterol and/or raise your LDL levels and/or lower your HDL levels, the higher your risk for serious ailments.

What to do about it: add a discussion of cholesterol to your checklist when visiting your doctor and nutrition specialist, and then simply stay away from foods that are going to cause trouble. There's no way around it.

Think about it. This is your life we're talking about here!

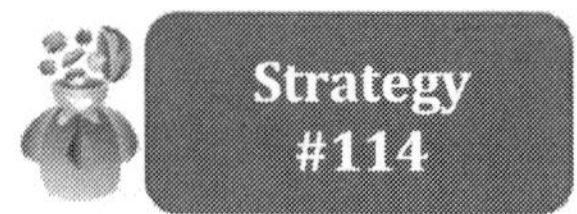

Think About Carbohydrates

With the popularity of low-carbohydrate diets, much confusion has arisen as traditional low-fat diets have been challenged by the low-carb programs. Because certain carbohydrates are primarily sugar, and other carbs turn to sugar, people are finding that controlling sugar intake is becoming more and more important, especially in the control and prevention of diabetes. Since the body burns carbs before it burns fat, the more carbs you eat results in the body having a hard time burning fat. There are types of carbohydrates:

- **Simple**. Most substances that end in "ose" are included here. Simple carbs are the least healthy for you, and include:
    - Sucrose – Table sugar, brown sugar, confectioners sugar, raw sugar and turbinado sugar
    - Glucose – Dextrose, corn syrup and glucose syrup
    - Fructose – found in many products
    - High fructose corn syrup (HFCS)
    - Honey – Made up of glucose, fructose and water
    - Sugar alcohols – Sorbitol, mannitol, xybitol
    - Lactose – milk and milk products
    - Maltose, dextrose – cereals and some baked goods
- **Complex**. These are the carbs that are most healthy for you.
    - Starches – Brown flour, dark breads, brown rice, oats, barley, sweet potatoes, legumes, fruits and vegetables
    - Fiber – Insoluble: whole-wheat breads and cereals, wheat bran, cabbage, beets, carrots, Brussels sprouts, turnips, cauliflower and apple skin (pectin)
    - Fiber – Soluble: oat bran, oats, legumes, citrus fruits, strawberries, apple pulp, psyllium, rice bran and barley

You've got to spend some time learning about carbs and determining with your doctor how important they are to your weight loss program. Doctors are starting to believe that carb control is as important as controlling fats. I've found that by being on a lower carb program, I not only lost weight, but had more energy and was sleepy less often than when I was on a low-fat regimen.

What to do about it: like with most of the advice in this section, discuss carbs with your doctor and nutrition specialist, and then construct your allowable food list accordingly.

Think about it. This is your life we're talking about here!

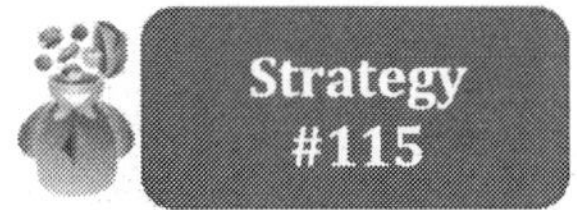

Think About Sodium (Salt)

Too many Americans consume about 3,300 milligrams of sodium daily, and that's more than DOUBLE what they should be! Many experts feel salt is a major factor in elevated blood pressure, which can lead to other complications, such as heart attacks and strokes. We get our salt in many ways:

- We add it to foods to give it more taste. We shake our salt shakers way too often and pour on too much salt.
- It's added to fast foods, particularly French fries. If you've ever seen how much salt is poured onto a batch of fries, then you know what I mean.
- The biggest loading up on salt is one that you may not even know. Manufacturers of processed foods often add large amounts of salt to improve the taste. For example, a half-cup of prepared spaghetti sauce can contain as much as 600mg of salt – almost half of your entire daily recommended intake!

In addition to these health risks, salt can increase water retention, which retards weight loss. Teenagers are among the biggest abusers of salt. By cutting salt intake by just 33%, there would be fewer teens subject to hypertension, heart disease, heart attacks, strokes and deaths. When combined with other elements in processed foods, sodium stimulates our appetites, leading to more weight gain. Dr. David Samadi of the Mt. Sinai Medical Center, indicates that too much salt can lead to kidney stones, present in 10% of all Americans (FOX News Sunday Housecall, 5/26/13).

Among the biggest contributors to salt intake are fast foods and snack foods. This is a particularly bad problem among kids and teens, and if you're a parent with children, severely limiting fast food and snacks is a very good idea. To give you an idea of how MUCH salt these foods contain, here are a few examples:

- Sizzling skillet steak fajita: 3 days' worth of salt in one dish
- Texas cheese fries with dressing: 2.6 days' worth
- Bone-in ham and eggs platter: 1.9 days' worth
- Signature pasta dish: 1.7 days' worth

In "7 Ways to Tame Your Salt Habit" at iVillage.com, here are some foods you might not expect to contain much salt but actually do:

- Bread
- Pizza
- Chicken soup
- Cheeseburgers
- Meat loaf
- Canned tomato sauce – the acid in canned tomatoes can cause a toxic chemical called BPA to leach, so stick with sauces in jars, not cans
- Pretzels
- Popcorn
- Miso soup
- Canned carrots
- Ketchup
- Italian salad dressing

Not only that. Dr. Marsha Gordon of the Mount Sinai School of Medicine says the worst thing to eat in terms of your skin is salt. Now you know one reason why people have bad skin. If you're an African American, you should know that you are likely to be more sensitive to the negative effects of salt, and should not be adding salt to food and avoiding processed foods and frozen foods that are high in salt. Check the label before you buy canned goods as many contain a lot of salt.

61% of us Americans think that "sea salt" is healthier than regular salt, reports the Tufts University Health & Nutrition Letter. In fact, it's the same as regular salt, except it comes from seawater as opposed to salt mines. Also, since most salt we ingest does not come from your salt shaker, removing the shaker does not solve the problem.

Do you really want to put that much salt in your system?

What to do about it: I know that weaning yourself off salt is one of the easiest things to do. If you must add something to enhance some of your food, fill your salt shaker with Mrs. Dash or some other salt-like substitute or herb blend that will add taste without the negative side effects of salt. Spices such as cinnamon, garlic, pepper and onion, available in powder form, make a great substitute, as do many other spices.

In restaurants, imagine that the salt shaker contains poison, and stay away from it. Bring a small bottle of onion powder to use instead of salt. Read food labels to see what foods contain more sodium than you expect...like pickles...and buy unsalted nuts instead of salted nuts. More foods that are high in salt: cottage cheese, salsa, dill pickles, croissants, corn bread, king crab and canned tuna. Ask your server which dishes are prepared with added salt, and if you want to order one, ask them not to add salt to it.

Think about it. This is your life we're talking about here!

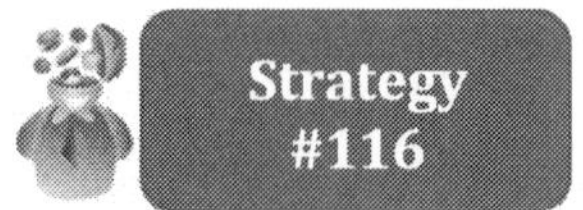

Think About Calcium

Calcium is a very important mineral, primarily for bone and teeth strength and to keep our muscles in tip-top shape. Many people do not get enough calcium on a daily basis. Best-selling author Deirdre Imus in her piece "Swap out soda to take control of your teeth" points out that both regular and diet soda are bad for your teeth, and suggests eating foods rich in calcium because calcium re-mineralizes damaged teeth. *Men's Fitness* outlines foods that are good and bad for your teeth:

Good Foods for Your Teeth

- Hard fruits like apples and peaches
- Hard vegetables like carrots
- Water

Foods That Attack Your Teeth

- Diet Soda, due to low pH and high acidity
- Sports drinks, because they contain sugar and acid
- Coffee and tea, because they are both acidic

One dieting problem that has arisen is that people eliminate or reduce dairy products in their diets in favor of foods that don't contain calcium. Calcium plays an important role in maintaining your weight. An April 2003 study done at the University of Tennessee found that people who included nonfat yogurt in the diet while trying to lose weight lost 22 percent more weight, 61 percent more fat, and 81 percent more stomach fat (an inch more off the waistline). Good sources of calcium include:

- Milk
- Yogurt

- Cheese
- Ice cream
- Beans
- Salmon
- Tofu
- Spinach
- Kale
- Broccoli

Plain and simple, your dieting choices cannot reduce or eliminate calcium to the point where it becomes dangerous. Reader comment: “I drink almond milk twice a day and have cut down on cheese and traditional milk products.”

What to do about it: when designing your diet program with your doctor and nutrition specialist, be sure to allow for enough calcium per day.

Think about it. This is your life we’re talking about here!

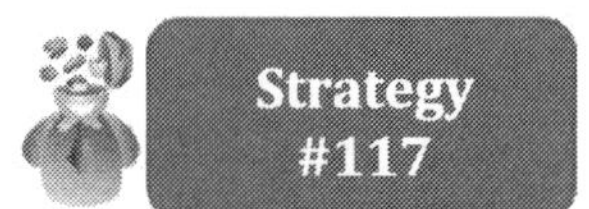

Think About Fat

I don’t think any topic has generated more discussion and debate than fat. For the longest time, a low-fat diet was the diet of choice, recommended by doctors around the world. Then along came Atkins and others who helped shift the emphasis away from fat, and onto carbohydrates and sugar. So what’s the deal with fat? First we need to look at the types of fat:

- **Saturated Fats**. The easy way to tell if a fat is saturated is if it is solid at room temperature. Butter and lard are two examples. Cream also contains saturated fat, but it is liquid at room temp because it also contains milk. Some oils like palm are also saturated fats. Stick margarine and shortening are also solid fats.
- **Monounsaturated Fats**. These fats are preferred because they lower cholesterol. The most common in this category are avocado and olive oils.
- **Polyunsaturated Fats**. These are found in most nut, seed and vegetable oils. They are traditionally combined with dairy foods to make margarine and cooking oils. Like saturated fats, they are also problematical.
- **Trans Fats**. These fats are produced through hydrogenation, a chemical process by which hydrogen is added to unsaturated fatty acids. You may have seen “partially hydrogenated oils” on the ingredients listed in various foods – that wording means trans fat. Health professionals have identified trans fats as being so bad for you, that they were added to food labeling years ago. Foods with high trans fat content

include commercially prepared and fried foods, such as chicken nuggets, donuts, cookies, crackers and pies. In fact, the FDA estimates supermarkets carry more than 42,000 items containing trans fats. A Harvard study showed that getting just 3% of your daily calories from trans fat increases your risk of heart disease by as much as 50% -- wow! Trans fat increases LDL cholesterol (the "bad" cholesterol) and lowers HDL, the good cholesterol. With the understanding that the goal is zero grams of trans fat consumption, here are a couple of foods and how much trans fat they contain (all at major fast food chains), courtesy www.bantransfats.com:

- Large fries: 8 grams
- Apple pie: 4.5 grams
- Popcorn chicken: 7 grams
- Chicken pot pie: 14 grams
- Chicken combo meal: 15 grams

I hope you get the picture: trans fat, like sugar, is toxic.

Getting enough of the right fat and reducing or eliminating the bad fats is critical for weight loss and health.

Good fats supply our bodies with energy, provide essential fatty acids (omega-3 and omega-6) and help the absorption of vitamins A, D, E and K.

What to do about it: stay away from saturated fats and trans fats. Learn what foods are high in trans fat – chicken pot pie, biscuits, French fries, cinnamon roll, fish sticks, nachos, margarine, cookies, etc. Beware of foods called "reduced fat" because they may be higher in sugar in order to compensate for the reduction in fat.

Think about it. This is your life we're talking about here!

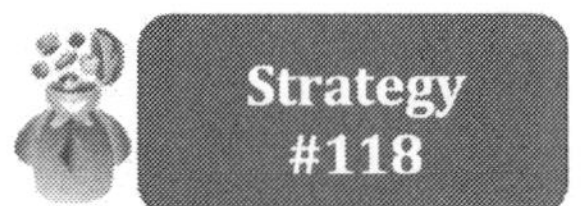

Think About Fiber

Fiber has been disappearing from the American diet at an alarming rate, leading to a deficiency of fiber in our population. Fiber is not only important for bodily functions (it helps with your bowel function), but it offers numerous benefits to those people who want to lose weight:

- Requires more chewing and therefore takes longer to eat.
- It provides you with fewer calories per serving.
- Fiber creates a sense of "feeling full."
- Decreases hunger between meals.

What's happened is that in the last decade or so, fiber has been all but eliminated from convenience products (Wall Street Journal, 10/22/2003) as cereals and "on the go" snacks and meal replacements have more fat and less fiber. The current recommendation is for 25grams per day for women and 38 grams per day for men, but the average American only gets 15grams. Many get a lot less.

Good sources of fiber include bran, oats, carrots, brown rice, pears, apples, whole wheat bread, Ezekiel brad and numerous types of beans.

What to do about it: you gotta get more fiber into your body. Before you nibble on the next breakfast bar that you <u>think</u> is good for you, check the fiber and fat content...the more fiber and less fat the better.

Think about it. This is your life we're talking about here!

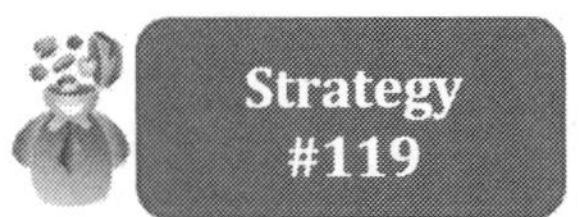

Think About Vitamins

With the advent of daily multiple vitamins, we'd all be getting enough vitamins. But unfortunately, that's not true. In fact, according to The Reader's Digest (6/2003), "We're living amid an unrecognized epidemic of vitamin D deficiency." And I think "D" is not the only one. Many researchers believe obesity actually causes vitamin D deficiency.

Back in 1982, the USDA surveyed over 20,000 Americans and found that not a single person obtained 100% of the Recommended Daily Allowance (RDA) of ten essential nutrients. And many think the RDA levels are set too low. The August, 2013 edition of *Life Extension* Magazine lists 15 conditions – many serious – that are associated with low Vitamin D levels, including multiple sclerosis, arthritis, several cancers, dementia and stroke.

Vitamins are essential to the healthy functioning of your body, and are instrumental in fighting off disease. Vitamin D, for example, can help reduce the chance of getting diabetes, hypertension, osteoporosis and others.

You can get vitamins in two ways: from food and vitamin pills. Typical pills contain 30 or more vitamins and minerals, and the labels on the bottles give you the amounts of vitamins and the percentage of the RDA. You can easily find out what vitamins are in various foods. Vegetables, for example, provide vitamins A and C, and minerals such as iron and magnesium.

If you don't get enough of the right vitamins and minerals, your body won't be able to fight off ailments, and you may have other problems as well. Vitamins help with nutrient absorption in our bodies.

What to do about it: if you're not taking a daily vitamin supplement, get your doctor's OK and start taking one religiously. It's the easiest thing you can do. But it's not enough. A good balanced diet, one that you should develop with your doctor and nutrition specialist, will give you the vitamins and nutrients your body needs.

Think about it. This is your life we're talking about here!

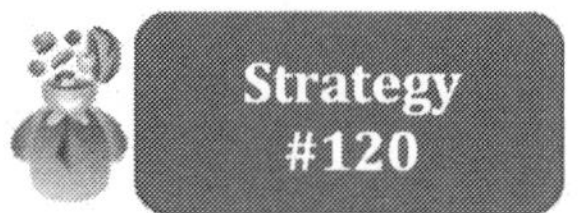

Think About Antioxidants

To understand the value and importance of antioxidants, we first need to understand and define "free radicals." No, they're not campus rabble rousers who are out of jail. Free radicals are natural by-products of processes that occur in the cells in your body, and they can also be created by exposure to tobacco smoke, radiation and other pollutants. Free radicals are bad for your body. If they're not stopped, free radicals can cause damage to cell walls, cell structures and genetic material within cells. Over time, this damage can lead to diseases such as cancer.

Antioxidants come to the rescue! They are chemical compounds that neutralize the effects of oxidation, and they get rid of free radicals within your body. Some of the best-known antioxidants are vitamins A, C and E, and the mineral selenium. These antioxidants are **not** manufactured by the body, so you've got to ingest them! Most people should get enough antioxidants from food, so this is another topic worth discussing with your doctors and nutrition specialist. High doses can actually increase risks, so be careful here.

Like vitamins, you can get them in two ways: food and pills. These foods are a good source of antioxidants: fruits, vegetables, whole grains, carrots and sweet potatoes.

What to do about it: same advice as in the previous section about vitamins. Make sure you get enough antioxidants in the diet you plan with your doctor.

Think about it. This is your life we're talking about here!

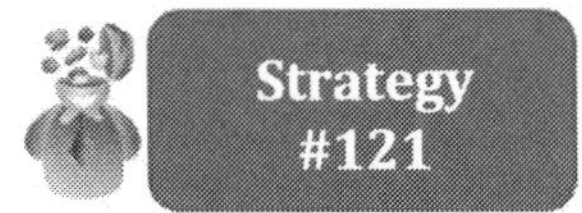

Think About Cooking Oil

There are numerous oils you can buy at the supermarket to use when you cook. As you can see from this chart, certain oils (at the top of the list) are much better for you than others at the bottom of the list.

You need to read labels carefully, because many oils labeled "vegetable oil" are actually soybean oil. Pure vegetable oil, as a liquid, has zero trans fat (bad for you) and is high in the good fats – polyunsaturated and monounsaturated.

Also, some oils are very healthy to consume, but are not good for cooking.

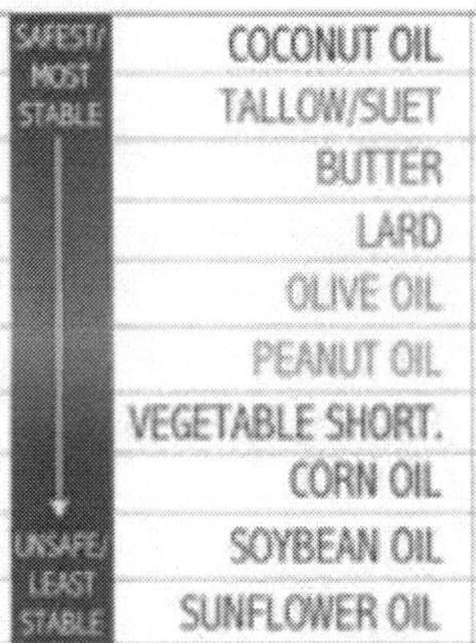

What to do about it: It's a must to read the ingredient list to see exactly what type of oil is in the bottle.

Think about it. This is your life we're talking about here!

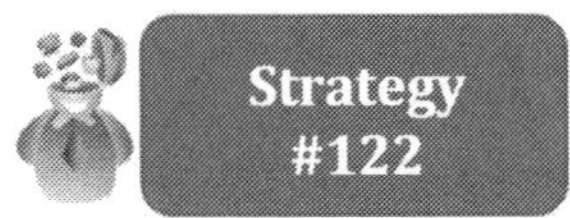

Think About Gluten

There's been a lot of people jumping on the "gluten free" bandwagon and with good reason. Gluten can cause havoc in people who have celiac disease.

But recent research shows that reducing gluten may be a good idea for most everyone, even if you don't have celiac. And reducing gluten may help you lose weight. Here's why.

Gluten is a protein found in wheat, barley, rye and many food additives. It's also found in processed foods like ready-made soups, soy sauce, candies, cold cuts, bread, pizza crust, pasta, cookies and pastries.

The connection is simple: gluten lurks in refined carbohydrates, which as we all know, is linked to obesity.

On the other hand, not all grains have gluten. Certain types of grains, seeds and flours are naturally gluten-free:

- Rice
- Corn (but only GMO free)
- Quinoa
- Sorghum
- Flax
- Amaranth
- Buckwheat
- Millet

Great article about Gluten on www.Mercola.com at: http://tinyurl.com/3lbd5aj.

What to do about it: Cutting out gluten may be a wise strategy, along the same lines as refined carbs. Check with your nutrition specialist.

Think about it. This is your life we're talking about here!

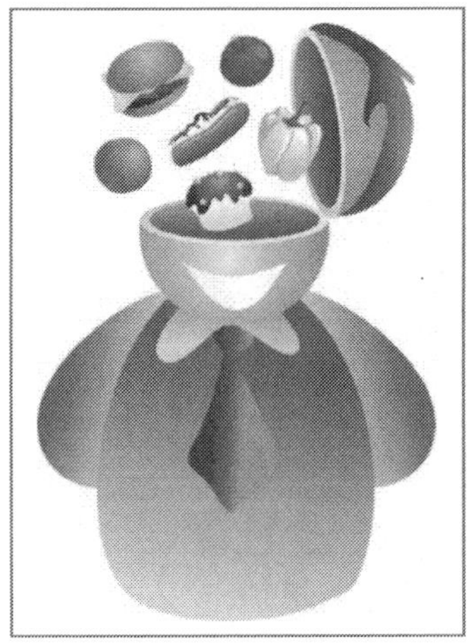

Guidebook #4

Tactics

After reading the first three sections – Truth, Beliefs and Strategies – you're probably expecting another similar section about Tactics, the fourth component of the "Success Pie" covered earlier:

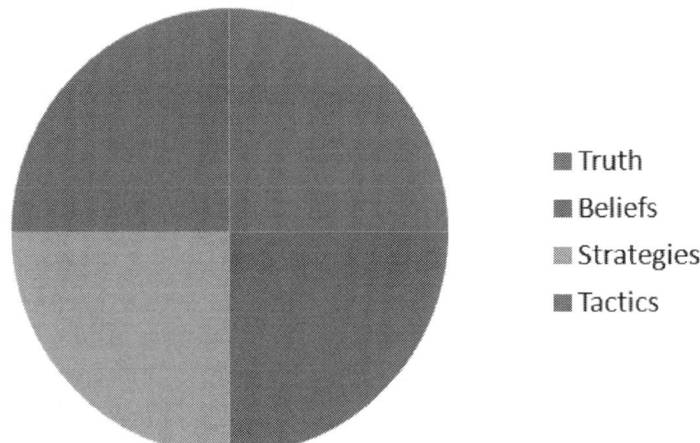

After you've found your Moment of Truth, embraced your set of beliefs, and absorbed the strategies, you're ready to identify and implement the tactics.

Most people think of tactics as the specific diet program you follow. And that's basically correct. But most people omit one important step that is the key ingredient for choosing and following the best program.

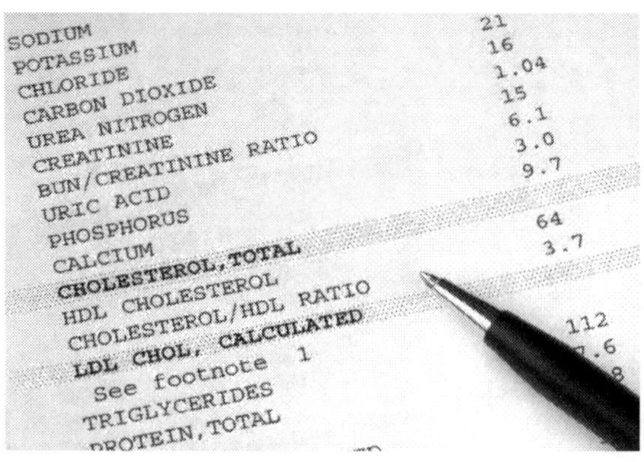

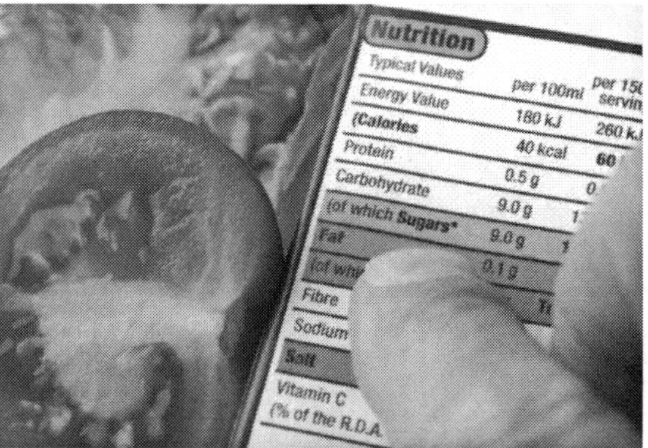

The first step is meeting with your medical doctor and nutrition specialist (a Registered Dietitian or a Certified Nutrition Specialist). Do NOT omit this step. Your MD should take a blood test and screen for abnormalities in:

- HDL cholesterol
- Triglycerides
- Abdominal circumference
- Blood pressure
- Fasting glucose
- Hemoglobin A1c

This basic information is the starting point. Depending on the educational level of your doctor in terms of obesity, you may want to seek out doctors who have been certified as specialists in the field of Obesity Medicine by the American Board of Obesity Medicine. Because obesity is so complex, a referral to an obesity specialist who will coordinate care with your primary doctor is certainly recommended.

Another important factor to discuss for women is whether or not you're in menopause. A large proportion of Dr. Lazarus' patients gain a lot of weight during menopause in spite of no change in eating habits. Weight control before and after needs to be part of this discussion if applicable.

These professionals will provide invaluable guidance based on your individual situation and background. They will help you choose the nutrition program to follow and the foods and drinks to both eat and avoid. Quoted in MensFitness.com, Kathleen Zelman, R.D., director of nutrition for WebMD.com's Weight Loss Clinic, said "Not every method of weight loss works with every person."

While there are many good programs of all flavors, most are created for the masses. You need a program that is designed just for you, and that can only be accomplished with input and guidance from your doctor and nutrition specialist. For example, a diet for a healthy young man in his 20's is not likely to be the best option for a pre-diabetic man in his 50's.

That's why diets created for the masses need to be adjusted or abandoned based on your unique medical profile.

Let's say that you're deficient in one or more nutrients. Dr. Michael Greger writes in the www.nutritionfacts.org blog, "98% of American Diets Potassium Deficient." A simple blood test will let you know your deficiencies, and the nutrition specialist will add foods to your diet to correct it. Vitamin D is right up there as well. Both are very important nutrients.

There's another very important reason to talk with your MD. Some foods, like grapefruit and other citrus fruits, interact poorly with some medications, like statins. Your doctor and nutritional specialist can advise you on certain foods to avoid based on your medications. Really important!

Today, make an appointment with your medical doctor.

Today, make an appointment with a nutrition specialist.

Leslie Goldman, writing in www.HealthLine.com suggests asking questions when you talk about your tactical diet plan, such as:

- What is day-to-day life on this plan like?
- How many daily calories will I be allotted, and will that change as I lose weight?
- What types of foods will I be eating most often?
- Are there any foods considered off-limits?
- Does the plan involve physical activity?

Dr. Ethan Lazarus writes about the second step in the tactical process, which is understanding all your options. Since 80% of people who diet do it themselves, that's where he starts:

When it comes to losing weight, there are many options available. The United States Preventive Task Force Services (USPSTF), an organization of independent, volunteer medical experts, recommends that primary care doctors screen all adults and children for obesity, and refer for or offer intensive multi-component behavioral interventions including:

- Behavioral management
- Improving diet and physical activity
- Addressing barriers to change
- Self-monitoring
- Strategizing how to maintain lifestyle changes

The most common things I see individuals use for the purpose of losing weight are:

1. Diet and Weight Loss Books
2. Web Sites
3. Join a Gym/Work with a Personal Trainer
4. Commercial Weight Loss Programs
5. Medical Weight Loss
6. Surgical Weight Loss

Let's discuss each briefly. My observations are based on working with thousands of patients as well as my colleagues who have written extensively about obesity. Since this book is about *truth*, here's my version of the truth about these options.

Diet and Weight Loss Books

Obesity is a tremendously complex problem. Most "diet" books villainize a particular macronutrient: "Don't eat fat!" "Don't eat carbs!" "Don't eat wheat!" "Don't eat....." "Detoxify with this 20-day cleanse and lose 30 pounds!"

Unfortunately, these sorts of books are oversimplifying and suggesting that by eliminating certain foods, we will achieve a lower weight. This rarely works out to be true. And, these sorts of diets rarely turn out to be long-term solutions. Significant sustained weight loss is rare for most individuals from reading a book about food restriction. If you don't believe me, ask the author or the publisher of the next book you intend to buy for scientific evidence that the book is an effective treatment strategy. Ask for number of patients treated, and total percentage sustained weight loss at 2 years.

Other books are more helpful. Some examine reasons why people eat - whether psychological, environmental, genetic, etc. Many of these can provide an individual a lot of insight in to where their unique challenges lie.

Web Sites

There is a new web site every day promising that by tracking your calories in and calories out, you will achieve a healthy weight. These web sites rely on the old "3500 calorie rule" stating that if you eliminate 3500 calories from your diet, or increase your activity enough to burn 3500 calories, you will lose 1 pound of fat.

This has widely been disproven. Because our bodies quickly adapt to changes, and because we tend to underestimate our caloric intake dramatically, the 3500 calorie rule is not helpful.

On the other hand, many individuals find that food and activity trackers are very helpful in being accountable to themselves or to people helping them with weight management. If you are one of those and enjoy tracking your food and activities, go for it! One of the habits most helpful in sustaining large amounts of weight loss is to continue to journal. So, for that reason alone, I recommend that you include them as part of an overall plan, but not solely depend on them.

Join a Gym/Work with a Personal Trainer

One of the most common efforts I see for weight loss is working with a trainer at a gym. Unfortunately, this doesn't generally result in a significant weight loss.

What? How could this be? Well, to date, there are no good studies showing that by itself, exercise is a useful weight loss strategy. We do not "burn" off the fat. We may burn calories, but our bodies are very good at getting them back.

Exercise has tons of health benefits - live longer, don't get diabetes or heart disease, improve your mood, sleep, and sex life. Feel better. Lose inches. Unfortunately, though, if weight loss was the goal, even with all these other benefits, when a person exercises and *doesn't* lose weight, they will typically say "That didn't work!" and stop exercising.

If signing up with a trainer, ask for the data! Ask for number of individuals treated, amount of weight lost on average as a percentage of total body weight, and amount sustained at 1 and 2 years.

On the other hand, individuals who combine exercise with other treatment strategies will lose weight more quickly, lose more weight, and most importantly, be far more likely to keep the weight off. So joining a gym and/or working with a trainer is great in general, but not the weight loss panacea that many think it is. What you eat and when you eat it is still the primary factor.

Commercial Weight Loss Programs

There are so many commercial weight loss programs out there that it is hard to summarize them in a few sentences. However, the theme of most is meal replacements and supplements. "If you eliminate your food and just eat our food and drink these shakes or take all these pills, you will lose weight."

In fact, meal replacement is a viable strategy for weight control and is endorsed by the Academy of Nutrition and Dietetics. But, is this a food plan you plan to continue long-term? If you are using a commercial product for weight loss, be prepared to use it for maintaining weight loss. For the rest of your life.

If it is not something healthy, something that you enjoy, do you really want to do that? Is the program asking you to take pills? What's in them? Why? There are NO over-the-counter supplements with good enough data to recommend that they are helpful for weight loss, in my opinion. If there are, please show me the data!

If you are considering commercial weight loss programs, ask to see the data! With the millions of clients, ask for data showing percentage of body weight, in all participants, lost and sustained at 1 and 2 years. If you are seriously considering one of these programs, discuss it with your doctor and nutrition specialist so you get both sides of the story.

Medical Weight Loss

In medical weight loss centers, there is a wide variety of different types of services offered. If you are considering medical weight loss, first make sure you are working with a medical doctor. Many "medical weight loss centers" in fact are not "medical" at all. Many "weight loss doctors" are not physicians. So, be sure you know what you are getting in to. Ask to see the credentials of the physician you are working with. Ask if the physician is a diplomate of the American Board of Obesity Medicine.

Medical Doctors can utilize meal plans, medications, and other treatments not available in any other setting. They can:

- Check for problems that may be contributing to obesity.
- Optimize treatment of diabetes, high blood pressure, insomnia, thyroid problems, and depression, all typically contributing factors to obesity.
- Coordinate treatment with primary care doctors and specialists.
- Develop an individualized treatment strategy appropriate for the individual.
- Utilize F.D.A. approved prescription medications to enhance weight loss and weight maintenance.

Unfortunately, many "medical weight loss doctors" recommend a lot of non-approved treatments. Some of the treatments commonly offered that we know do NOT help with weight loss are:

- HCG (a hormone that cannot be sold legally in the U.S. as of 2013)
- Vitamin B12 shots
- Lipotropic injections (compounds that can purportedly break down fat, but are not long-lasting)

So, know who you are working with. A good medical weight loss doctor will get to know you, individualize your treatment plan, and try and piece together the components that will help you be successful, whether it is a diet plan, partial meal replacement, management of other medical problems, weight loss medication, structured exercise program, or a little bit of each! As with any entity, there are top-shelf medical weight loss professionals and others that have questionable methods – always get references before you start.

Weight Loss Surgery

For an individual with significant medical problems from their weight who has been unsuccessful with medical weight loss for at least six months, surgery may be the only other treatment option.

Weight loss surgery has been around a long time, but has improved significantly in the last 10 years. These days, there are 3 common procedures being used:

- Gastric Bypass
- Lap Band
- Sleeve Gastrectomy

Gastric Bypass

In this surgery, a portion of the stomach is removed, and a portion of the small intestine is bypassed. Thus, there is restriction - less food can fit in the small stomach pouch that remains, and malabsorption - much of the food that the individual eats is not absorbed. After gastric bypass, patients lose an average of 35% of their total body weight. At 5 years, they sustain 25% weight loss on average.

Lab Band

In this procedure, a band is placed around the stomach. The tightness of the band is adjustable with a simple office procedure. The band restricts the stomach so less food can fit in. The procedure is safer than gastric bypass with less complications, but also has less weight loss and a higher failure rate. The numbers I've seen published are that the average weight loss after lap band is 20% of total body weight, but that a high percentage of individuals regain all of what was lost.

Sleeve Gastrectomy

This is the newest procedure. In this surgery, a large part of the stomach is removed, but the intestine is not bypassed. It offers a similar amount of weight loss as a gastric bypass, but may be somewhat safer. Long term data is not yet available.

If you are considering surgery, I recommend seeking out a hospital and surgeon that does a lot of these procedures. Learn the pros and cons of each procedure. And, discuss it with your medical obesity doctor to help you make a decision. Ask for references of patients who have been through these procedures to get first-hand input on their effectiveness, complications and ask "if you had it to do over, would you make the same decision?"

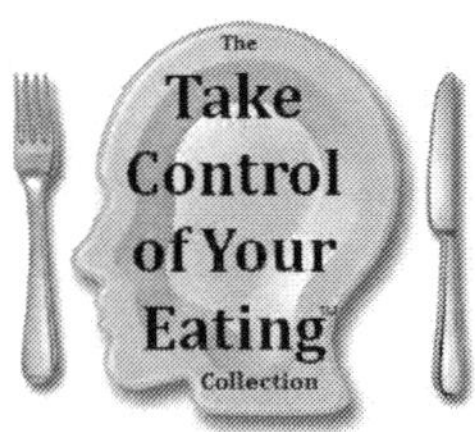

Summary & Conclusions

After reading these first four sections of *The Mind Diet,* you should be ready, willing and able to lose weight successfully. Because you've read so much, I thought it would be of great value to summarize what I consider to be the eight most important lessons, ones which impacted me the most in my successful weight loss.

Eat Right. Live Right.

It's not just a phrase. It represents exactly how you have to look at eating and lifestyle. It's not as simple as eating less and moving more. It's about what, when and why you eat. It's about how you live your life.

Timing is Everything.

Most people eat big meals at dinner, and have little or nothing for breakfast and/or lunch. Eating 90% of my food for breakfast and lunch was the single most important change I made in my weight loss efforts.

Substitution is King.

Eating healthy food is not that hard. When you substitute good and tasty foods for unhealthy and evil foods, drinks and ingredients, you lose the desire to eat junk.

Take Responsibility.

Successfully losing weight and keeping it off starts with you taking personal responsibility. It's entirely up to you. The time for "trying" and making excuses is over. Take charge of your life and you'll succeed.

It's for life.

The *Mind Diet* way of dieting does not have an ending. The changes you need to make are for life, and will benefit you in every aspect of your life.

Knowledge is Power.

The more you know, the easier it is to succeed. The first four sections and the balance of *The Mind Diet* present the realities of the world of food and drink today. Spending the time to learn about food choices is a must.

Failure and Success Pies.

Spending time to think about Truth, Beliefs, Strategies and Tactics equally is critical. They are all critical components to weight loss success.

It's About Making The Right Choice.

Everything I've written in this book and the others in the *Take Control of Your Eating* collection boils down to one choice.

You either want to live a healthy and active life or you don't.

Every food and drink choice you make must be tied back to the choice between a healthy life and the opposite. The more junk you eat, the less healthy your life will be, and more importantly, the shorter your life expectancy will be.

It really is just this simple. Make the right decisions, starting right now.

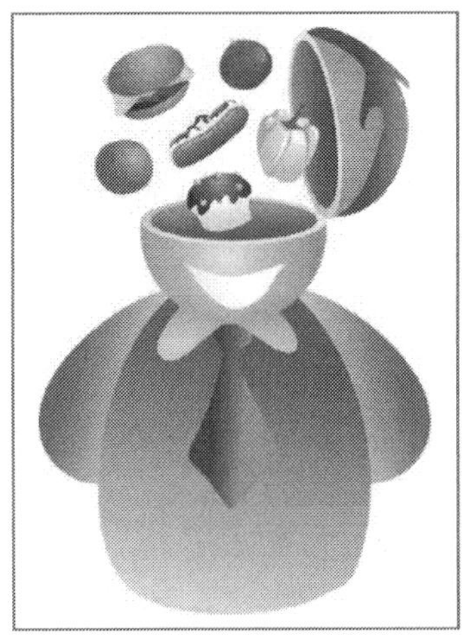

Guidebook #5 *Why People Don't Lose Weight*

You should recall that earlier in the *Mind Diet Collection of Guidebooks*, I talked about the fact that there are only two reasons to eat and drink:

- Sustenance – in order to live
- Everything else – a wide variety of reasons, both good and bad

Our bodies do not need much food to live and be healthy, certainly not nearly the amounts we consume. If we all ate only what our bodies need, we'd all be thin. So let's concentrate on "everything else" – all the other reasons we eat. Here is my list of the top 20 reasons why we don't lose weight and can't keep it off.

#1: Medical Reasons

Situation: there are numerous medical reasons for weight gain, including an underactive thyroid, a specific ovarian syndrome, Cushing's syndrome, medications and family history of obesity.

Solution: if you have a medical issue that is causing weight gain, suspect you do, or haven't thought about it, the first step is to consult with your doctor. Ask him/her about potential causes for weight gain, and should it turn out that you are impacted by one of these, what to do about it.

#2: Celebrations

Situation: we love to celebrate all kinds of positive outcomes, and we've become conditioned to celebrating by eating. And while I've done my share of eating to celebrate, those dining out or eating in occasions always result in weight gain, simply because we tend to overeat when we're in a celebratory mood.

Solution: between birthdays, anniversaries, graduations and other events, let's say you have 20 occasions a year to celebrate something. Why not take 25% of them and do something other than eating. Celebrate by going to a concert, show, comedy club, bowling or anything else you enjoy doing instead of eating. And when you do eat, be aware that we all tend to eat more during celebrations, so make up your mind ahead of time to take small portions, drink plenty of water first, and stay away from sugary desserts.

#3: Frustration

Situation: when we are frustrated by other people or events, we often turn to food because it's "instant gratification," tastes great and is readily available. When I sold advertising in my first job, I was guilty with a capital G of this. When I got turned down by a store owner, I found a snack to make myself feel better. I'm sure we've all done this over and over without really thinking about it.

Solution: the key here is to think not about food but the root cause of what frustration that resulted in eating. In my example, I should have focused on **why** I didn't sell the ad and find a way to reverse that, rather than thinking about eating as a reaction to my particular frustration.

#4: No Self-Control

Situation: you feel like you have no control over eating, as if someone has hijacked your mind and told it to eat now.

Solution: well, that's bunk, and here's why. You DO have self-control over most things in your life. There are thousands of situations where you exhibit self-control. What's going on here is that you choose NOT to exert self-control, and then blame your out-of-control mind for your eating. If you think you have a self-control issue coming on, snap out of it and remember that you do have self-control over when and what you eat.

#5: Peer Pressure

Situation: we all know how tough peer pressure can be, especially if you enjoy being with your friends/colleagues/classmates. Whether it's simply an invitation to join a group at a restaurant, or a more forceful peer who loves food, peer pressure is something you need to learn to deal with.

Solution: I've indicated during the discussion about reaching your Moment of Truth that it is extremely important for you to get the support and cooperation of friends and family. The best way to do this is tell everyone that's close to you that you've made a very important decision, to once and for all lose weight…and that you would greatly appreciate their support. This means that they should not push food on you and give you the option of passing on an outing to a buffet. When people who support you do this, they remove or reduce the effect of peer pressure. Peer support is a very important aspect of weight loss success. If your friends are all food-focused, consider making new friends that are more into a healthy lifestyle.

A reader says, "No one if forcing you to eat bad foods. If you go out with a group or a friend, plan ahead to make the right choices, no matter what they do. I used to want to blend in, but I decided my health was much more important."

#6: Widespread Availability of Food

Situation: food is available everywhere! Not just restaurants, supermarkets, convenience stores and drug-stores. Food – especially snacks and candy loaded with sugar – are in Home Depot, Office Max, gas stations, airport stores and kiosks, and on and on. You can't escape the constant presence of food.

Solution: keep healthy snacks, such as nuts and fruits, with you, so you have something to munch while you're waiting for gas, waiting for your flight or waiting just about anywhere. And whenever you see candy, cakes and other sugar-laden foods, visualize a skull-and-crossbones as part of the packaging, as a reminder to stay away from them.

#7: Appeal of Food

Situation: images of food make them so appealing. High-definition TV, mouthwatering air-brushed pictures in magazines and on menus, and sensory stimulating copy that describes food makes them irresistible. Displays on buffets and in stores also are designed to get you to buy without tasting first.

Solution: chances are that your experience with food images is a lot like mine: the actual food never lives up to the photos, copy and video. Bake that thought into your mind, so that when you see food images, you instantly remember that you'll most likely be disappointed when you consume the food, and therefore, it's not worth it!

#8: Strategic Placement of Food

Situation: I'm sure you've noticed the racks of candy bars at supermarket checkout lanes, right? And when you go to pay at a department store, you might find chocolates right next to the register. Or, every time I buy something at Walgreens, the clerk points to candy bars and asks if I want to buy them. You won't see veggies in checkout lanes or next to registers. Food, especially food that's bad for you, is in full view almost everywhere you shop, strategically placed to catch your eye.

Solution: develop an association with food that's designed to be impulse buys, by associating them with a big red circle and line that denotes "no" – like this:

This technique will reinforce that these are foods, usually laden with sugar, are no good for you.

#9: Emphasis on Big Dinners

Situation: for most of our lives, we've been conditioned to eat big dinners. Families usually eat dinner together more so than any other meal. While you always hear people say "I'm looking forward to a nice big dinner," you rarely hear people say that about breakfast or lunch. And many people look forward to a big dinner as a reward after a long day's work.

Solution: I've learned (after being a "big dinner" guy for more years than I'd like to admit!) that going small for dinner is a big, big reason for my weight loss. Many nights I have nothing more than a delicious salad for dinner, and by having a lot less food in your stomach before you go to bed, it makes a huge difference. If you don't eat breakfast and lunch, do so. And reduce the size of your dinners.

#10: Eating vs. Other Activities

Situation: "let's go out to eat" seems to be one of the first choices when we want to celebrate something or just get out of the house. We don't hear "let's go for a hike" or "let's go play basketball" in these situations. And in most cases, it's "let's go out for dinner." Since the appetizing menus and oversized portions served in most restaurants almost always lead to weight gain, thinking of eating out as a first choice is not the right one if you're really serious about losing weight.

Solution: the key here is not to make a quick spur-of-the-moment decision at the last minute to go eat out. It's better to take some time to think of a more meaningful way to celebrate an event that doesn't revolve solely around food. Maybe it's going bowling, where food (i.e. a pizza) is secondary would be a better (and more fun!) choice. Plan events in advance when there is time to think about what to do, instead of relying on the old standby of eating out.

#11: Stress

Situation: it's my personal belief that stress is one of the top reasons people eat when they're not hungry, and eat bad foods. Eating as a reaction to stress is clearly the wrong response, even though it gives one instant gratification.

Solution: in the same way you've reached your Moment of Truth and made a serious commitment to losing weight, you need to make the same commitment to eliminating stress. This process starts with making a formal statement to yourself and others in your circle of family and friends: "I am going to eliminate stress from my life because it's unhealthy and results in my eating foods that are not good for me." I don't mean to over simplify this issue, but I have learned that almost any decision starts with a commitment to YOU!

#12: Conflict

Situation: you have a disagreement or fight with your boss, spouse, sibling or friend, and you immediately go for the junk food. In my mind, conflict is simply another form of stress, and the response you choose to a conflict directly impacts your eating pattern.

Solution: the preceding paragraph on stress is pretty much the same advice for conflicts. Learning how to deal with conflict is critical, and junk food can't be the response every time there is conflict in your life. I'm sure you know that communication is the key to dealing with conflict. Figuring out an ability to deal with conflict without food is the correct response to this situation.

A reader offers this viewpoint: "Remember, eating junk just adds another problem to the original problem."

#13: Disappointment

Situation: another reason why people turn to food is to deal with disappointment. Life is full of them, and how you deal with things that don't go your way is critical.

Solution: Eating is the wrong response of disappointment. Turn your source of disappointment around, not by eating, but by dealing directly with the cause.

#14: Eating When Not Hungry

Situation: one of my basic beliefs is that you should not eat unless you're actually hungry. I'm convinced because I used to do this, that most people do in fact, eat when they are not hungry. Perhaps they imagine they're hungry or talk themselves into believing they are hungry. In any event, eating when you're not hungry, especially at night, is not going to help your weight loss efforts.

Solution: I've asked you on several occasions to make commitments to yourself. This is no different. Simply make up your mind that you're not going to eat unless you're hungry. And, if you have friends or family that like to push food on you, let them know you're not going to eat if you're not hungry.

One reader said "I used to binge, but then I started planning to eat healthy snacks that were enough to prevent me from binging."

#15: Portion Sizes

Situation: the operators of restaurants realized a long time ago the value of large portions and buffets, because people like getting a lot of food for their money and in the case of buffets, they like to talk about how much food they ate which in turn benefits the restaurant. With food being plentiful and inexpensive in the U.S., big portions and buffets have become the norm. That creates a big problem for people who want to lose weight.

Solution: buffets are really enticing, so the best way to avoid eating too much is by not going to them in the first place. If someone wants to go to a buffet, just say no. And be firm – just don't go. In terms of restaurants, decide **ahead of time** what you're going to eat. Check out their menu online, and make your wise choice ahead of time, instead of being influenced by the menu, photos, descriptive copy, etc.

#16: Eating 3 Meals a Day

Situation: we've been conditioned, pretty much from birth, to eat three meals a day. The phrase "three square meals" has been around forever. And in so many situations, we don't have time for a good breakfast, often skip lunch, and then have big dinners. And some people key in on the word "square" as meaning plentiful, giving them the thought that they need to eat three big meals.

Solution: our bodies don't need much food. They certainly don't need a lot of food, three times a day. Plus, our eating habits are backwards. Perhaps the most important change I've made is to simply reverse my former eating habits:

- I eat a healthy breakfast, but not a large one.
- I eat a smaller lunch
- I usually eat a much smaller dinner – in fact, dinner is the smallest meal of the day

#17: Food Exposure

Situation: we are all presented with waves of food eating opportunities all day long. This includes food advertising, invites to dine out, snacks co-workers bring to work, scheduled meals, passing by snack machines at work, and on and on. The temptation is always great, especially when there are home-baked cookies in the office or candy bars on colleague's desks.

Solution: as you know, the main goal of *The Mind Diet Collection* is to give you the ability to get motivated to truly lose weight by adhering to the beliefs that were presented in guidebook #2. **Resisting bad foods and drinks must be top-of-mind all day long**. You must need to say "no" when you're offered food, and you must associate snacks with the dozens of diseases and conditions that being overweight causes or impacts.

#18: Group Binge Eating

Situation: you've heard of binge drinking, but how about binge eating? It's where a bunch of people go to a restaurant or tailgate at a football game, and they encourage each other to eat and eat and eat. They order a lot of food, way more than is prudent, and everyone ends up pigging out because they don't want to be embarrassed.

Solution: while these kinds of get-togethers may be fun, one of them can set you back a couple of weeks. Simple solution: if you hang with people who do this, just don't go. Peer pressure combined with good-smelling food is hard to resist...unless you're not there.

#19: Because It's "Free"

Situation: when you're at a party, basically the food is free. Yes, you may have brought a dish, but the rest of the food was paid for by someone else. As we all know, the word "free" is extremely powerful, and I believe people overeat when they aren't paying for food.

Solution: have a "party plan" that is top-of-mind before you arrive. Drink a lot of water ahead of time or when you get there. That will fill you up. Concentrate on conversation, not food. It's easier than it sounds.

#20: Because You're "Trying" to Lose Weight

Situation: whenever I hear "I'm trying" about anything, but especially about weight, that's a dead giveaway, always leading to failure. When someone says "I'm trying" they are actually giving themselves a way out in case their weight loss efforts don't work.

Solution: if you find yourself "trying" to lose weight, then you need to reread the first guidebook, *Truth.* If you find your willpower is eroding, reading *Truth* will be like a refresher course to help you get back on track.

Experts and authors have identified other common reasons why people don't lose weight – all from various issues of *Prevention* Magazine:

- Christine Gerbstadt, MD, RD and author of *The Doctor's Detox Diet*, writes that if you really cut calories and have less than 1,200 per day, your body slows down your metabolism in order to hold onto the few calories you've ingested, so this can actually harm your weight loss efforts.

- Heidi Skolnik, author of *Nutrient Timing for Peak Performance*, says that if you reward yourself after a workout that burned 300 calories with a high-calorie treat, all that work is negated.

- A University of Pittsburgh study found that people who used a digital app that monitored their diets and exercise, and provided daily feedback, lost more weight than those who used paper and pen. Another study showed that dieters who recorded meals online as infrequently as once a month were three times more likely to keep off the weight compared with those who did so less frequently.

- Dean Ornish, MD and author of *The Spectrum* says that some people are good all day but blow it in the evening when they lose self-control. He suggests doing a "chocolate meditation" – take a single piece of the best chocolate you can find and let it dissolve very slowly in your mouth, so you get a lot of pleasurable taste without the added calories of eating additional pieces!

A massive study with over 120,000 people tracked over 12 to 20 years, concluded that people who were basing weight loss on common beliefs that people hold (everything in moderation, avoid fatty foods, etc.) is not optimal. NY Times Personal Health columnist Jane E. Brody reports in "Still Counting Calories?" that **counting calories is not enough – understanding the type of calories is critical**. As I've pointed out, 100 empty calories is a lot different than 100 nutritious calories. And Jane's dinner favorite, a big salad with protein and lite dressing, is what I have for dinner on many nights!

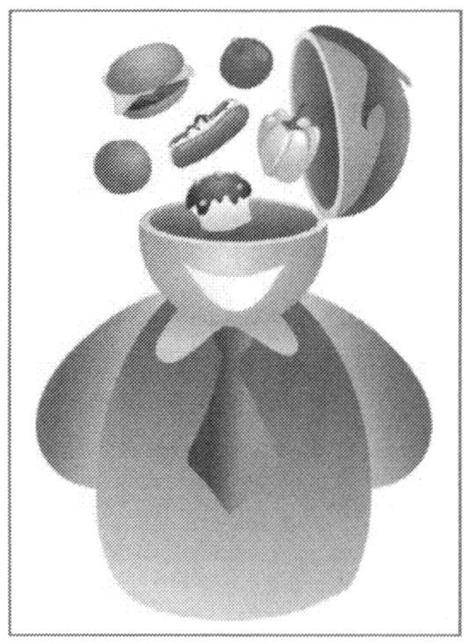

Guidebook #6 *Marriage and Weight Loss*

Successful, Long-Term Weight Loss is Exactly Like a Successful, Long-Term Marriage or Relationship

As I thought more and more about losing weight and the formula I had created to do so, the more the process was like my successful marriage to a wonderful woman named Nadine.

Hopefully what you learned in the first three *Mind Diet Guidebooks* will get you well on your way to losing weight and keeping if off. Consider this guidebook another way of looking at weight loss, in the context of a great relationship. And it could be almost any relationship: mother/daughter, father/son, brother/brother, etc.

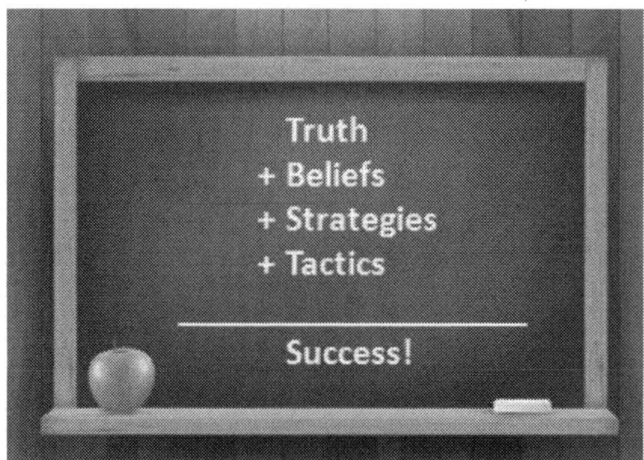

This is the weight loss formula that I created, which happens to be the same one that works in every successful marriage or relationship. To review:

- **Truth** is the moment where you make up your mind once and for all to accomplish a goal, such as losing weight or getting married.

- **Beliefs** are the ideals you see as absolutely necessary to achieving that goal.
- **Strategies** are ways of approaching situations that enable you to reach your goal.
- **Tactics** are specific things you do to lose weight and keep it off.

Truth

If you are happily married or in a solid relationship, or have been, you may recall that in the beginning, you most likely gave the potential relationship a lot of thought. You may have said these kinds of things to yourself:

- "I'm going to do everything possible to have a great relationship."
- "I really want this marriage to work."
- "I love this man and will do anything for him."

These kinds of statements closely parallel what I've suggested you do with regards to weight loss, in the *Truth* guidebook:

- "I will do everything humanly possible to lose a lot of weight and keep it off permanently."
- "I will not fail in my quest to lose weight."
- "Losing weight is the most important thing I will do for myself and my family."

See how close these "truth" statements are? Whether you thought about it or not, you reached a Moment of Truth when you first decided to have a relationship. The parallel is identical when it comes to weight loss.

Beliefs

If you ask happily married people, or those in happy relationships, they will list numerous beliefs they have about their relationships. Once you decide to enter into a meaningful relationship, you need a set of beliefs that support that major decision, that support the truth. In a happy marriage, the most basic beliefs are:

- Honesty
- Kindness
- Communications
- Respect
- Affection
- Laughter
- Listening
- Fun
- Shared Values
- Education

In the same fashion, you recall the 26 beliefs I identified in the second *Mind Diet Guidebook*. You need to formulate your beliefs for losing weight as you would for a relationship. If you think about the 26 beliefs, you'll see that they fill the same role as the beliefs you have for a successful marriage!

Strategies

Once you have truth and beliefs, layering in strategies are the day-to-day ways to have a happy marriage or lose weight and keep it off. Strategies are based on your belief system. For relationships:

- Honesty – always telling the truth
- Kindness – being empathetic and caring
- Communications – always talking through issues
- Respect – seeing the other's point of view
- Affection – holding hands, cuddling, etc.
- Laughter – making each other laugh every day
- Listening – not responding until the other is finished talking
- Fun – finding fun things to do together
- Shared Values – on the same page about issues that matter
- Education – stressing the importance of learning

In the same vein, here are a handful of strategies pertaining to weight loss with the corresponding action:

- The Power of Substitution – replacing bad foods with good foods
- Honesty & Sharing – being honest with yourself and sharing what you're doing with family and friends
- Knowledge Makes All the Difference – spending the time to learn and educate yourself about foods and diets
- Visualize Your Way to Success – picturing yourself thinner, happer and in better shape
- Tricks & Cheats Never Work – recognizing that cheating never works
- Teach Your Children Well – passing on healthy eating values to your kids

There you have it.

Successful weight loss really is like a successful marriage or relationship.

Use that knowledge to achieve greater success in both!

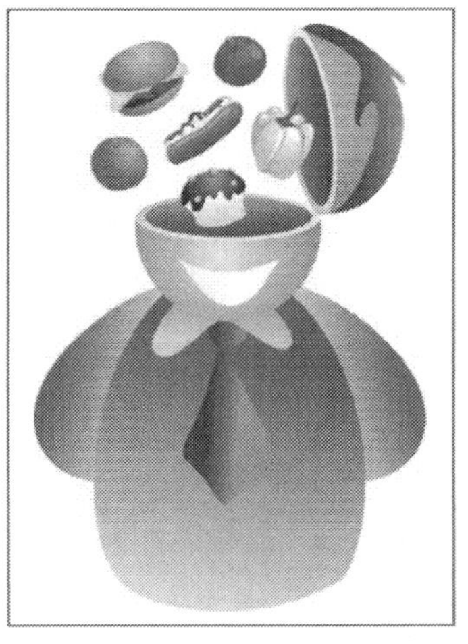

Guidebook #7
100 Great Reasons to Lose Weight

Most of us can name a dozen or so reasons to lose weight. Well, here are one hundred. Every one of them should serve as additional motivation to make sure you put everything else in life ahead of food – forever.

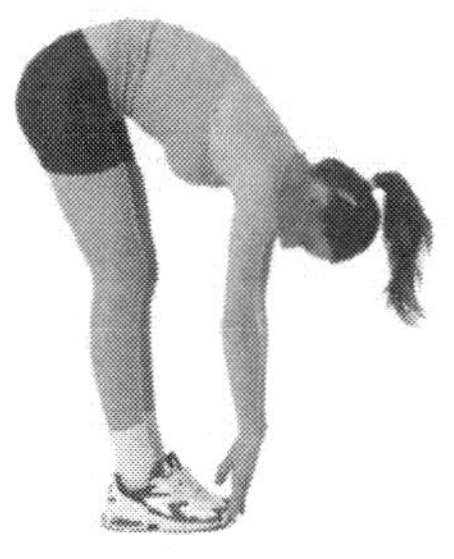

#100: Being able to touch my toes without falling over.

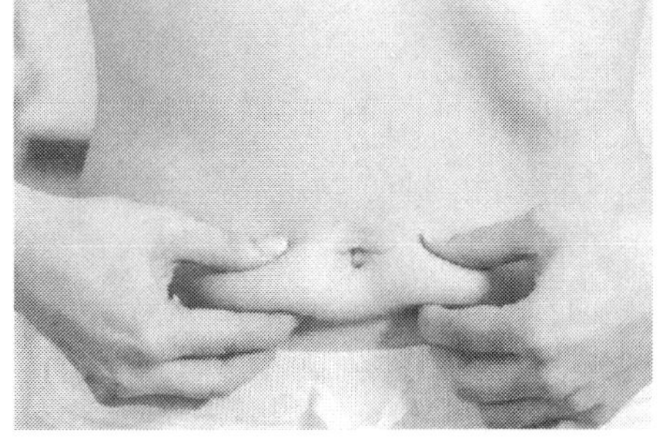

#99: No more love handles.

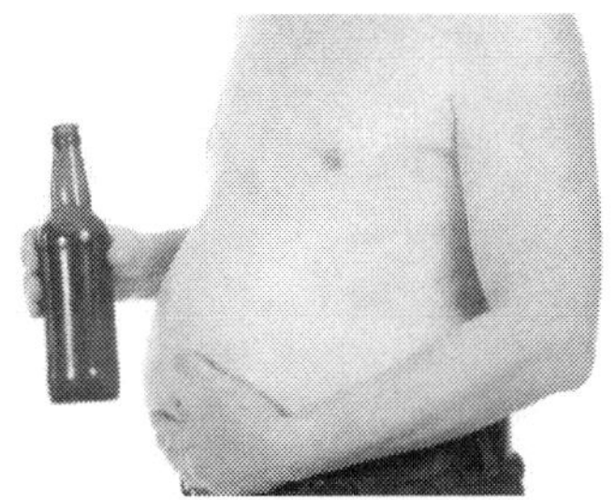

#98: No more beer belly.

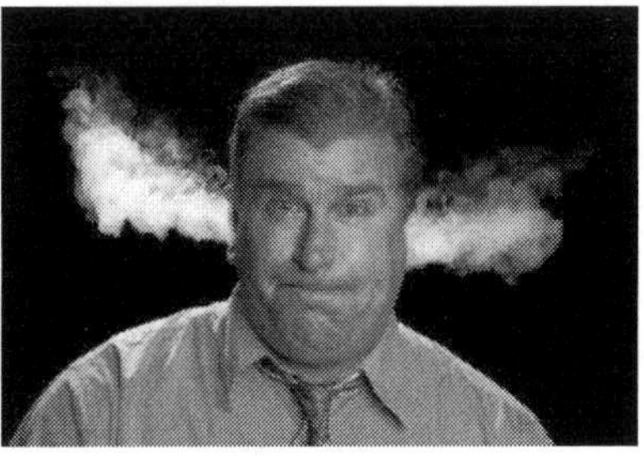

#97: No more anger over being fat.

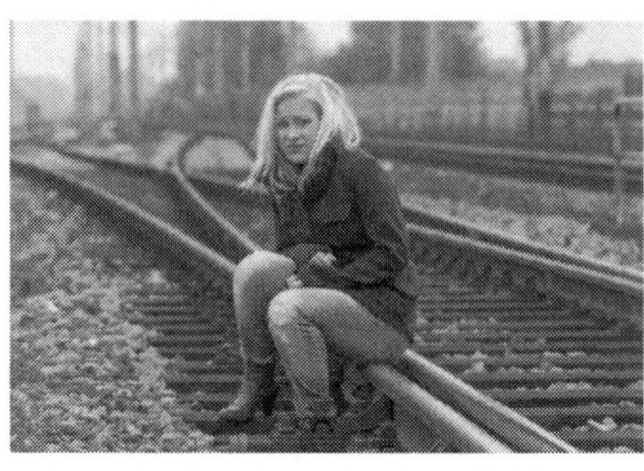

#96: No more feelings of loneliness due to being isolated as overweight.

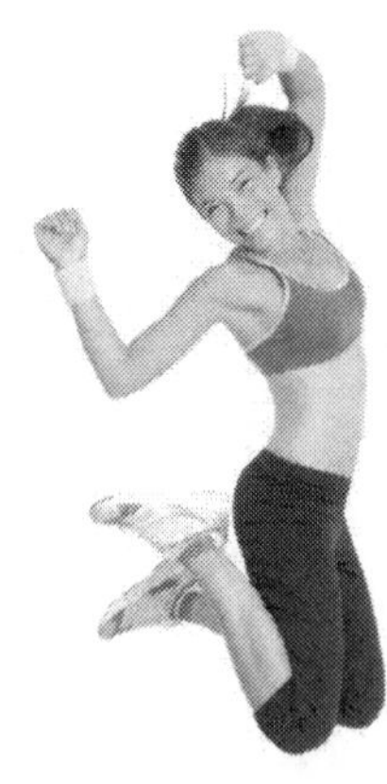

#95: Jump without hurting myself.

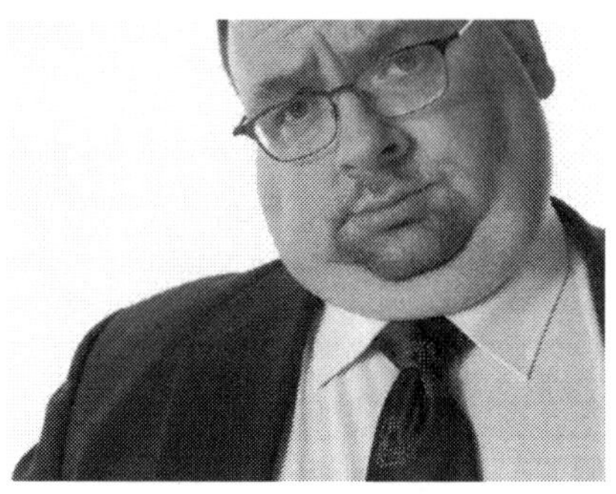

#94: No more double chin.

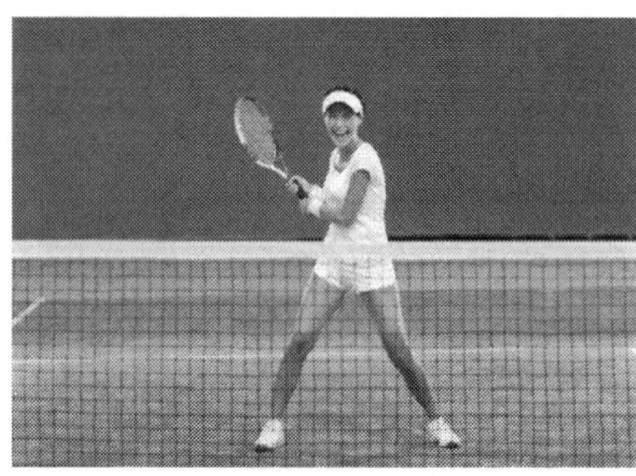

#93: Look great in shorts.

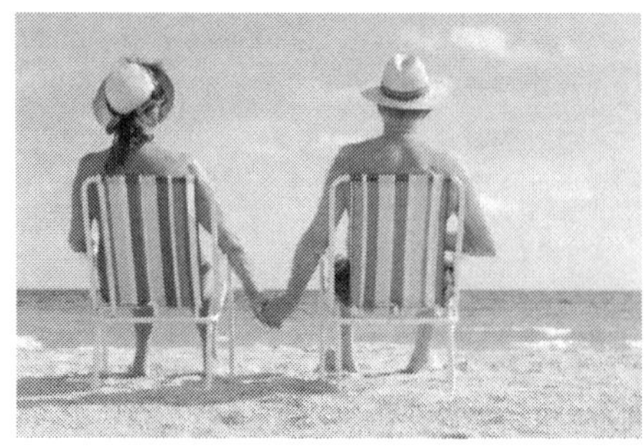

#92: Sit on a lounge chair without it sagging.

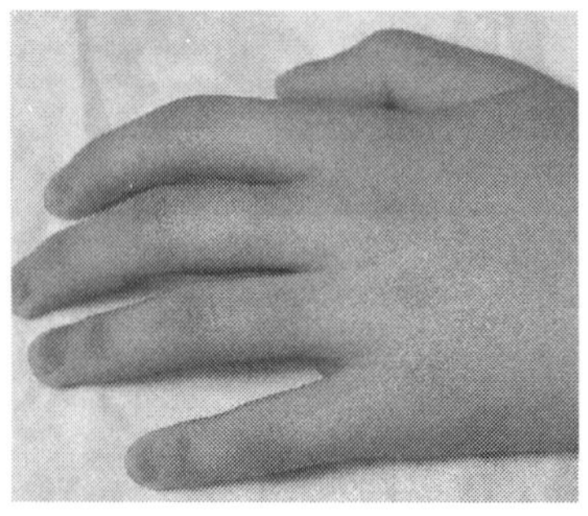

#91: No more fat fingers.

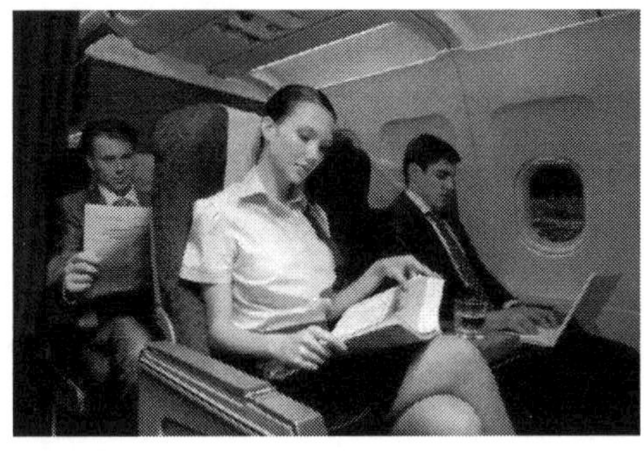

#90: Sit comfortably on a plane.

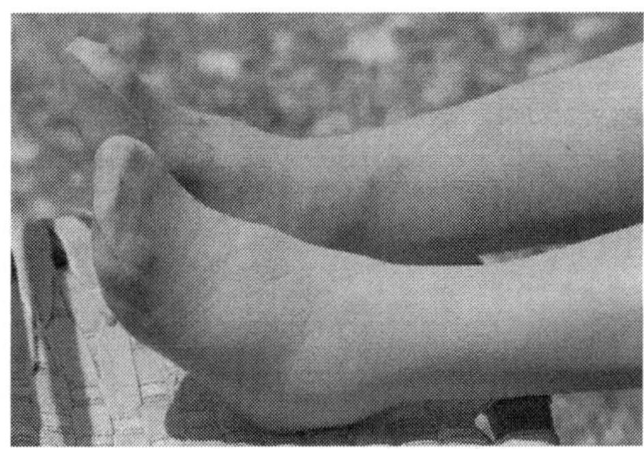

#89: No more swollen ankles and stubby toes.

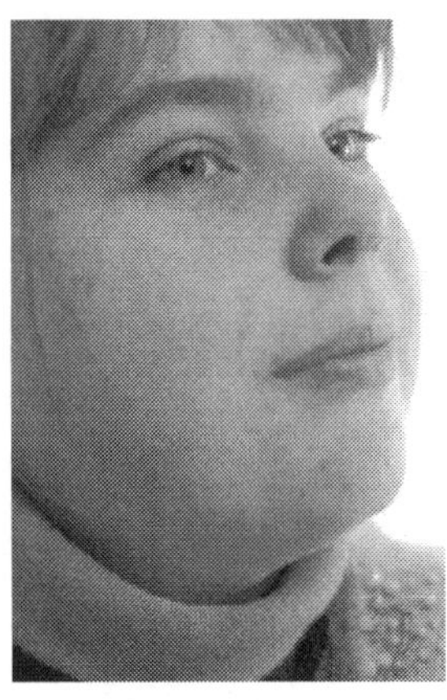

#88: No more pudgy face.

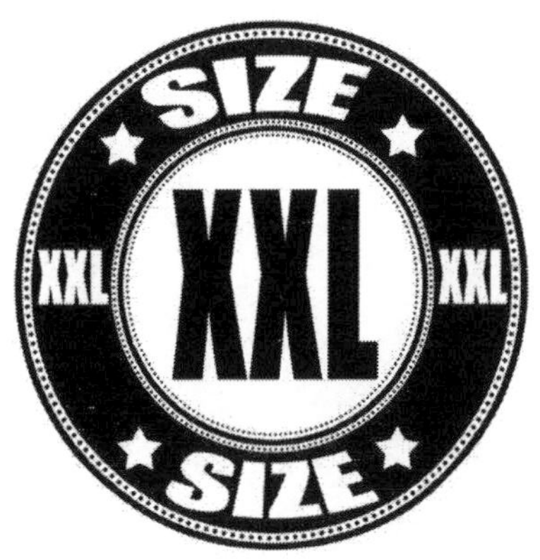

#87: No more having to buy large-sized clothing.

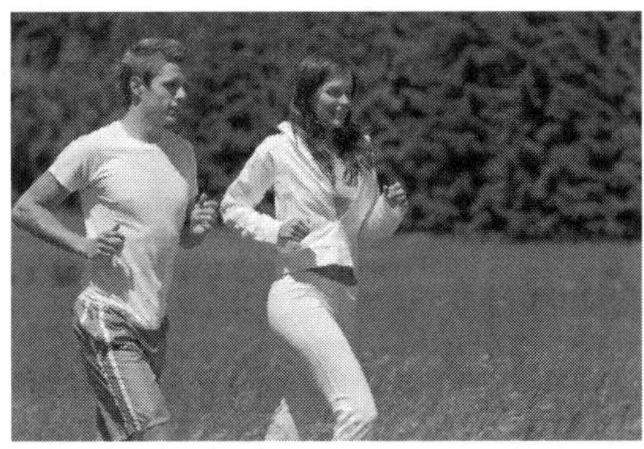

#86: Run or jog without huffing and puffing.

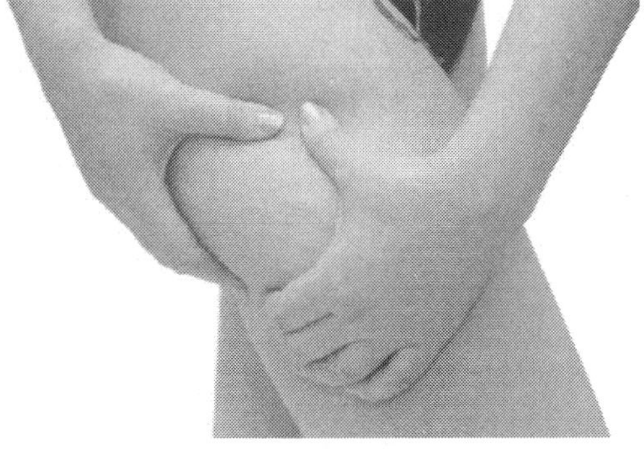

#85: No more fat legs.

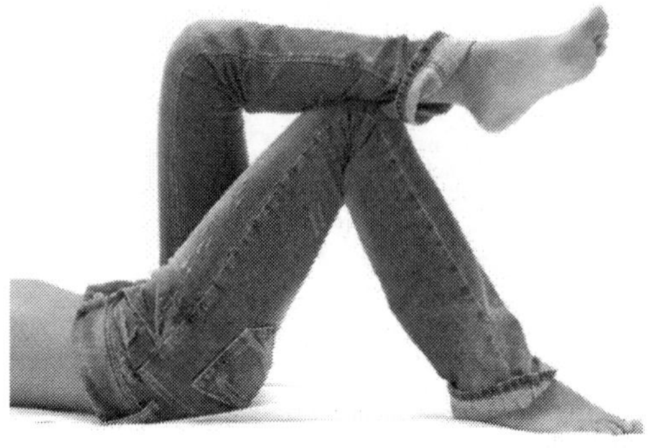

#84: Look good in tight jeans.

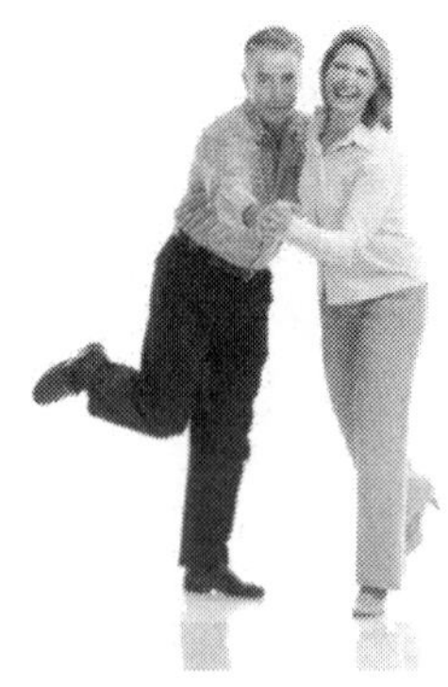

#83: Be able to dance like a star.

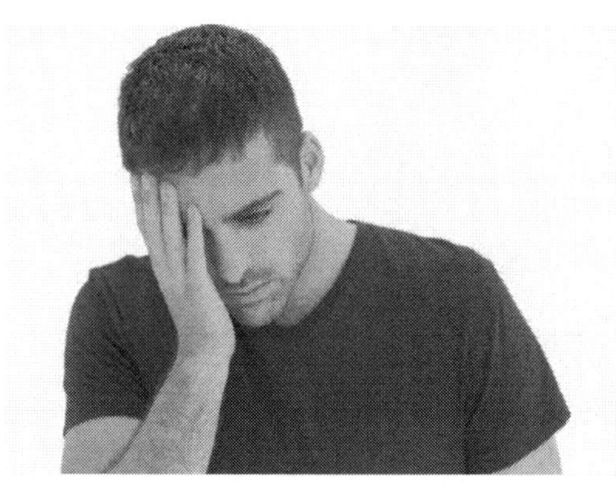

#82: No more feelings of frustration.

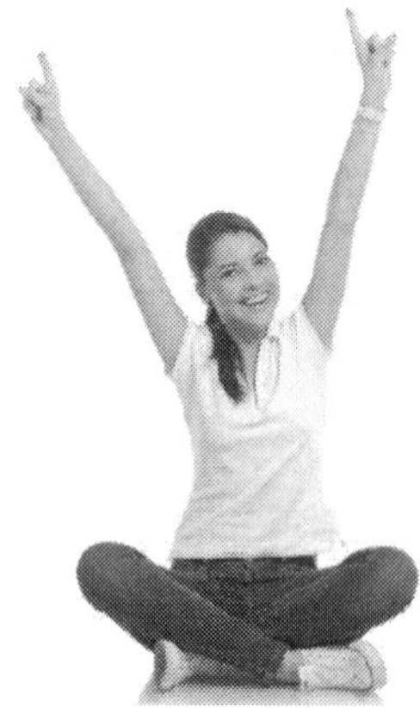

#81: Cross my legs easily and without pain.

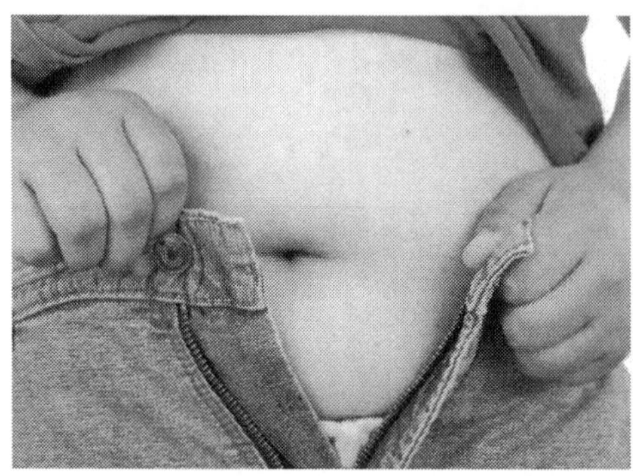

#80: No more battles zipping up pants and buttoning shirts.

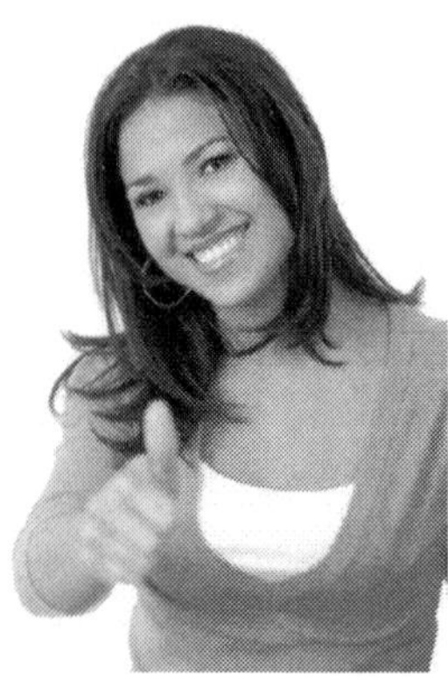

#79: Being proud of myself and the way I look.

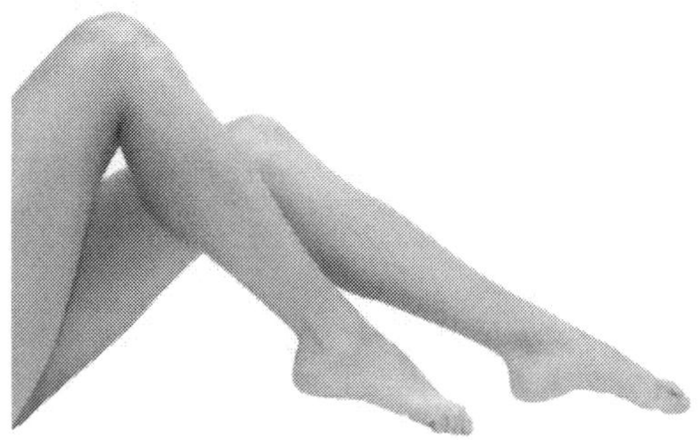

#78: Have great legs that I don't have to cover up.

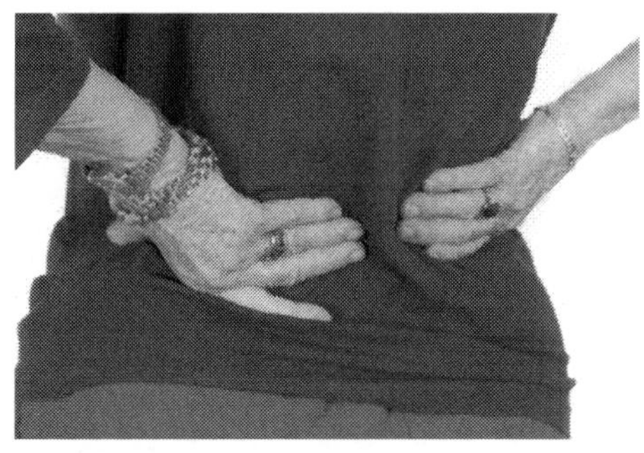

#77: No more back pain.

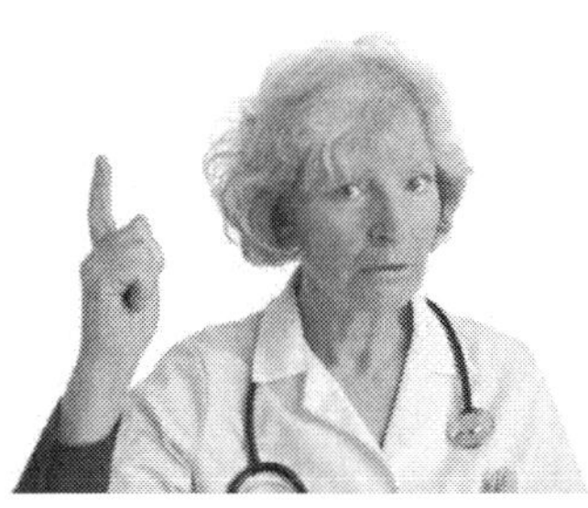

#76: No more scolding words from my doctor about losing weight.

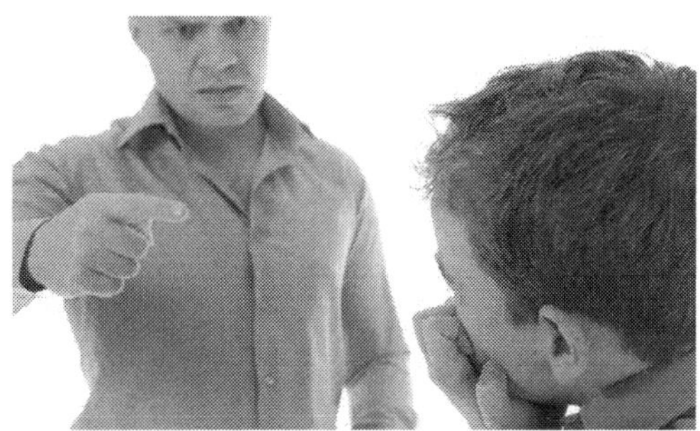

#75: No more lecturing kids that are overweight.

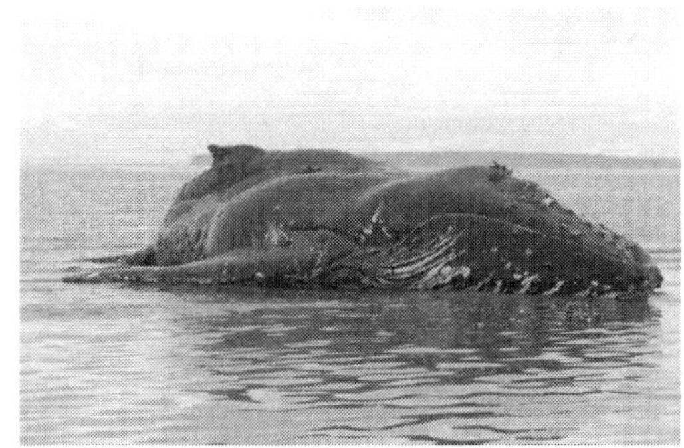

#74: No more "beached whale" remarks and other taunts.

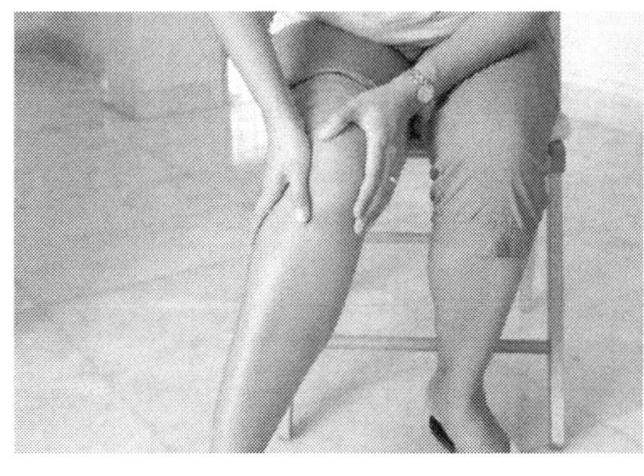

#73: No more aching joints.

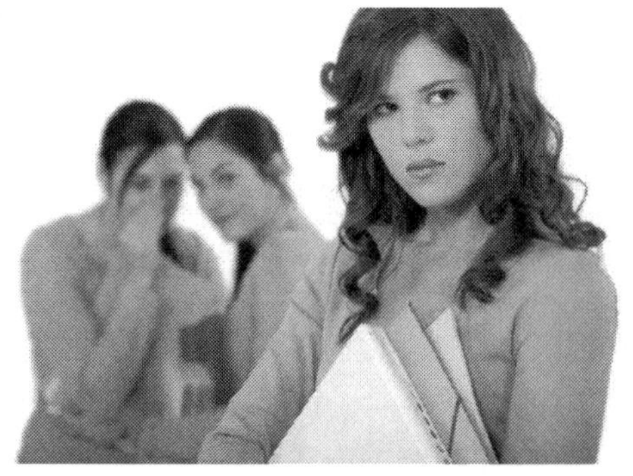

#72: No more embarrassment and exclusion by others.

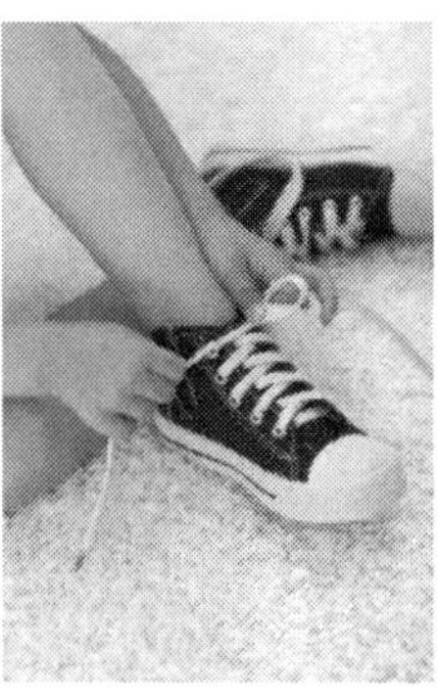

#71. Be able to tie my shoe laces easily.

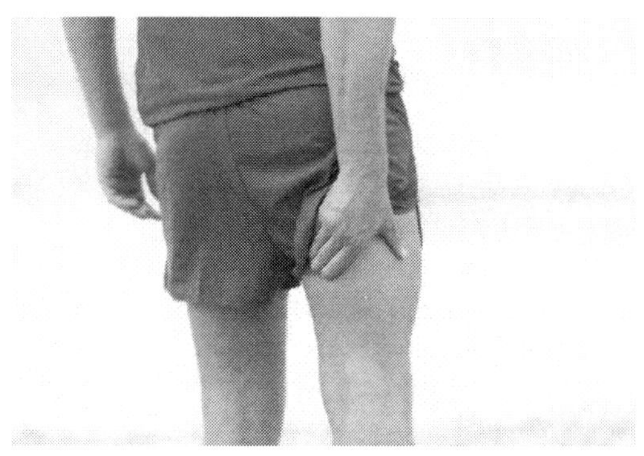

#70: No more aching thighs

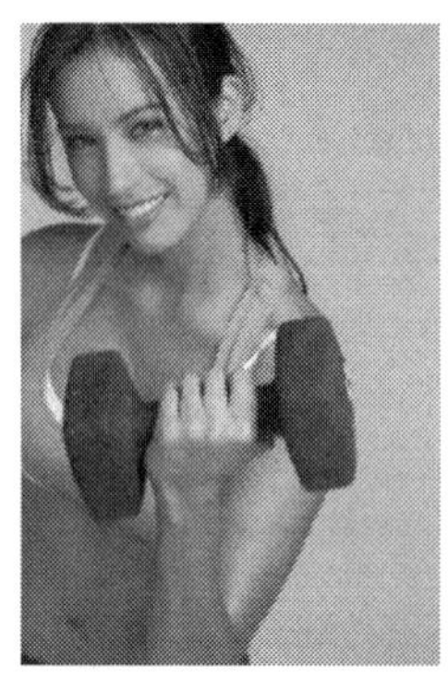

#69: Lift weights easily and develop strong muscles.

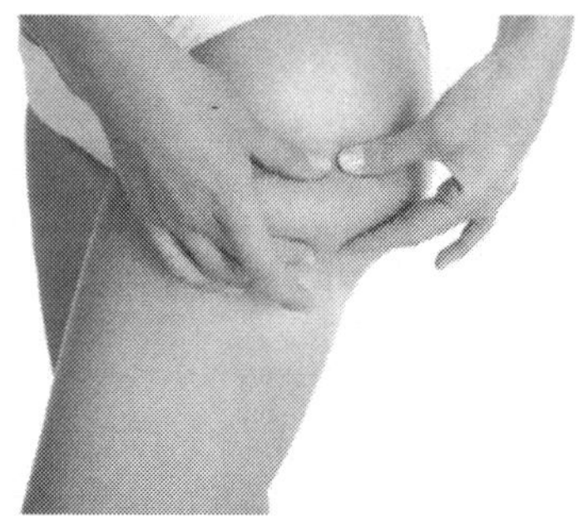

#68: No more cellulite.

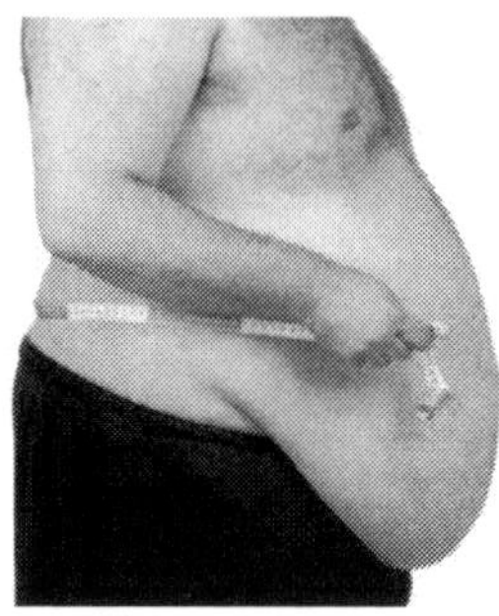

#67: No more sagging belly.

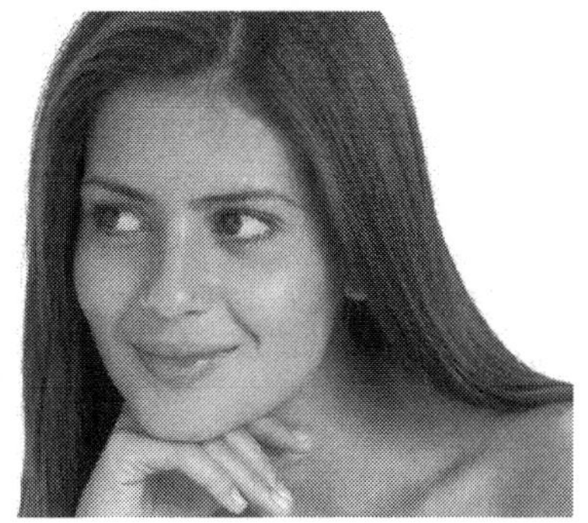

#66: Have great healthy skin.

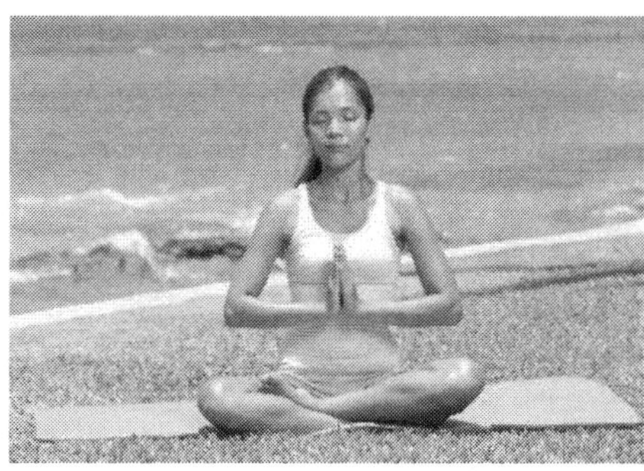

#65: Do yoga easily.

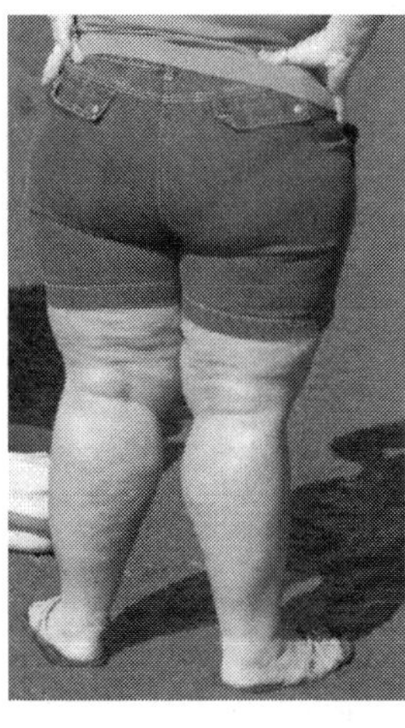

#64: Never look like this.

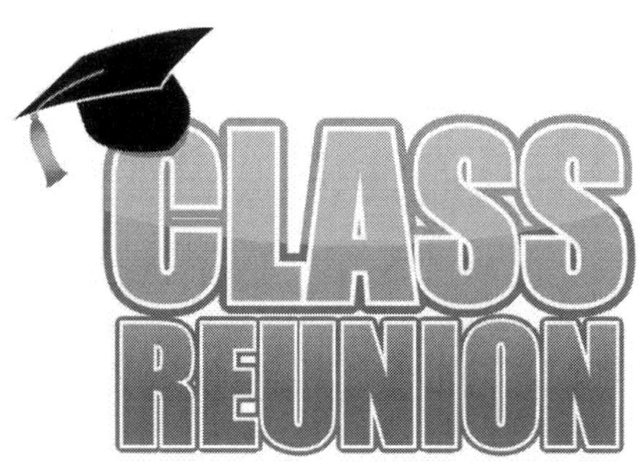

#63: Never avoid a class reunion due to being fat.

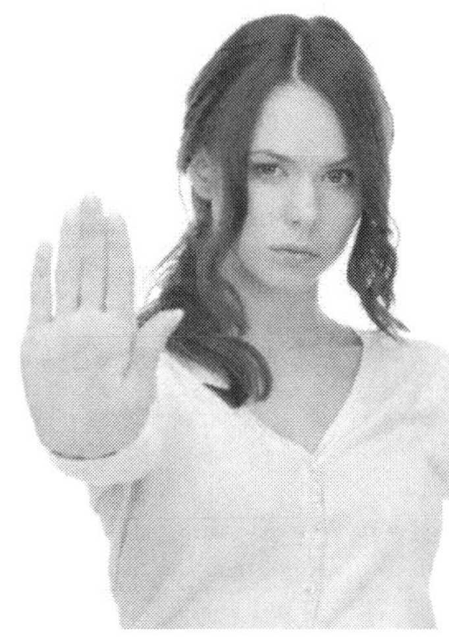

#62: No more rejection by others.

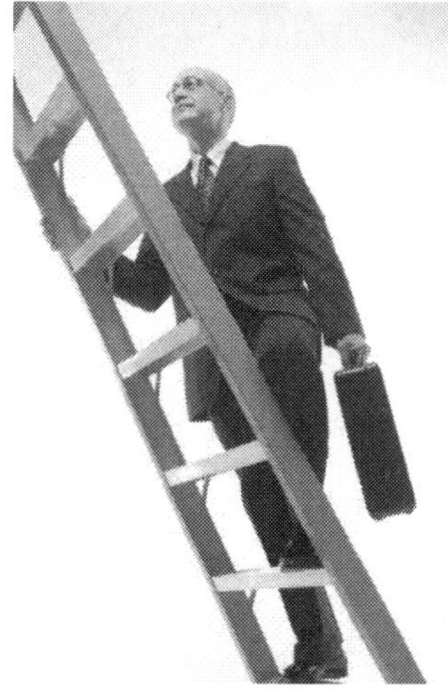

#61: Get ahead in my career without "fat discrimination."

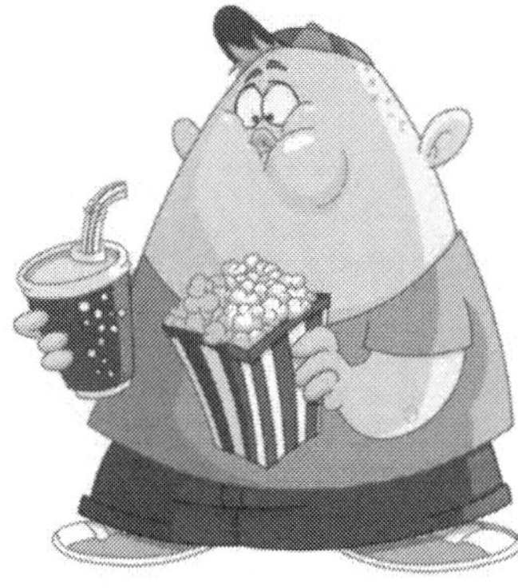

#60: No more fat jokes and insults.

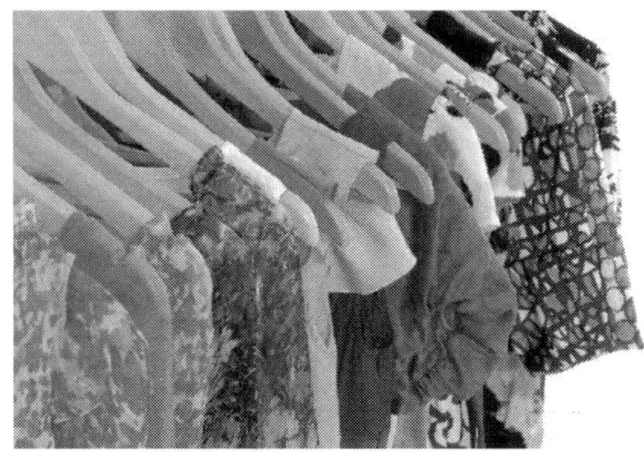

#59: Buy and wear clothes that look great on me.

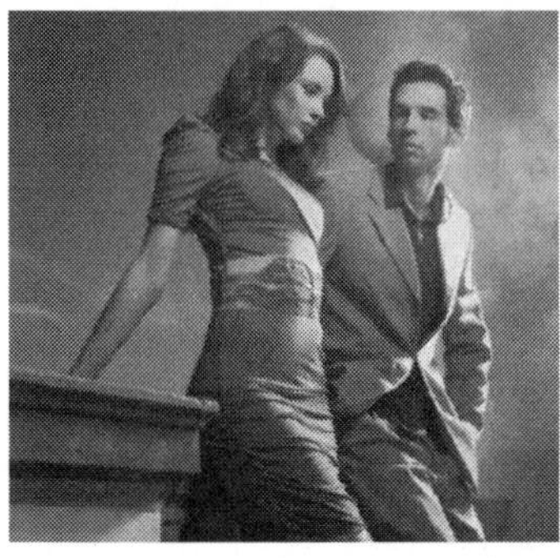

#58: Look great for my partner.

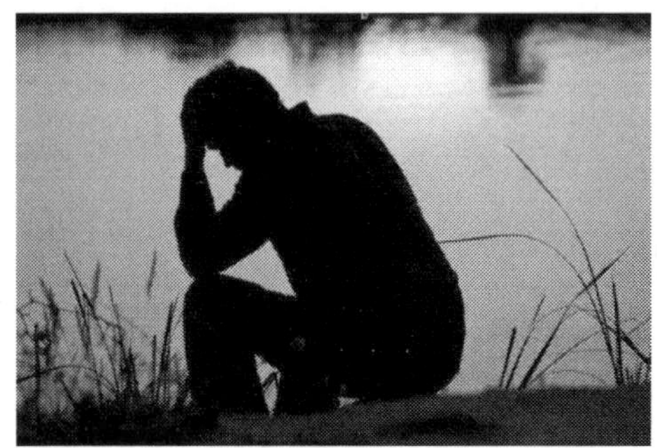

#57: Relieve feelings of depression due to weight.

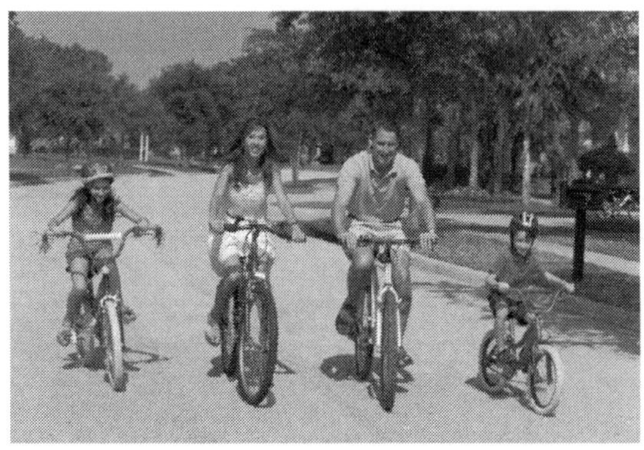

#56: Set a great example for my kids.

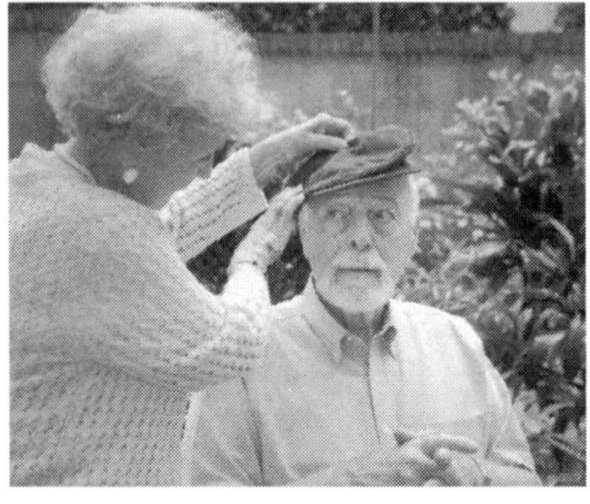

#55: Reduce risk of dementia.

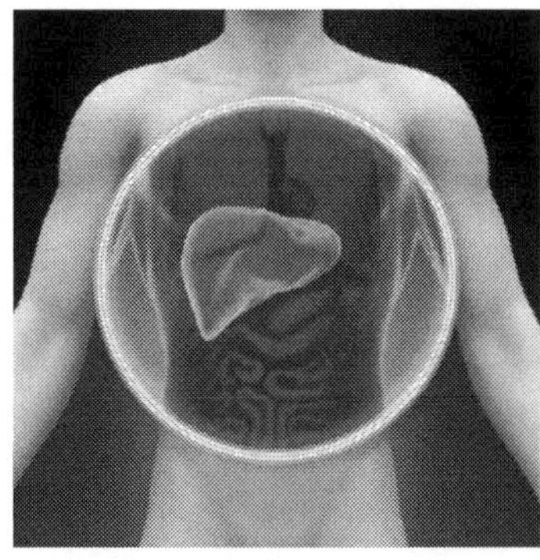

#54: Reduce risk of liver disease.

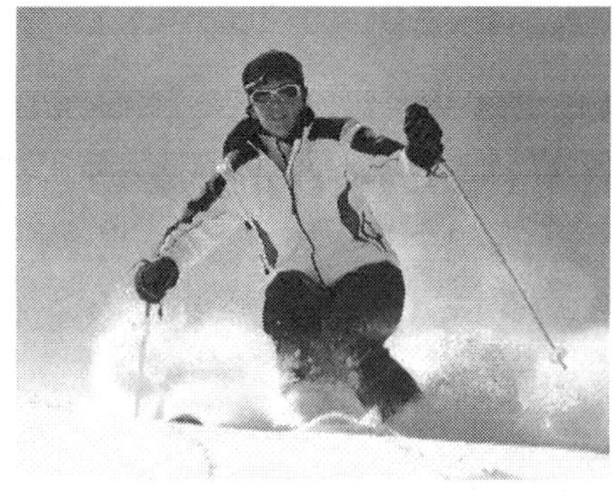

#53: Ski with ease.

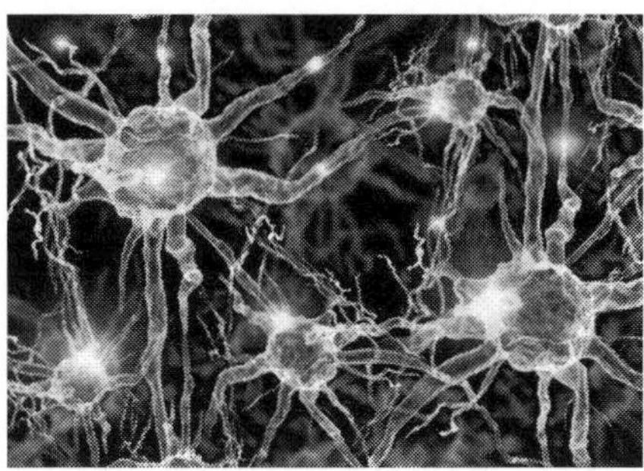

#52: Reduce risk of nerve damage.

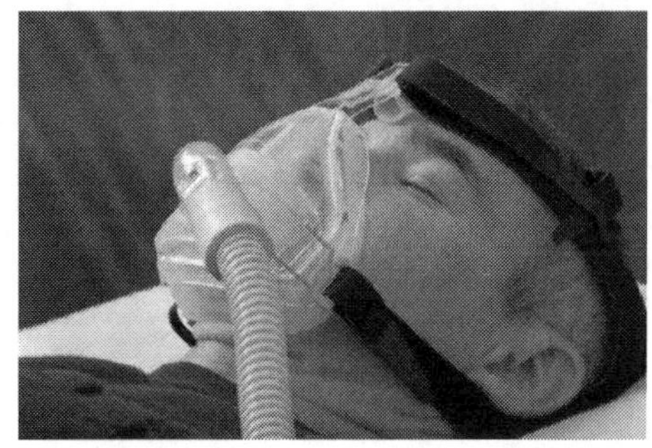

#51: Eliminate sleep apnea.

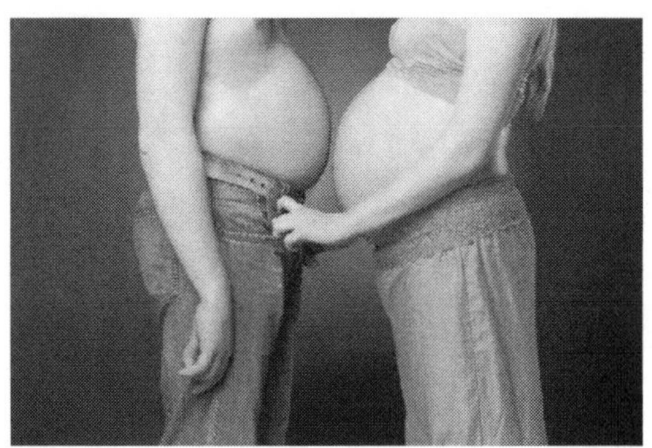

#50: Not look like my pregnant wife!

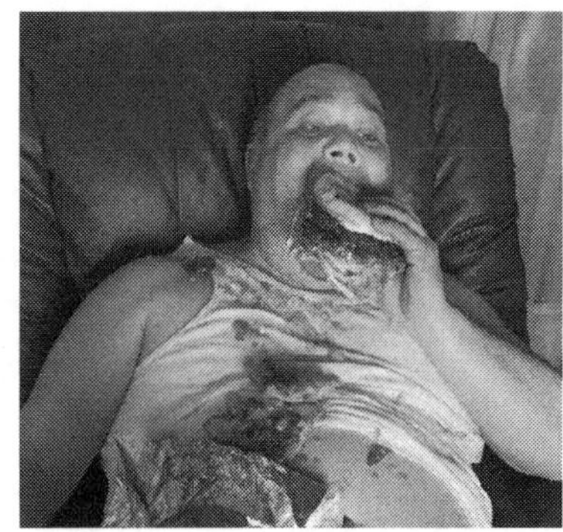

#49: Never look like this!

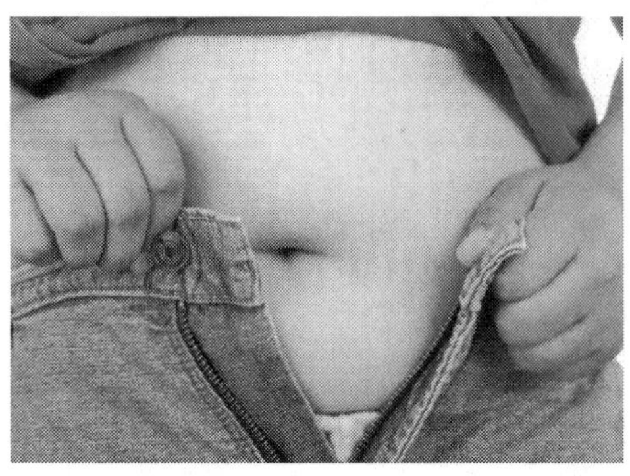

#48: Be able to button my clothes.

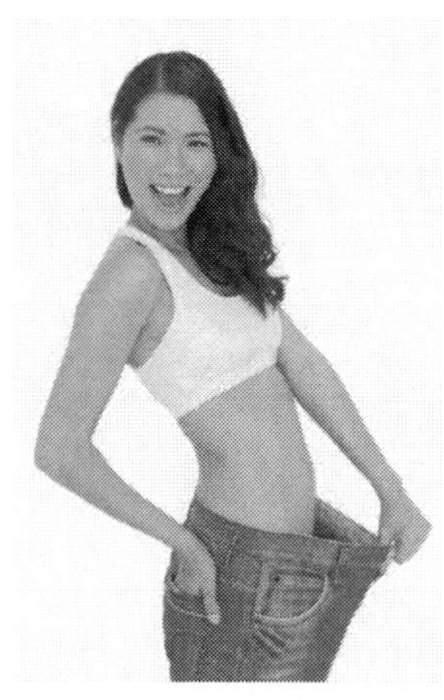

#47: Having pants too big to wear.

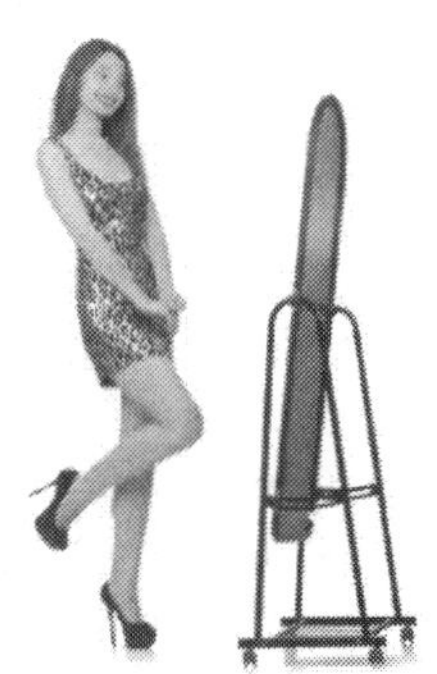

#46: Liking what I see in the mirror.

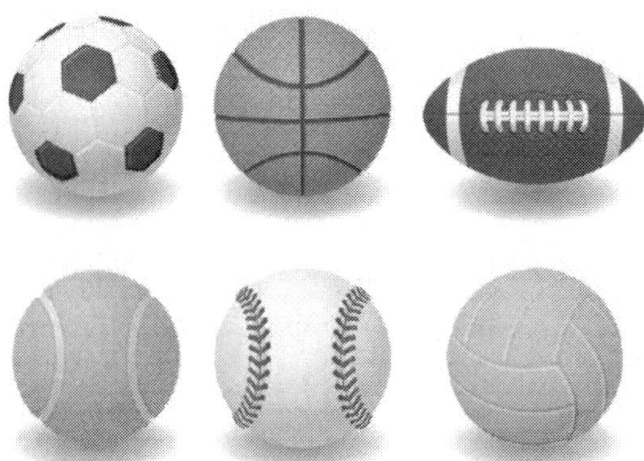

#45: Play sports instead of being a spectator.

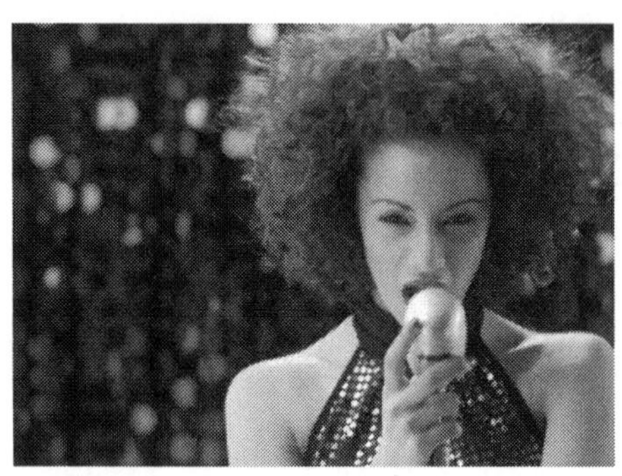

#44: Sing (and dance) easily.

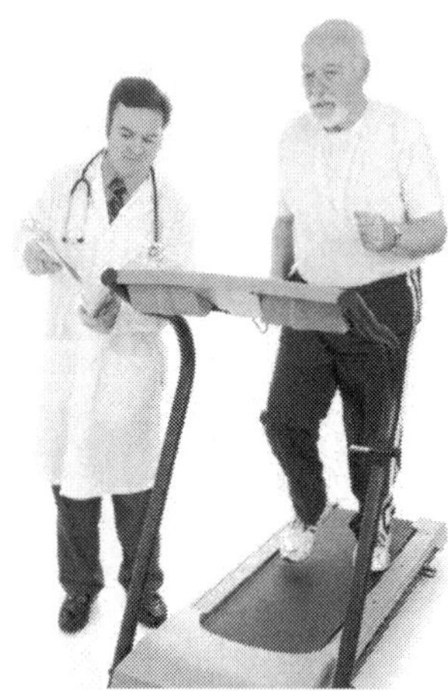

#43: Pass a fitness test.

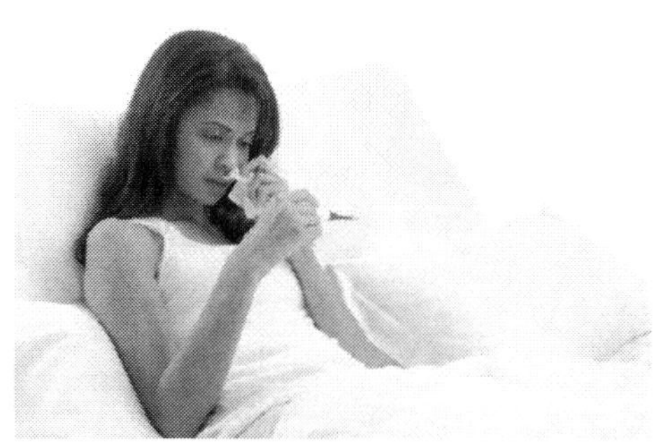

#42: Have more resistance.

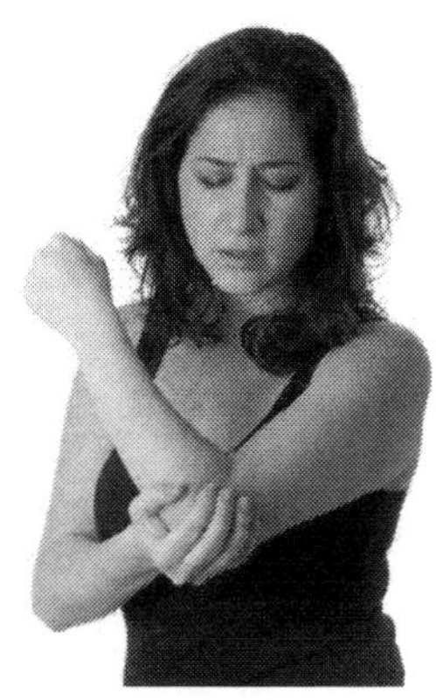

#41: Reduce joint and bone pains.

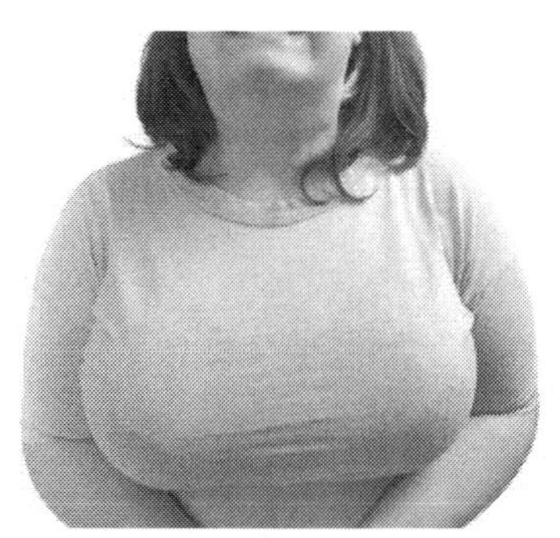

#40: Reduce chest size.

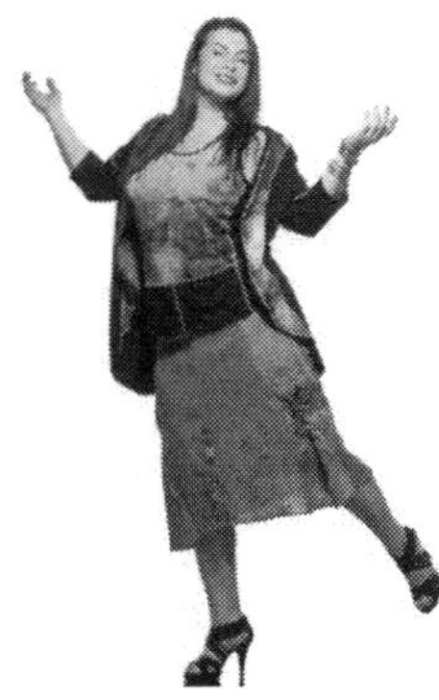

#39: Not spend a fortune and time shopping for fashionable clothing.

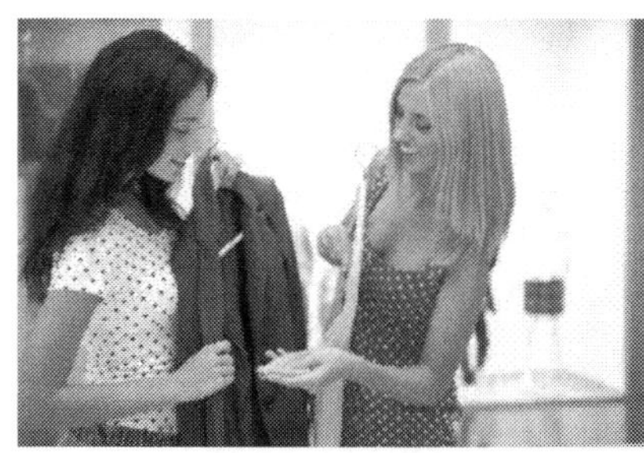

#38: Share clothes with my best friend.

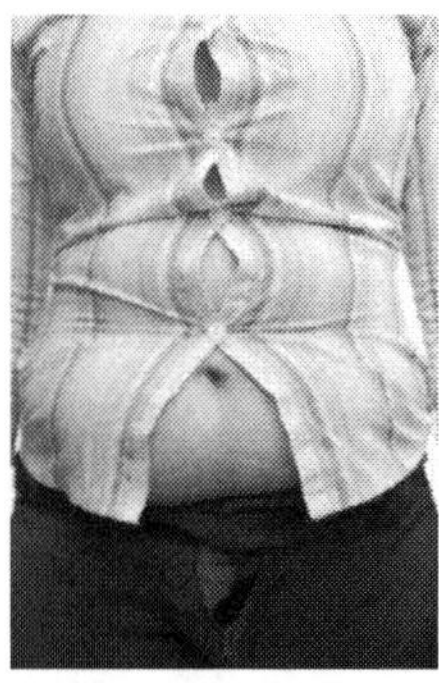

#37: Be able to tuck my shirt into my pants.

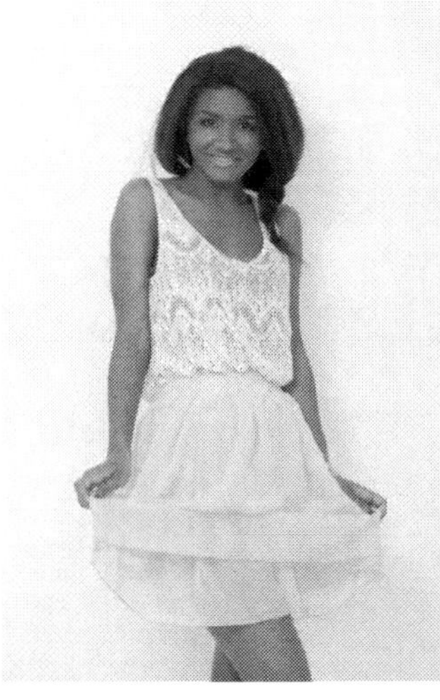

#36: Look great in a skirt or dress.

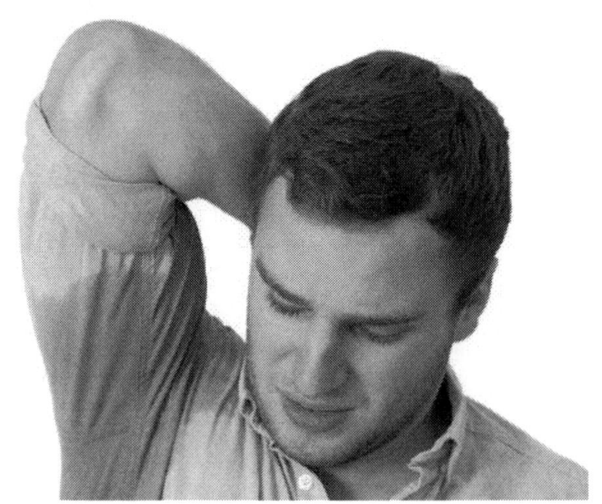

#35: Reduce sweating.

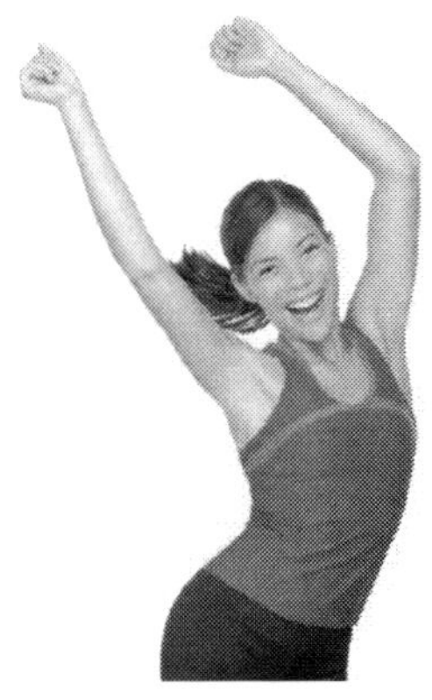

#34: Feel lighter and happier.

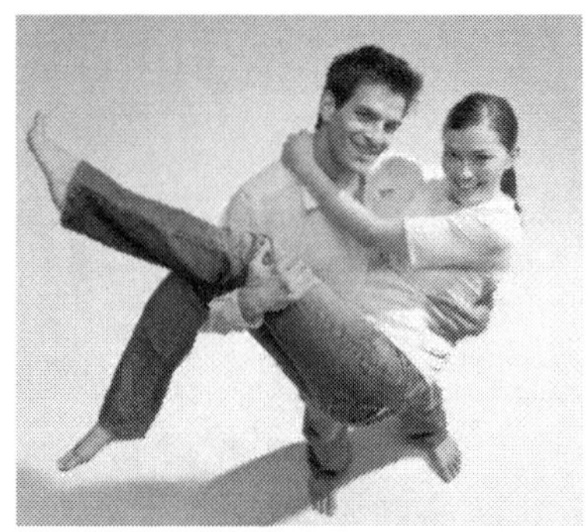

#33: Be so light that my guy can pick me up!

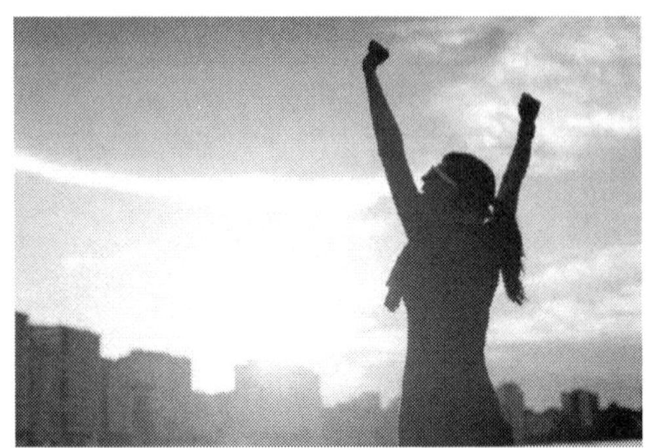

#32: Feel alert and sharp.

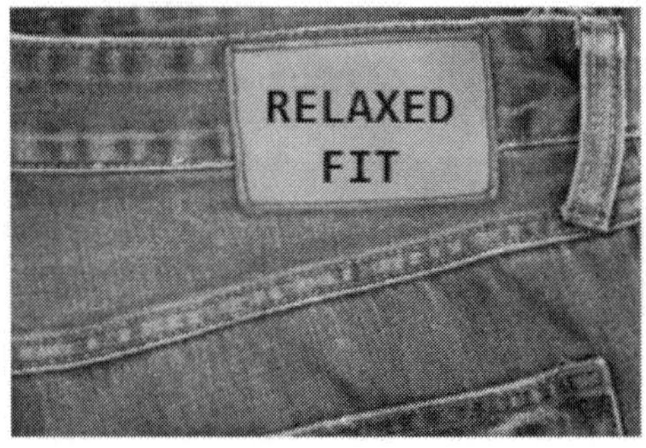

#31: Not having to buy clothes made for overweight people.

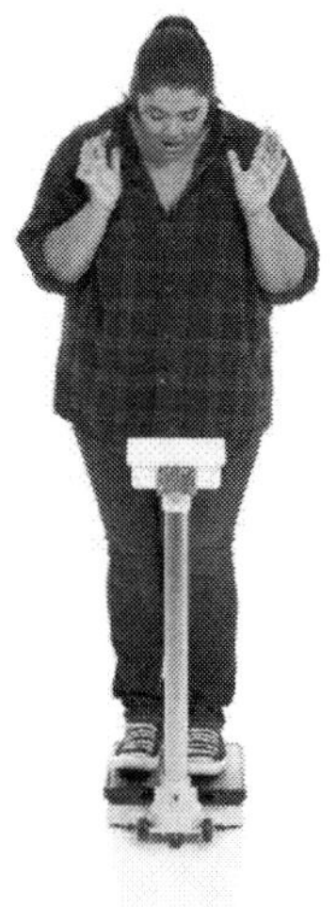

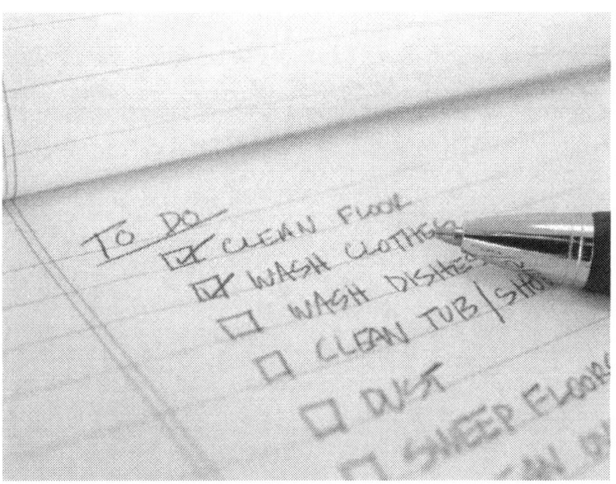

#30: Not having to constantly worry about being heavy so that I can fit in at school.

#29: So that household chores are easy to do.

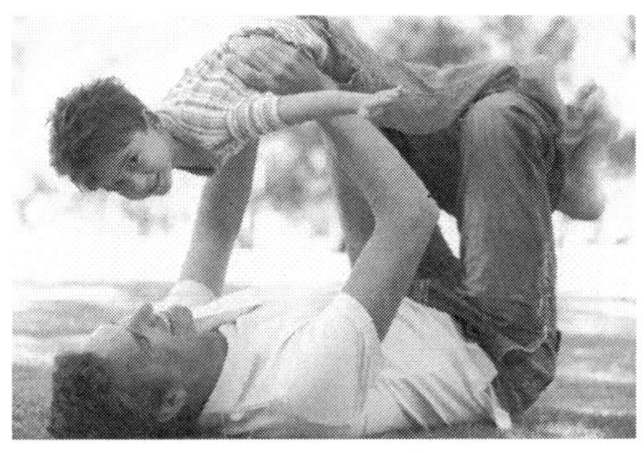

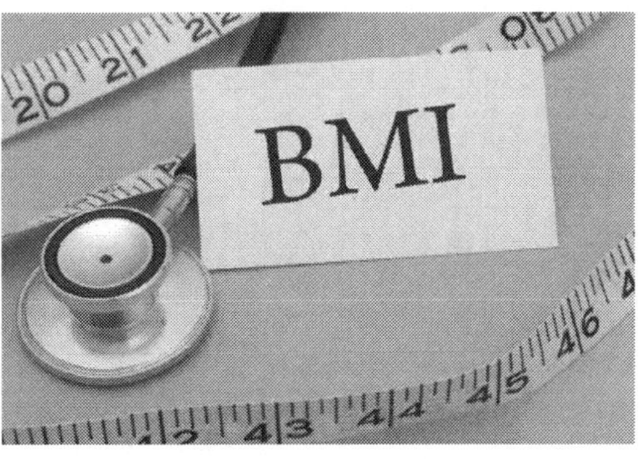

#28: Have energy to play with my kids.

#27: Lower my Body Mass Index.

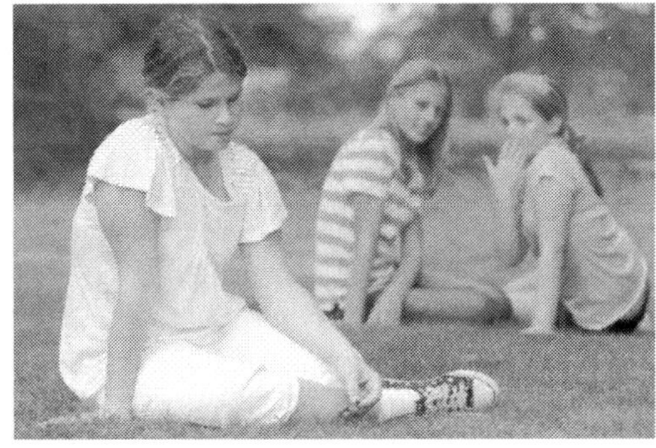

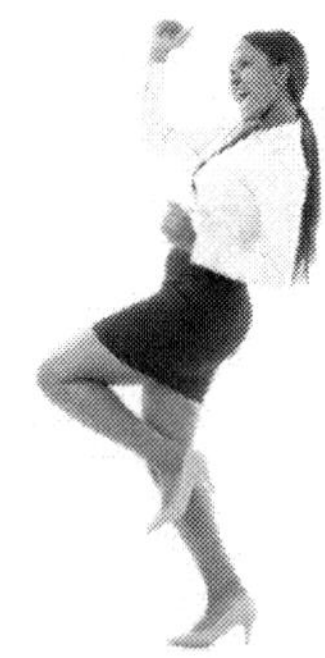

#26: Stop being taunted and laughed at.

#25: Getting complimented on how I look.

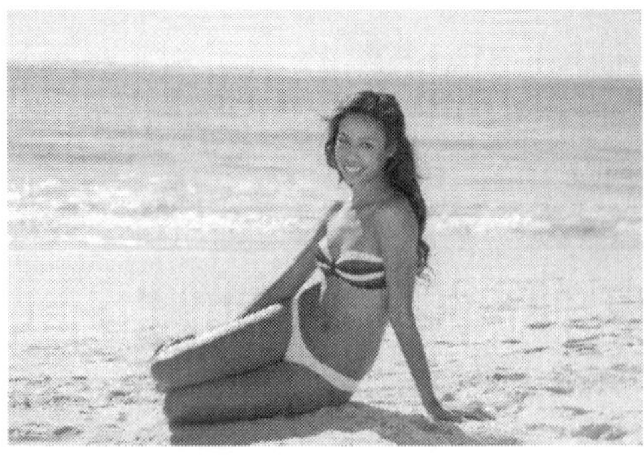

#24: Look great in a bikini.

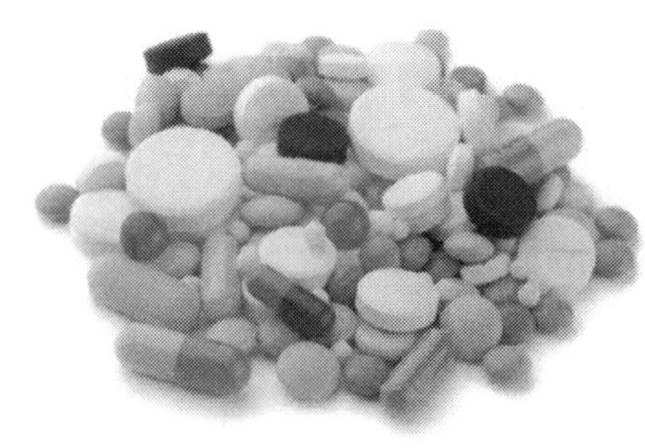

#23: Eliminate the need for pills and drugs.

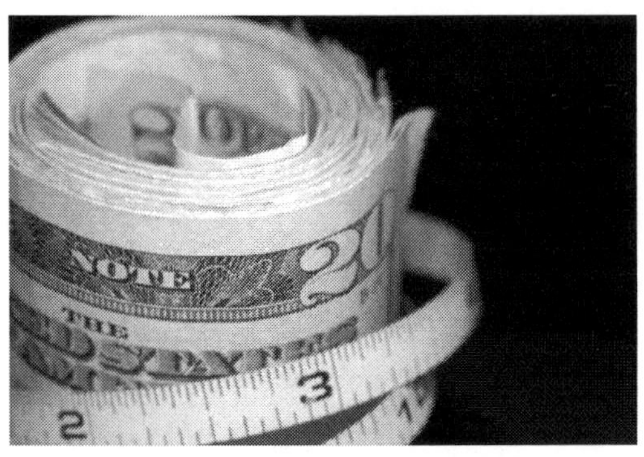

#22: Save money by not constantly buying diet products.

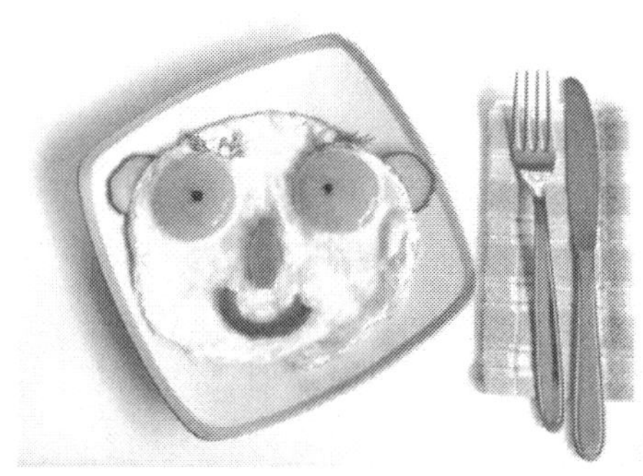

#21: Be happy with the food I eat.

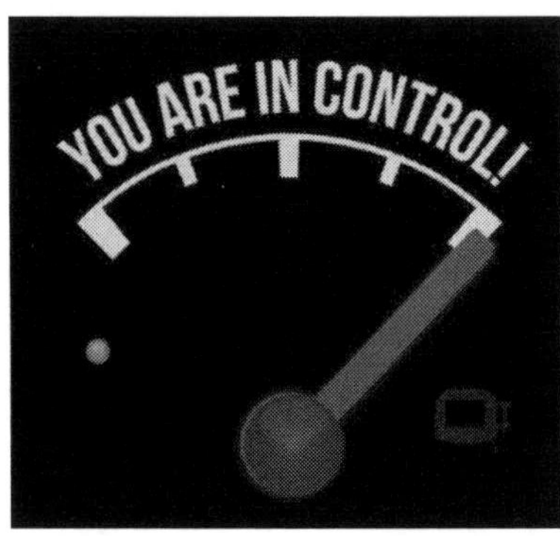

#20: Be in control of my weight.

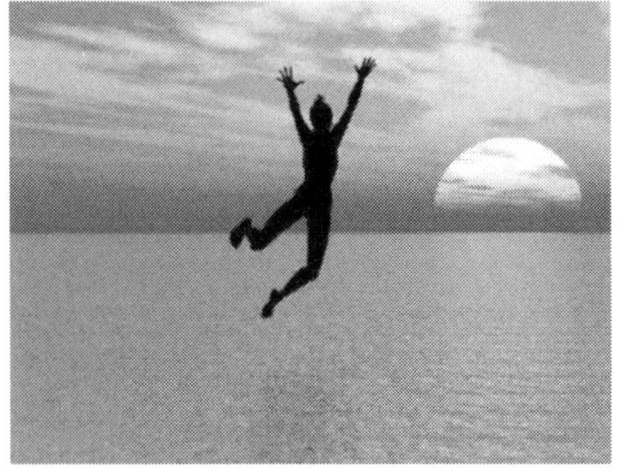

#19: Have a lot of self-esteem based on the way I look.

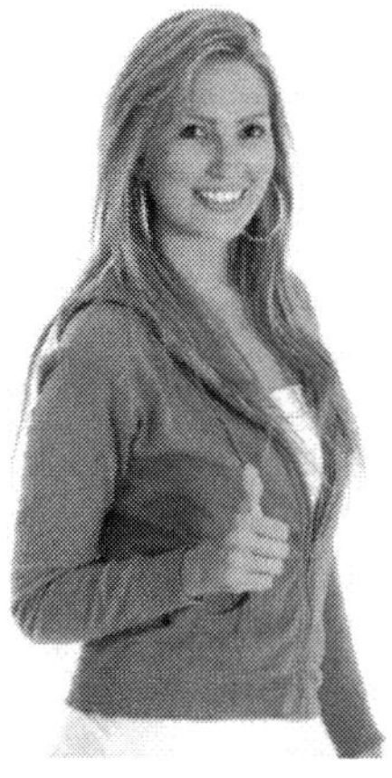

#18: Have plenty of self-confidence based on the way I look.

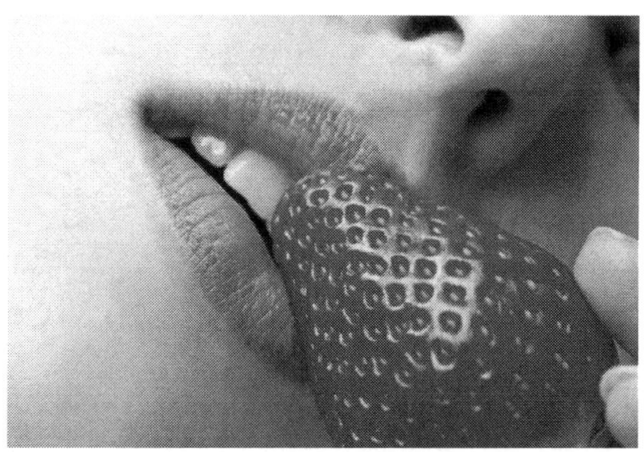

#17: Really enjoy the taste of food.

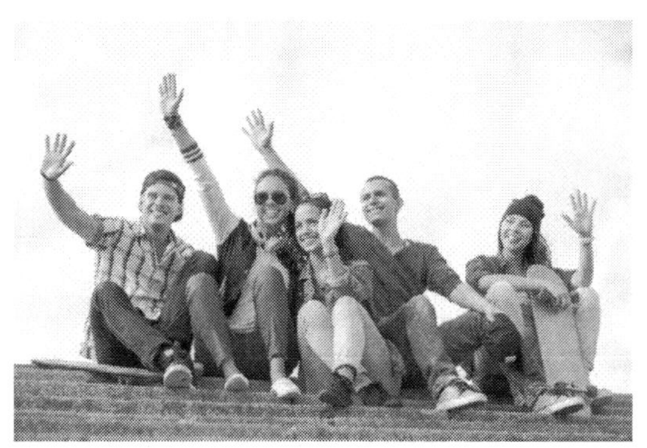

#16: Have more friends.

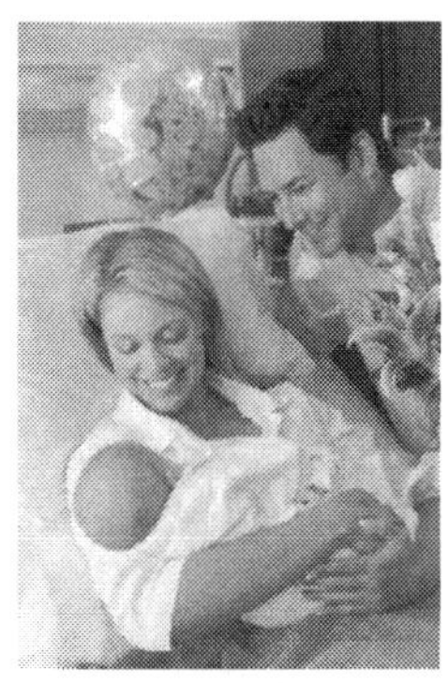

#15: Have healthy babies.

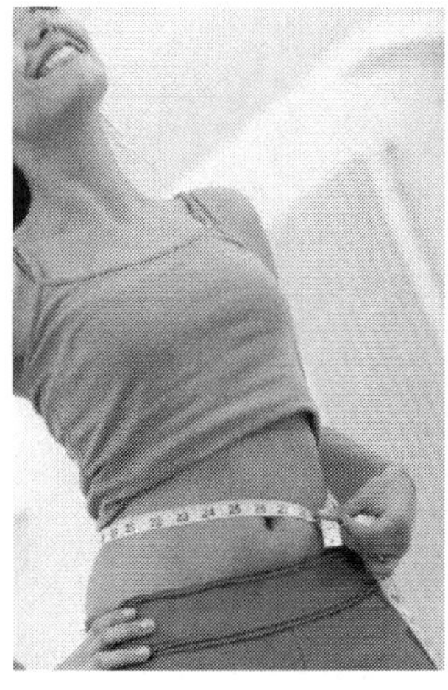

#14: Fit into my favorite clothes.

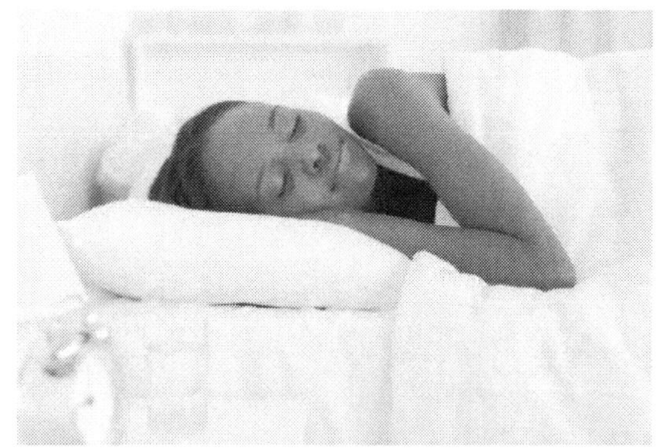

#13: Get a good nights' sleep, every night.

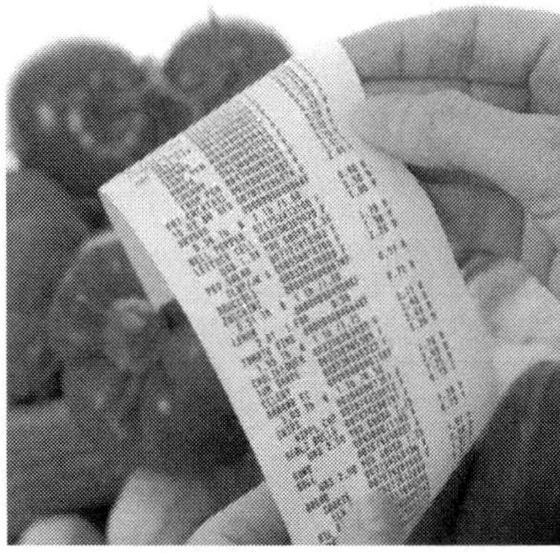

#12: Save money by buying less food and less expensive food.

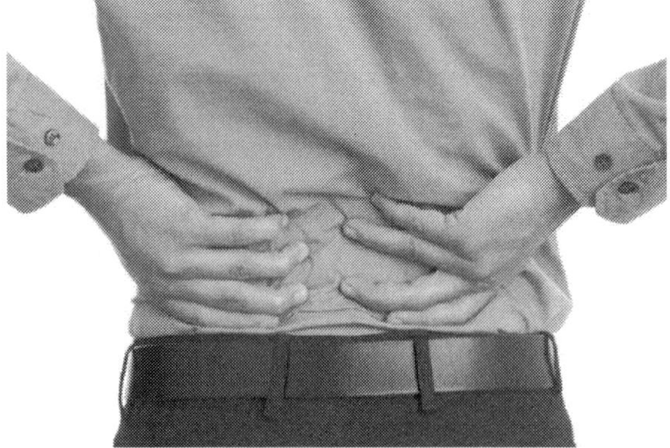

#11: Wake up with fewer or no aches and pains.

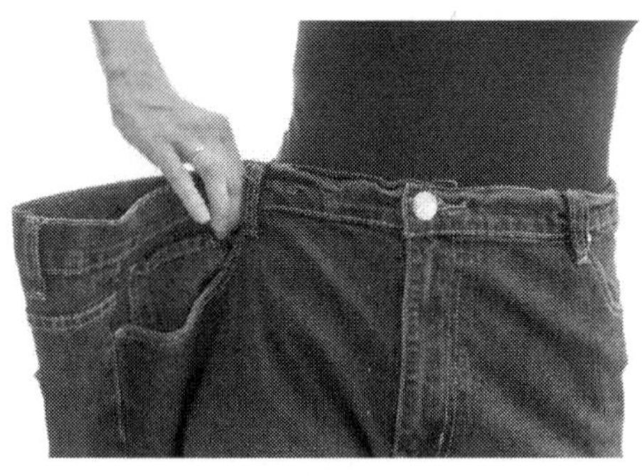

#10: Drop clothing sizes and inches.

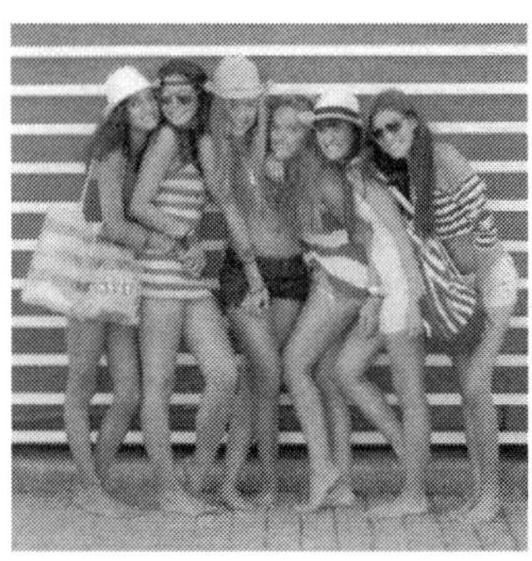

#9: Wear trendy clothes.

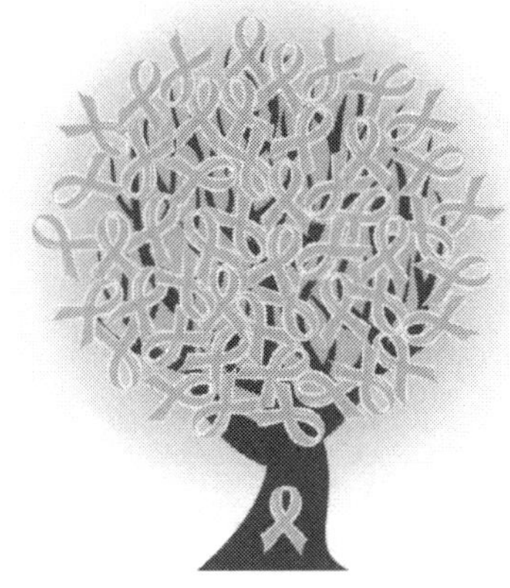

#8: Decrease the chance of getting breast and other cancers.

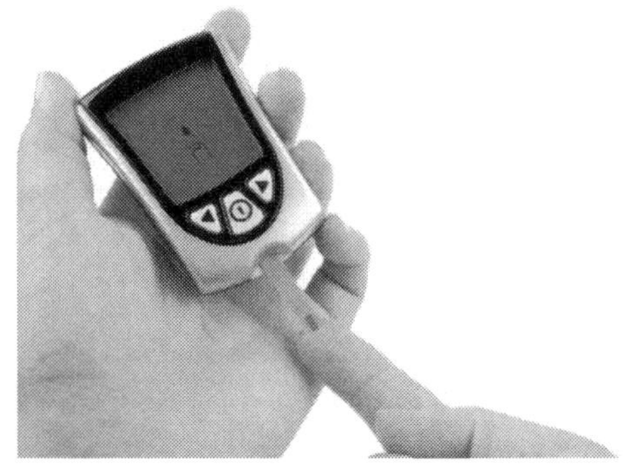

#7: Reduce the risk of getting diabetes.

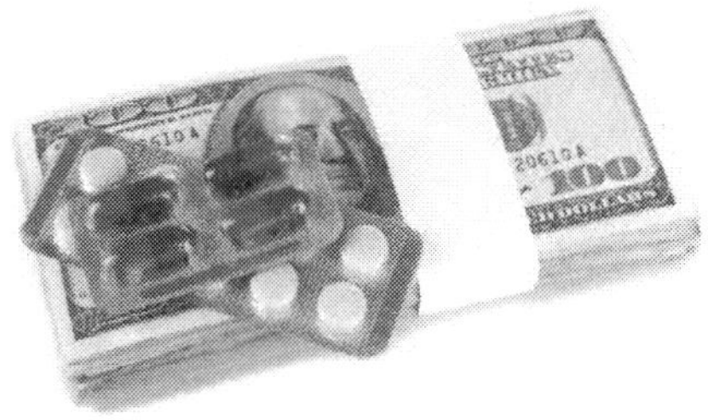

#6: Reduce the amount of money I spend on expensive medications.

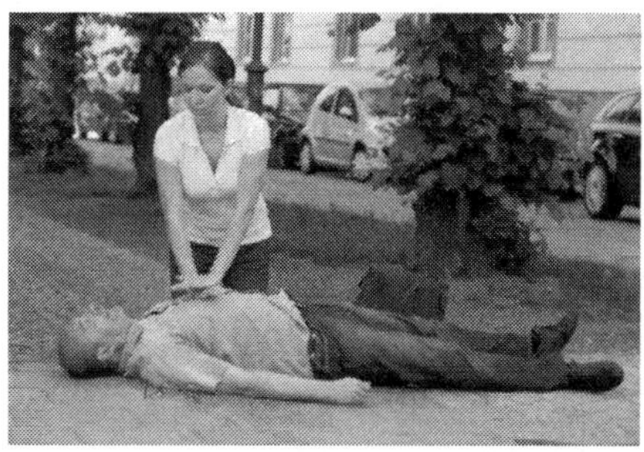

#5: Lower the risk of having a heart attack.

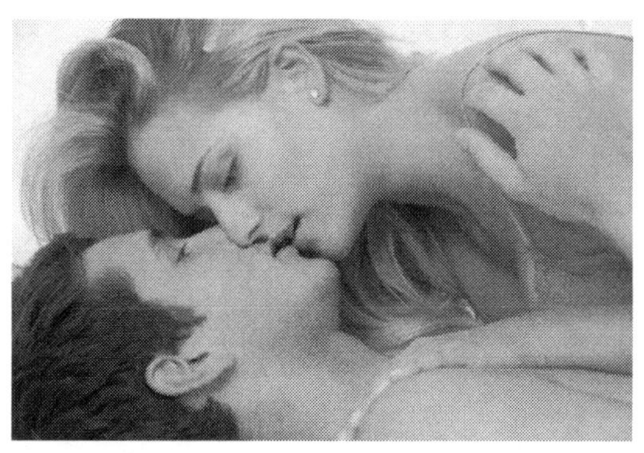

#4: Have great sex and more of it!

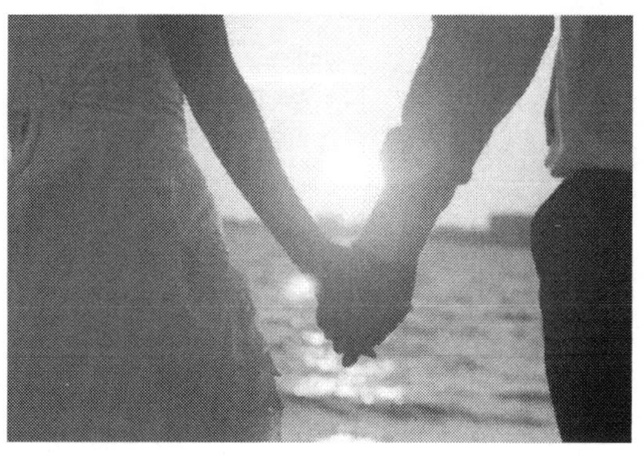

#3: Find love.

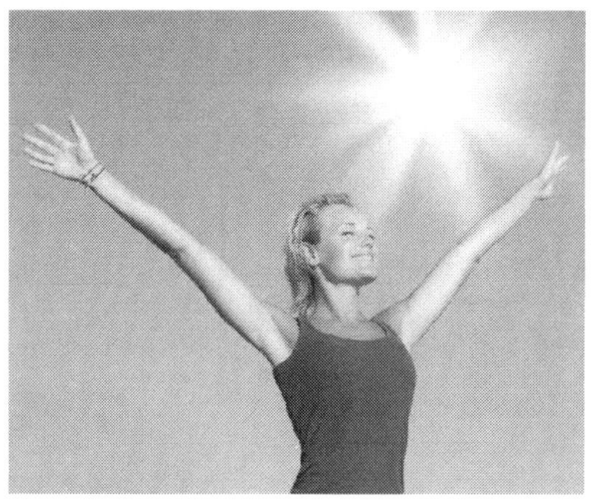

#2: Have a happy and healthy life.

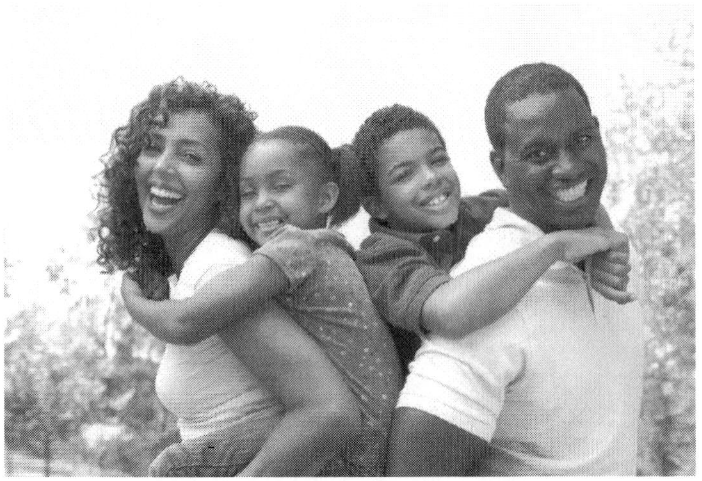

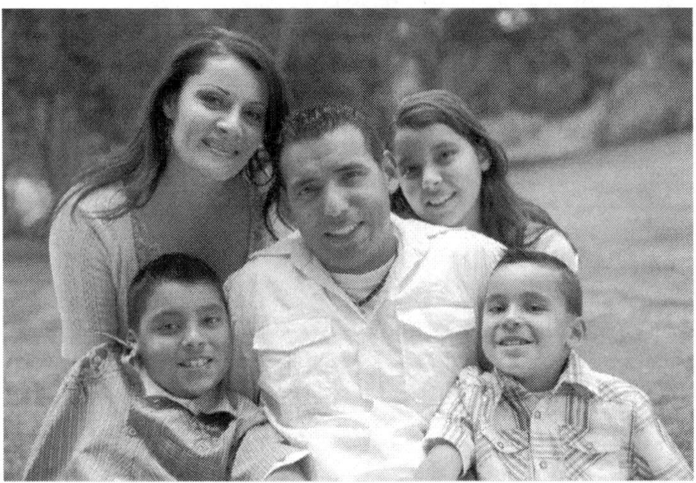

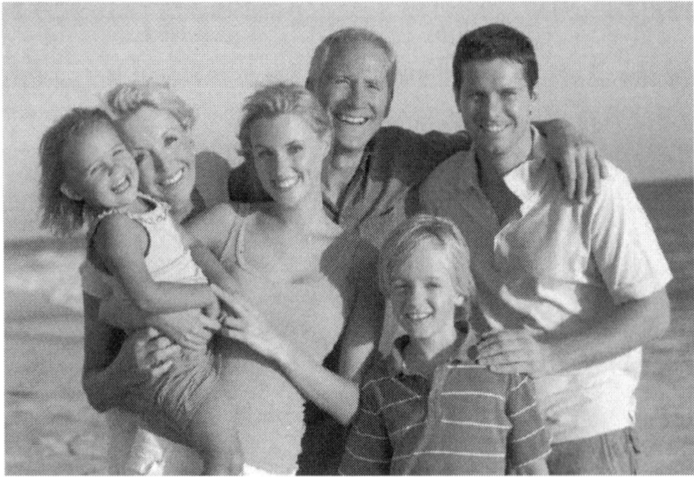

#1: Live longer so I can partake in everything good life has to offer and enjoy those I care about and love.

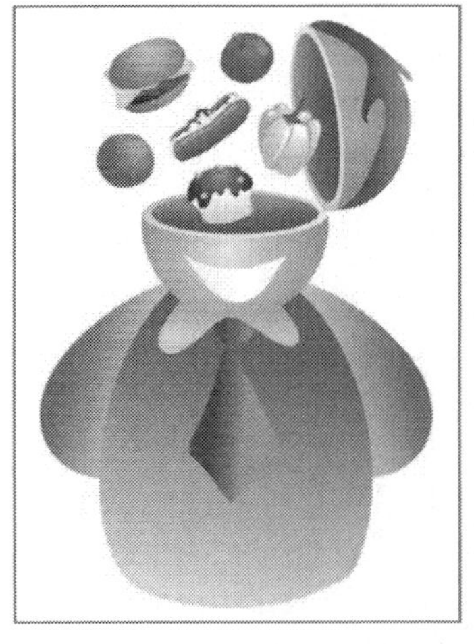

Guidebook #8
Sugar Is Evil

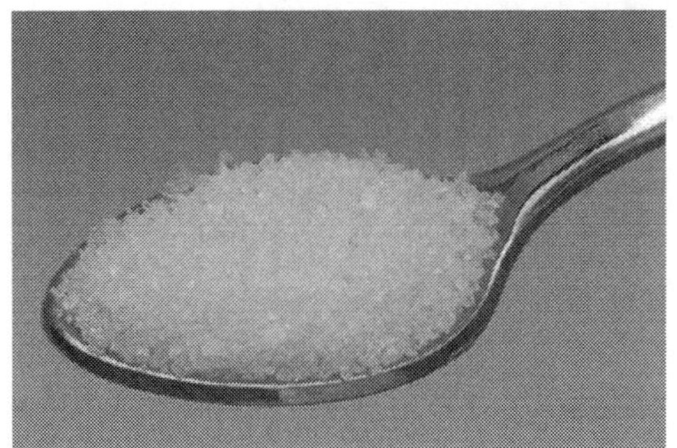

Guess how many teaspoons of **added** sugar (not naturally occurring in fruit) the average American consumes every month.

Turn pages slowly.

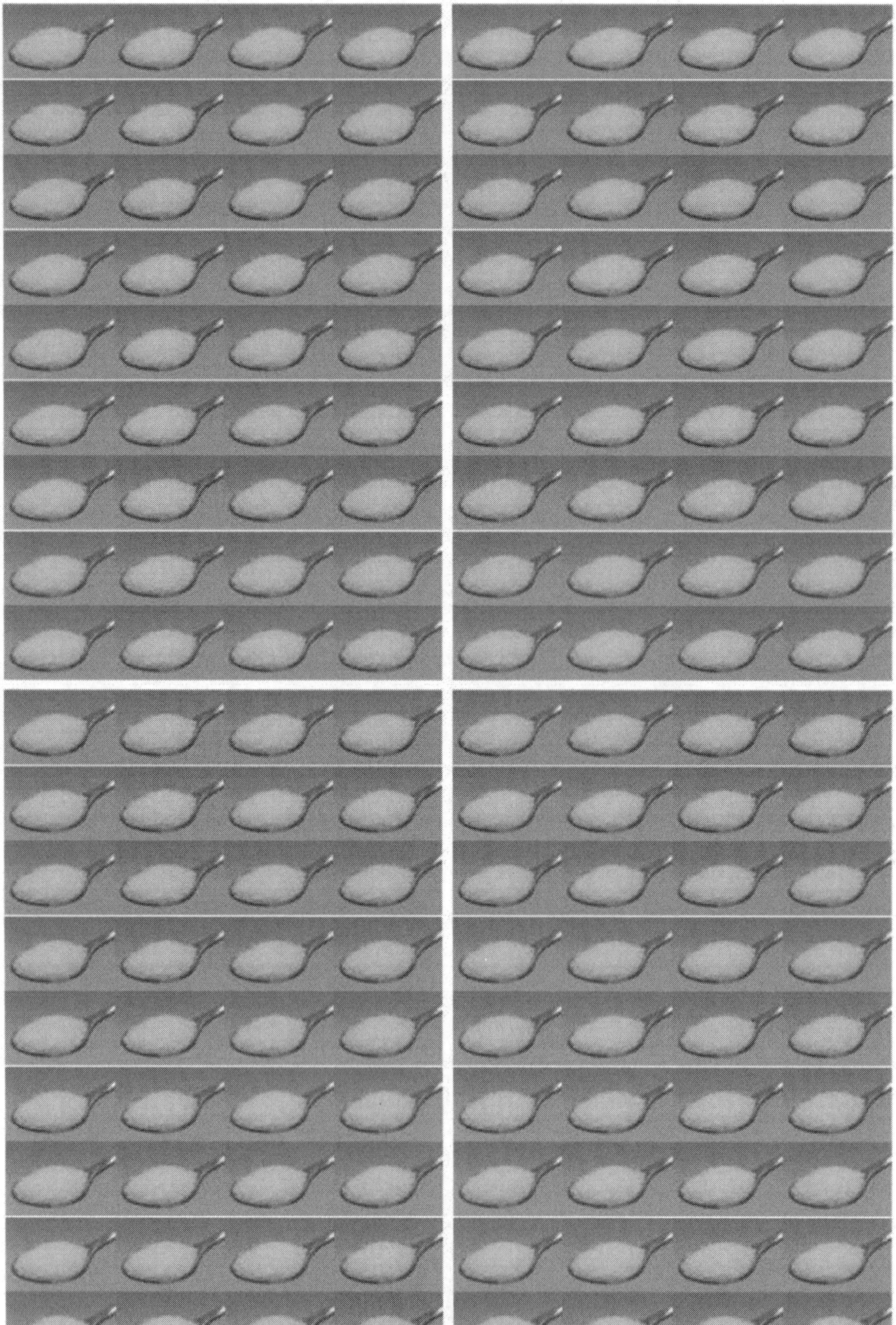

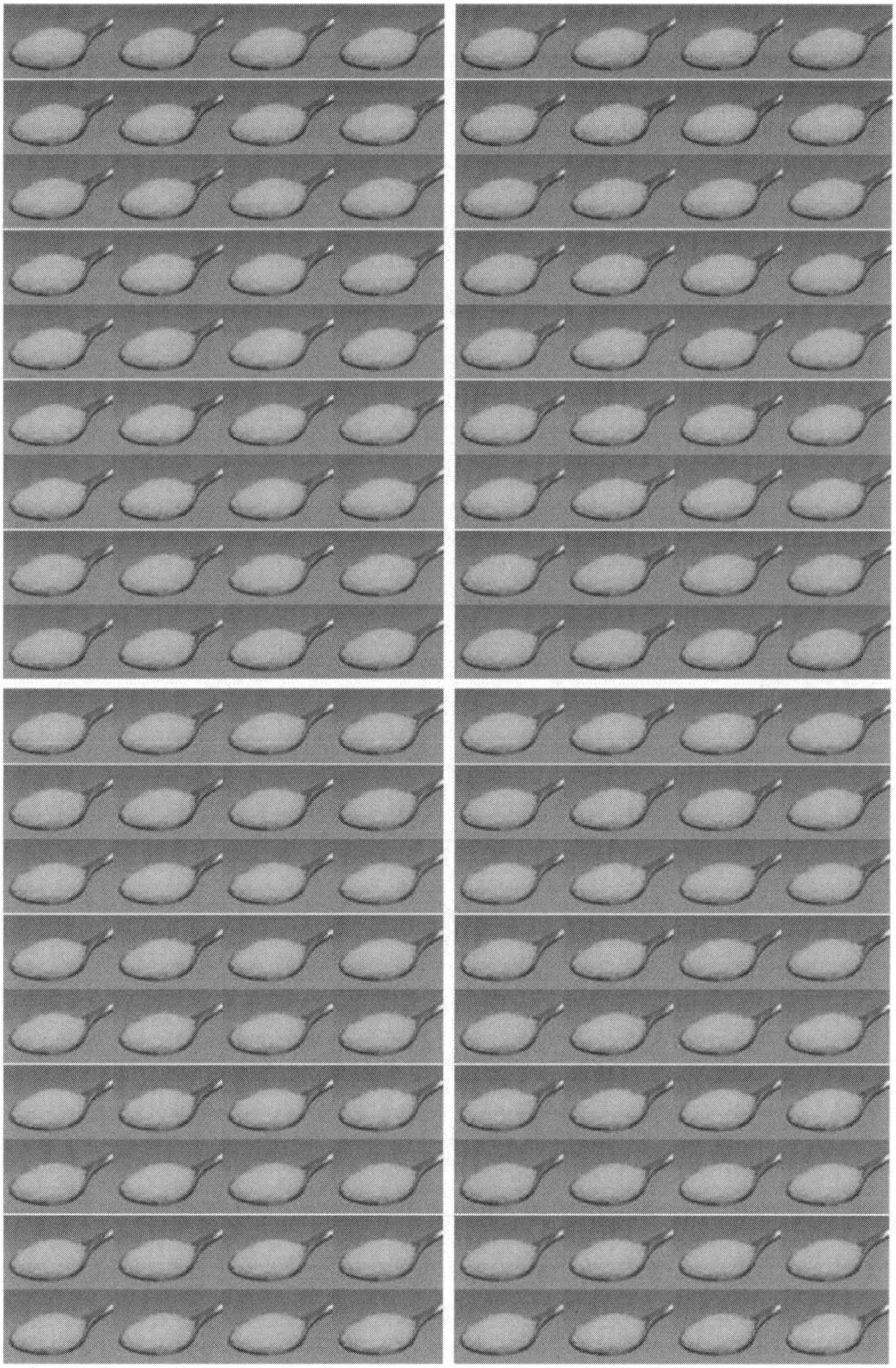

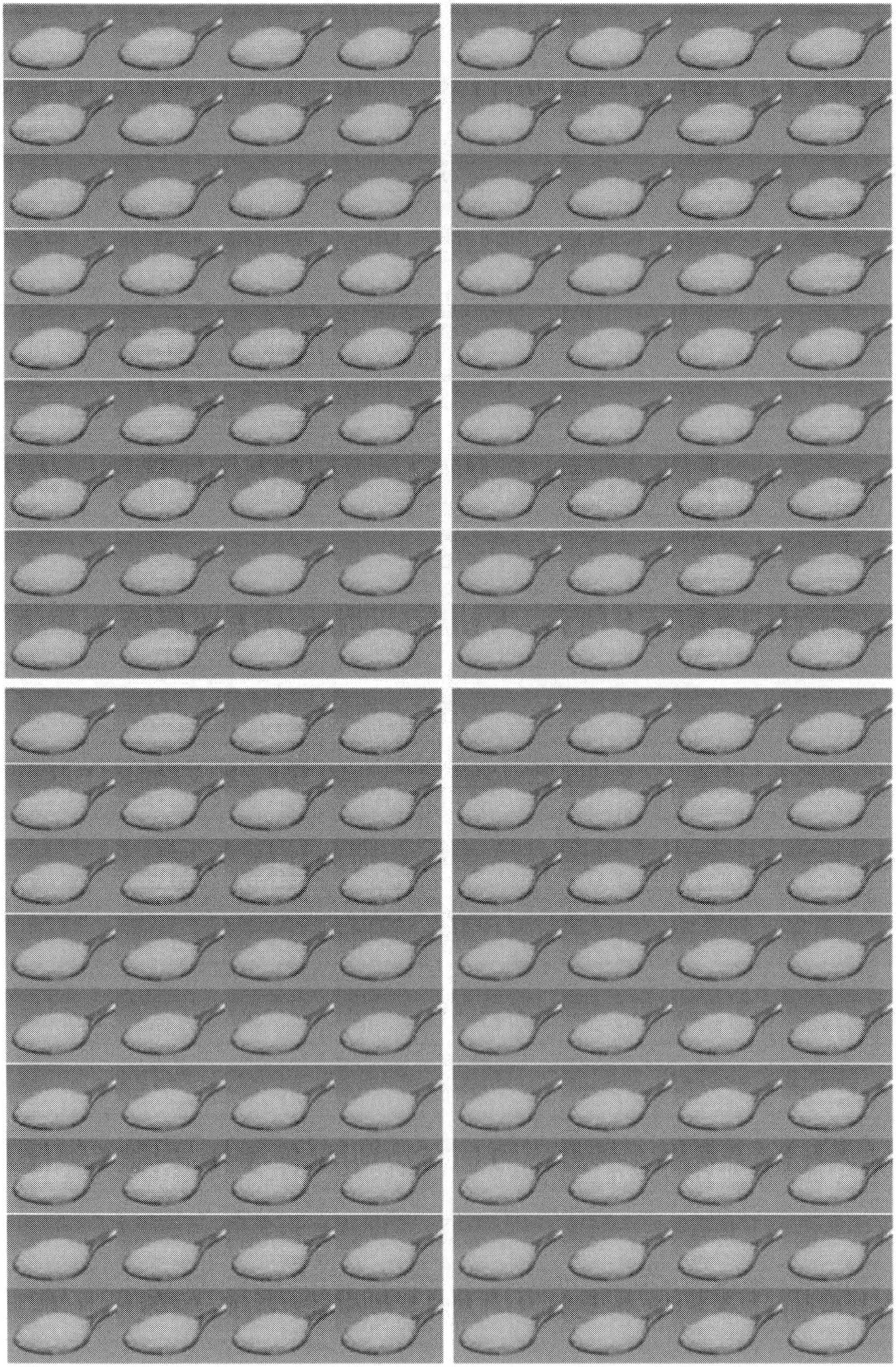

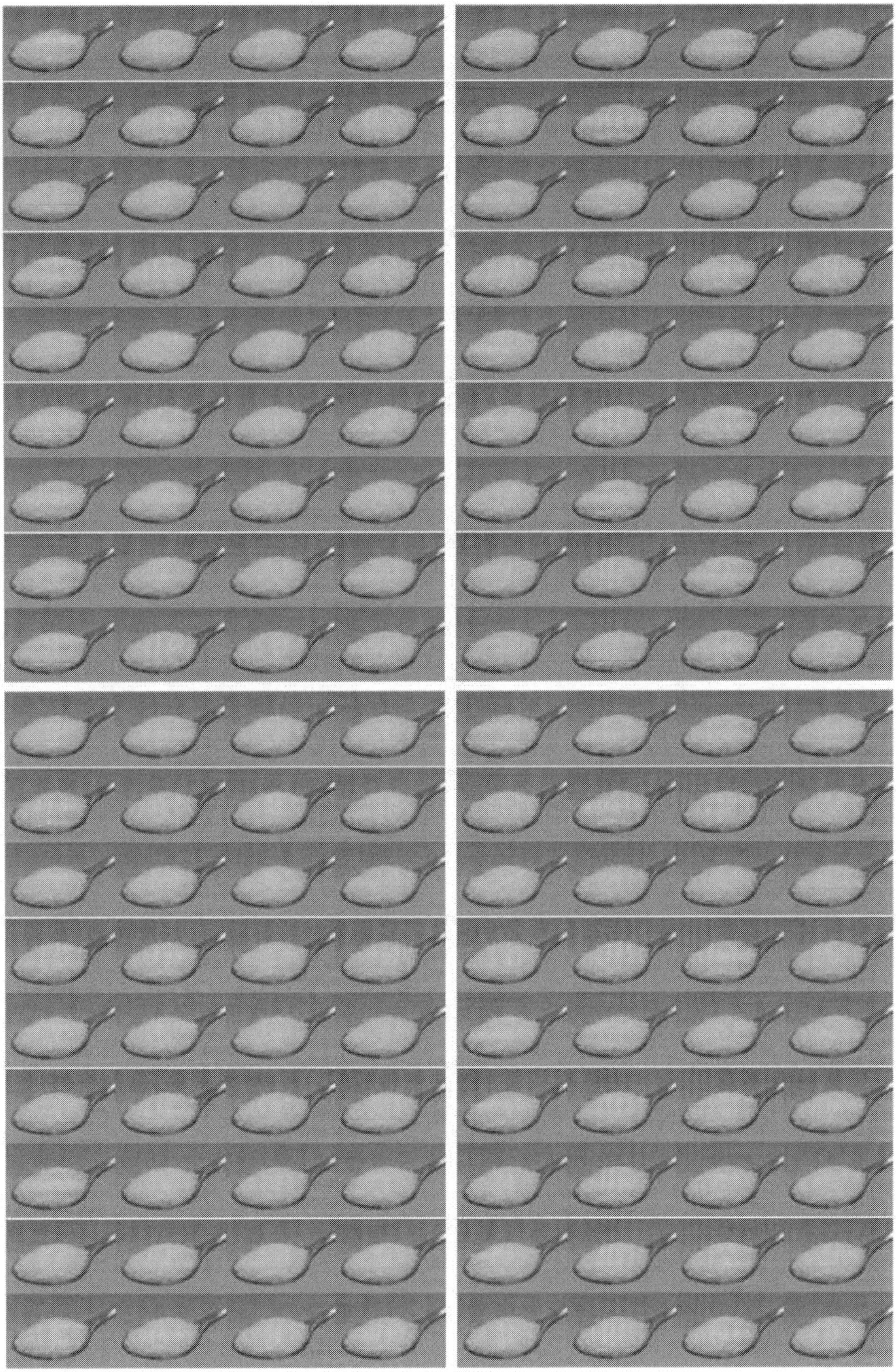

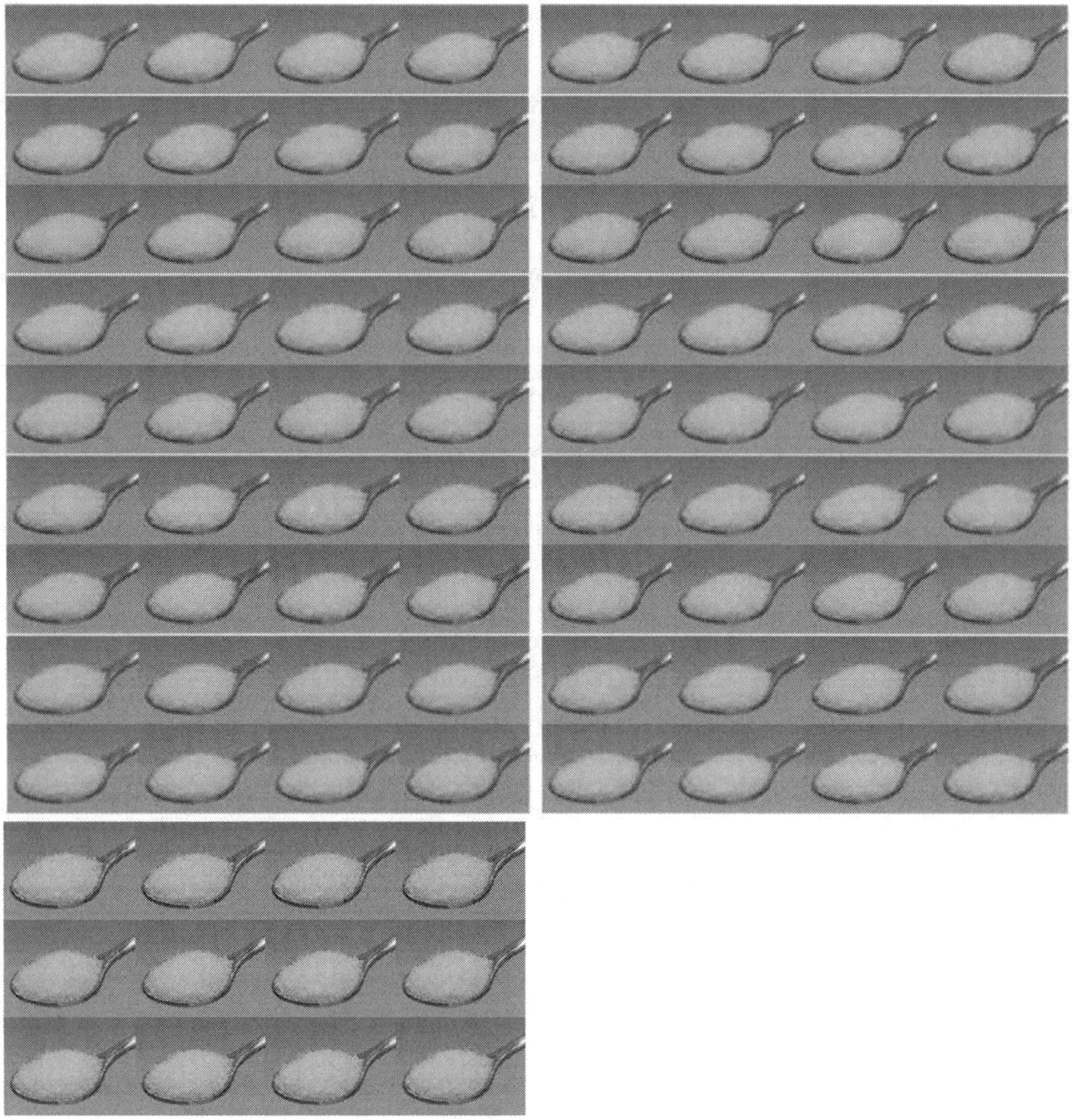

That's 660 teaspoons per month or 7,920 per year. Teens on average consume 1,020 teaspoons a month, or over 12,000 a year. **Any wonder why we're so fat?**

I came across a fascinating infographic about sugar consumption from Trendhunter.com: http://tinyurl.com/kkm35hh.

Dr. Robert Lustig gave a lecture titled *Sugar: The Bitter Truth* that was posted on YouTube (http://tinyurl.com/ldgu9k). Since being posted in July, 2009, this relatively unentertaining video has been viewed over 3.5 million times. It's worth watching for an in-depth understanding of why he also calls sugar "evil" as I do, as well as toxic and poison. *Advertising Age* called sugar "Public Enemy No. 1."

A "must watch" video called "Sugar is Killing Us" helps everyone understand the toxicity of sugar and high fructose corn syrup. Here: www.youtube.com/watch?v=Yda8RtOcVFU.

Part of the nitty-gritty explanation includes the fact that refined sugar and high fructose corn syrup "don't come with any protein, vitamins, minerals, antioxidants or fiber, and so they either displace other more nutritious elements of our diet or are eaten over and above what we need to sustain our weight, and this is why we get fatter," according to an April, 2011 New York Times article *Is Sugar Toxic?* authored by Gary Taubes.

This Truth Will Set You Free

I've learned a lot over my successful weight loss journey, and there is one thing that stands out far and above all else when it comes to eating:

Added sugar is the most evil, toxic, destructive food ingredient there is.

We're the fattest country because of all the sugar in food, both the obvious (cake, candy, ice cream, soda, etc.) and the not-so-obvious (processed foods, tropical fruits, juices, etc.).

I took the time to learn about the different forms of sugar and their relative toxicity, and how much you should have every day. I would venture to say that less than one percent of us understand how bad sugar is.

By drastically reducing my sugar intake, I was able to lose 40+ pounds and keep them off for years. And I know deep down inside that if there was only one thing you do to get healthy and lose weight, it's dealing with sugar in all its forms.

Note that not all brands that are sweetened contain a lot of sugar, but many or most do. Check the labels to be sure before you buy.

In a 2012 article in the journal *Nature,* **the conclusion is that sugar is a toxic substance that should be regulated like tobacco and alcohol**. Now that's quite a statement that should bring home just how bad sugar, especially added sugar and High Fructose Corn Syrup, really is. *Bottom Line Personal* reports that just one can of soda per day increases male prostate cancer risk.

One of the best articles I've found was written by Kris Gunnars and appeared on AuthorityNutrition.com. Titled "Top 9 Reasons to Avoid Sugar as if Your Life Depended on it" presents a very concise and powerful summary at: http://tinyurl.com/cy2k3ts. Here's a quick condensation:

#1: Added Sugar Supplies a Large Amount of Fructose

Sugar and its evil cousin High Fructose Corn Syrup are half glucose and half fructose. Glucose is essential and is good for your body. Fructose has no value to our bodies and most of it gets turned into fat.

#2: Sugar Doesn't Contain Any Vitamins or Minerals (Empty Calories)

Not only are foods with added sugars bad for you, they contain little or no essential nutrients. Fruit, on the other hand, has natural sugar as well as vitamins and minerals that are good for you.

#3: Sugar Causes Deposition of Fat in the Liver

Consuming a lot of sugar leads to increased fat in the liver, which can lead to Non-Alcoholic Fatty Liver Disease.

#4: Sugar Harms Your Cholesterol and Triglycerides

Consuming fructose can lead to these bad occurrences:

- Increases in blood triglycerides.
- Increases in small, dense LDL and oxidized LDL (very, very bad).
- Higher fasting glucose and insulin.
- Decreased insulin sensitivity.
- Increased fat in the abdominal cavity (visceral fat).

#5: Sugar Causes Insulin Resistance

The main function of insulin is to drive glucose from the bloodstream into cells. Our "Western" diets lead to insulin resistance, leading directly to obesity and diabetes. Excess fructose consumption leads to insulin resistance.

#6: Sugar Raises Your Risk of Western Diseases

Excess sugar consumption is associated with many diseases that plague people who have fallen into Western diet traps, including obesity, diabetes, heart disease and many more. You may recall the long list of obesity caused conditions found earlier in *The Mind Diet* guidebooks.

#7: Sugar Doesn't Cause Proper Satiety

Consuming glucose makes you feel full. Consuming fructose does not.

#8: Sugar is Addictive

Eating sugar is like using cocaine. Let that sink in. When we eat sugar, dopamine is released into the brain, giving us a feeling of pleasure. That's how we get addicted to the feeling that added sugar creates.

#9: Sugar Causes Resistance to a Hormone Called Leptin

Leptin resistance, found in people who are obese, is a major reason why people eat more calories than they burn. When leptin is working, it sends a signal to our brains that we're full, to stop eating. But the fatter you get, the greater the chance that leptin isn't doing its job.

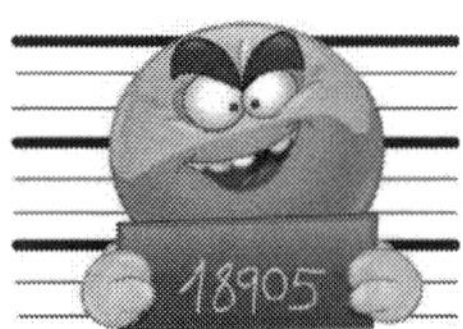

So Just Who Are The Bad Guys?

Sugar is a subset of a large group of ingredients in food called sweeteners, including naturally occurring (i.e. fruit) and man-made (i.e. aspartame). There is a lot of confusion about sugar in general and a lot of misinformation on how bad it is for you. To simplify matters, here are the definitions of the sweetener family. Those in **bold** are really bad for you:

Fructose	Naturally occurring sugar in fruit
Sucrose	Commonly called "table sugar"
Sugar	Catch-all name for variety of sweeteners
High Fructose Corn Syrup	Found mostly in processed foods Has replaced table sugar in the manufacturing process
Natural Sugar	Found in **unprocessed foods:** fruit, milk, vegetables and some grains.
Artificial Sweeteners	Many believe that artificial sweeteners are just as harmful as table sugar

Other commonly used names for sweeteners include brown sugar, cane juice, cane syrup, confectioner's sugar, corn sweetener, corn syrup, dextrose, glucose, granulated sugar, honey, invert sugar, lactose, maltose, malt syrup, molasses, raw sugar and turbinado. For an in-depth discussion of sugar substitutes, check out: http://tinyurl.com/mr457w7.

There is a "double whammy" to eating too much food that has added sugar and high fructose corn syrup:

- Too much sugar of all kinds leads to obesity, diabetes, tooth decay, bad cholesterol and heart disease.
- The more you eat and drink foods/beverages that contain sugar, the less likely you are to eat healthy foods.

It's just that simple!

20/36/12

The American Heart Association's recommended intake of added sugar on a daily basis is:

- 20 grams for adult women (5 teaspoons)
- 36 grams for adult men (9 teaspoons)
- 12 grams for children (3 teaspoons)

Most people get much more, and many experts believe that these guidelines, especially for men, should be even lower. I've seen surveys that say that the average American consumes over 22 teaspoons (88 grams) of added sugar every day! Here's an example of how fast sugar intake occurs:

Just one 20 ounce bottle of regular soda contains about 16 packets of added sugar, which is 43.4 grams. That is more than **double** the recommendation for women, almost **quadruple** for children and **25% more** for men. *And that's if you consume zero sugar from any other source – all day long!*

iVillage.com put together a list of foods that surprisingly are high in sugar. When you look at these, keep in mind the maximum daily amount of sugar recommended for men (36 grams), women (20 grams) and children (12 grams):

• Dried cranberries	1/3 cup	30g
• Canned baked beans	1/2 cup	12g
• Bran muffin	1 muffin	22g
• Packaged fruit cup	1 cup	16g
• Instant oatmeal	1/2 cup	13g
• Canned tomato soup	1/2 cup	12g
• Chocolate sorbet	1/2 cup	30g
• Apple sauce	1 serving	20-25g
• Iced green tea	12 oz	20g
• Orange juice	1 cup	20g
• Ketchup	2 tbs	7g
• BBQ sauce	2 tbs	7g

The biggest surprises on this list: bran muffins, iced green tea and dried cranberries!

The problem is that we don't know how much sugar there is in any given item. The next few pages are eye-openers in terms of the amount of sugar you consume without realizing it!

Thanks to Dr. Patricia Farris, a clinical professor at Tulane University, here's a quiz about your sugar I.Q.

1. Which one contains the most sugar?
   A. Snapple Lemon Tea (16 oz bottle)
   B. Coca Cola (12 oz can)
   C. Starbucks Vanilla Latte (Tall, 12 fluid ounces)
2. True or false: humans naturally prefer the taste of sugar from birth.
3. True or false: Sugar toxicity causes liver damage.
4. True or false: Sugar substitutes help control weight gain.
5. Which of these foods is hiding the most sugar (half-cup serving)?
   A. Tomato sauce
   B. Salsa
   C. Tomato soup
6. Reduced-fat packaged foods often have...
   A. Less sugar than the full-fat version
   B. More sugar than the full-fat version
   C. The same amount of sugar as the full-fat version
7. True or false: eating too much sugar causes wrinkles.
8. True or false: natural sugars, such as honey, have less of an effect on the body than refined sugar does.
9. True or false: Natural sugars, such as honey, have fewer calories than refined sugar.
10. True or false: People with high blood sugar generally look older.

Answers:

1 B
2 True
3 True
4 False
5 A
6 B
7 True
8 False
9 False
10 True

Dr. Farris also writes that in addition to all the harmful effects of sugar, it also triggers the production of a chemical that accelerates skin aging, making us look older! Yikes!

For a real good visual comparison of the amount of sugar in various foods and drinks, check out: www.sugarstacks.com.

Dr. Robert Lustig points out in an article in *The Atlantic* that one could make the case for regulating sugar as our government does with alcohol. Substances are regulated when they meet four distinct criteria:

- Be ubiquitous (found everywhere, readily available)
- Be toxic (I and many others certainly believe it is!)
- Be addictive (no question here)
- Have a negative impact on society (for sure!)

Even if the government does not regulate sugar, YOU need to!

Now I'll show you the added sugar content for common foods and drinks, and most importantly, what percentage of the recommended daily allowance that is. The American Heart Association offers these general guidelines for daily added sugar intake:

- Men: 9 teaspoons
- Women: 6 teaspoons
- Children: 3 teaspoons
- Teenagers: 5-8 teaspoons

The key point is that one serving of one food, or one drink, can blow your entire day's allowance!

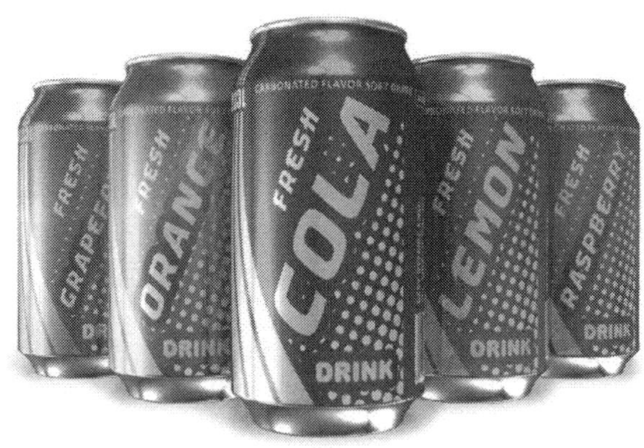

One 12oz can of soda

40 grams = 10 teaspoons of added sugar

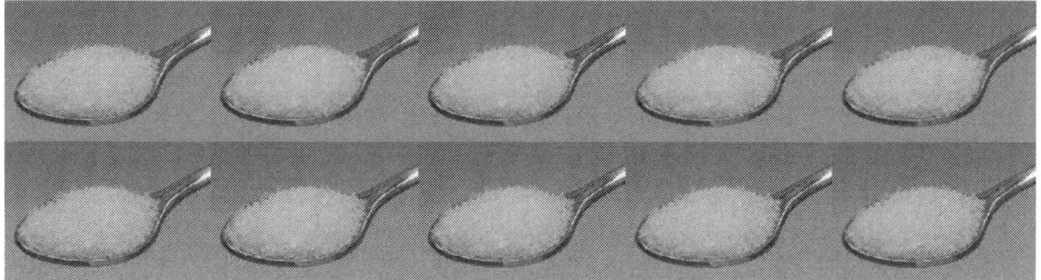

Men: **Equal to your entire daily sugar allowance**
Women: **1.5 times your entire daily sugar allowance**
Children: **3 times your entire daily sugar allowance**
Teens: **Up to 2 times your daily sugar allowance**

Find out what happened when polar bears drank soda.
Watch the video at: TheRealBears.org

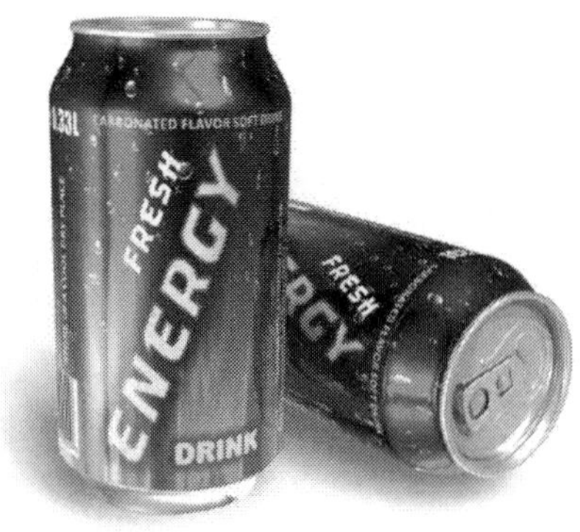

One 16oz can of energy drink

42 grams = 10½ teaspoons of added sugar

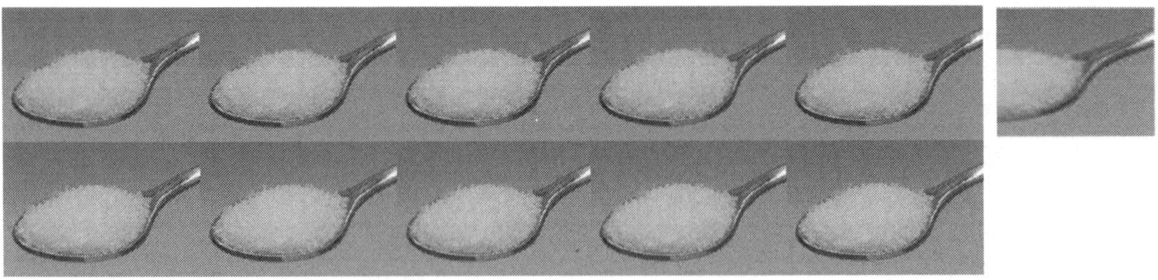

Men: Equal to your entire daily sugar allowance
Women: 1.5 times your entire daily sugar allowance
Children: 3 times your entire daily sugar allowance
Teens: Up to 2 times your daily sugar allowance

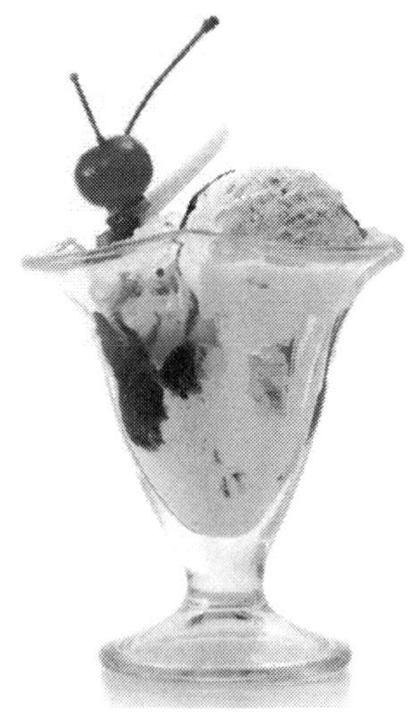

One cup of ice cream

30 grams = 7½ teaspoons of added sugar

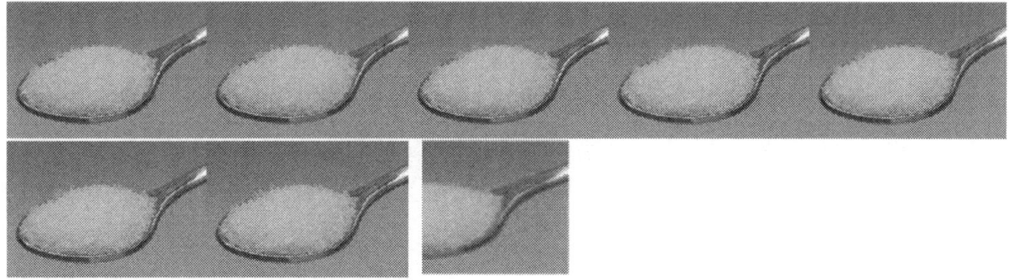

Men: 80% of your entire daily sugar allowance
Women: 25% more than your entire daily sugar allowance
Children: 2 times your entire daily sugar allowance
Teens: About equal to your daily sugar allowance

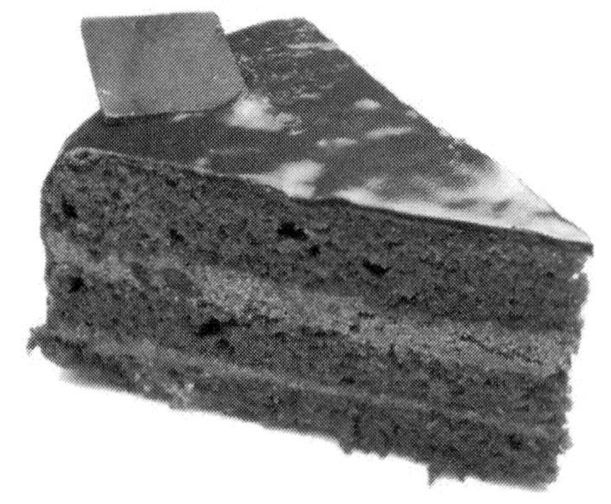

One slice of chocolate cake

60 grams = 15 teaspoons of added sugar

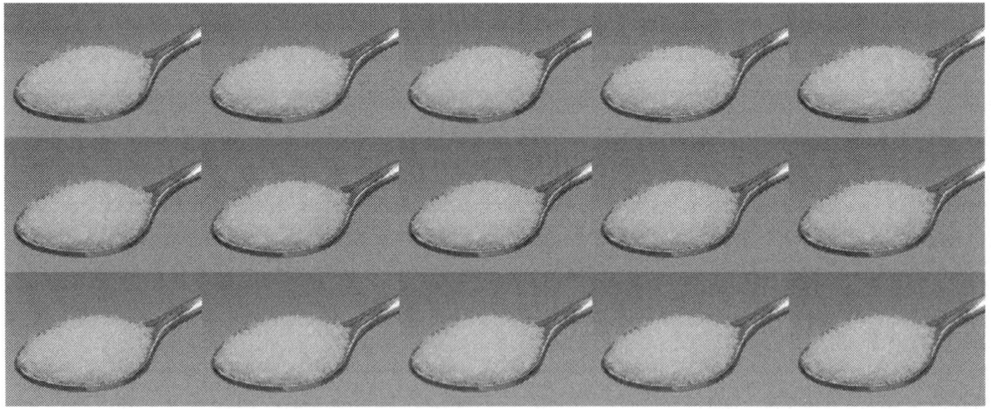

Men: 50% more than your entire daily sugar allowance
Women: 2½ times your entire daily sugar allowance
Children: 5 times your entire daily sugar allowance
Teens: 2 to 3 times your daily sugar allowance

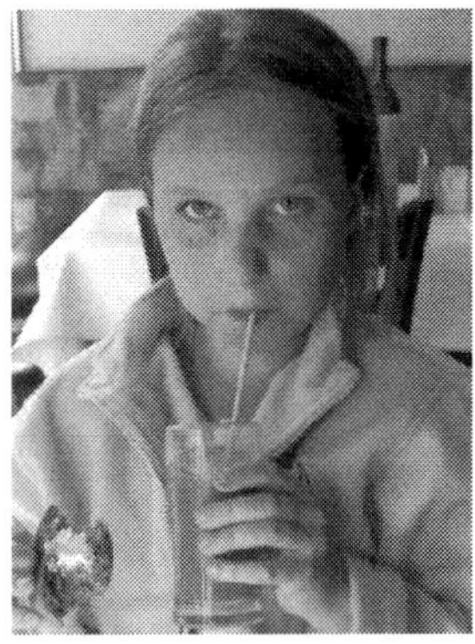

One glass of fat-free chocolate milk

54 grams = 13.5 teaspoons of added sugar

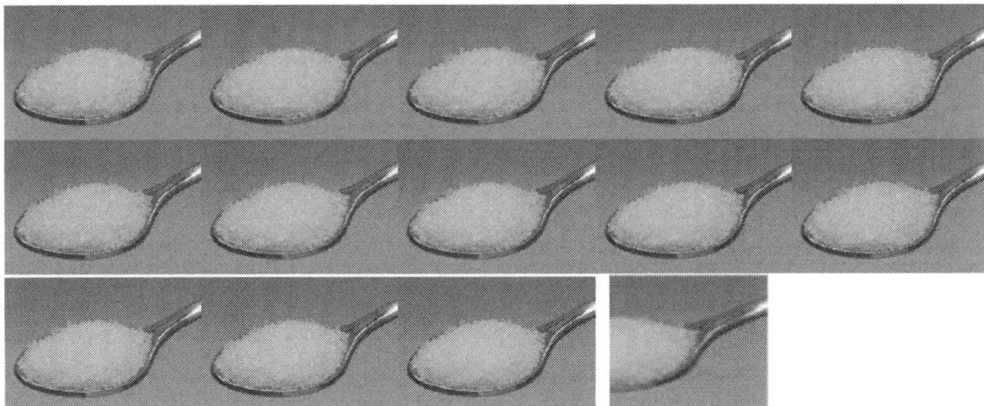

Men: 50% more than your entire daily sugar allowance
Women: Over 2 times your entire daily sugar allowance
Children: 4 times your entire daily sugar allowance
Teens: 2 to 3 times your daily sugar allowance

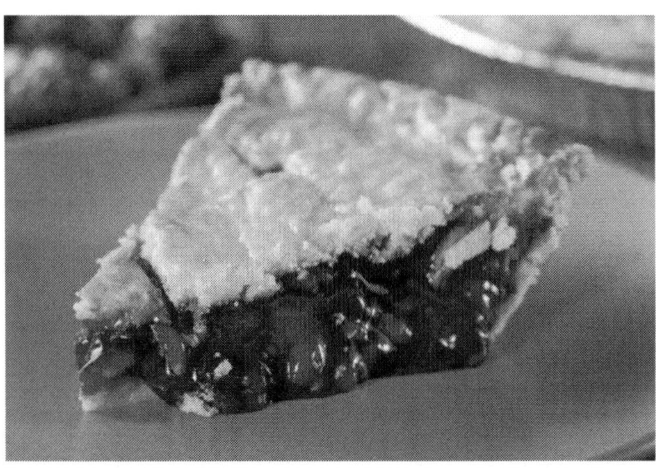

One slice of fruit pie

36 grams = 9 teaspoons of added sugar

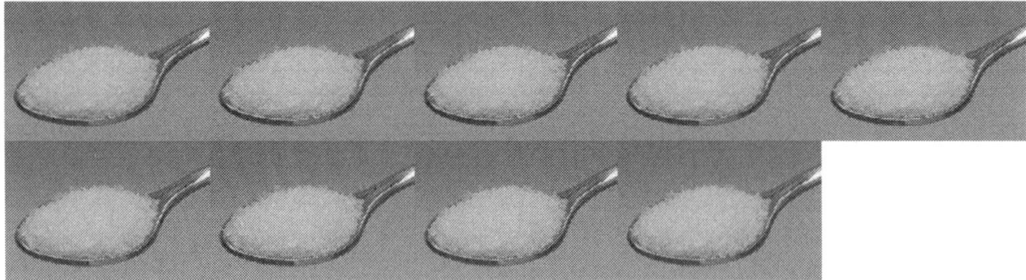

Men:	**Equal to your entire daily sugar allowance**
Women:	**1½ times your entire daily sugar allowance**
Children:	**3 times your entire daily sugar allowance**
Teens:	**1 to 2 times your daily sugar allowance**

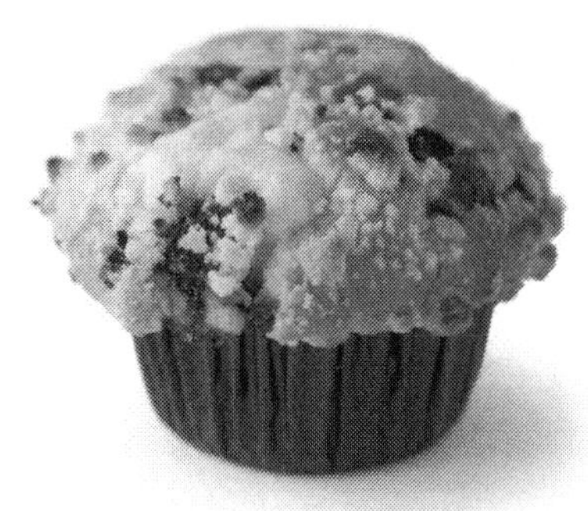

One blueberry muffin

38 grams = 9.5 teaspoons of added sugar

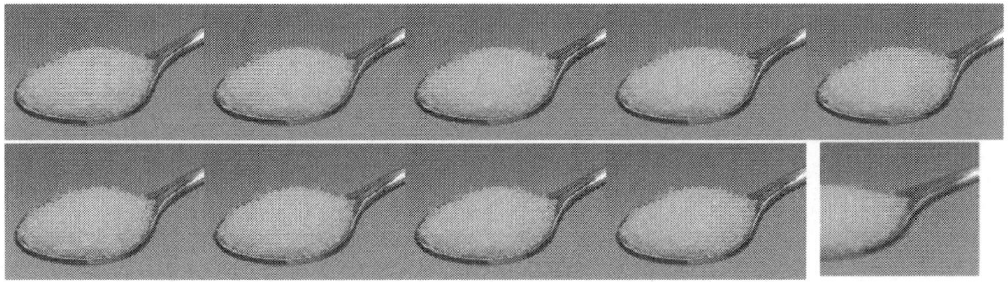

Men: Equal to your entire daily sugar allowance
Women: 1½ times your entire daily sugar allowance
Children: Over 3 times your entire daily sugar allowance
Teens: 1 to 2 times your daily sugar allowance

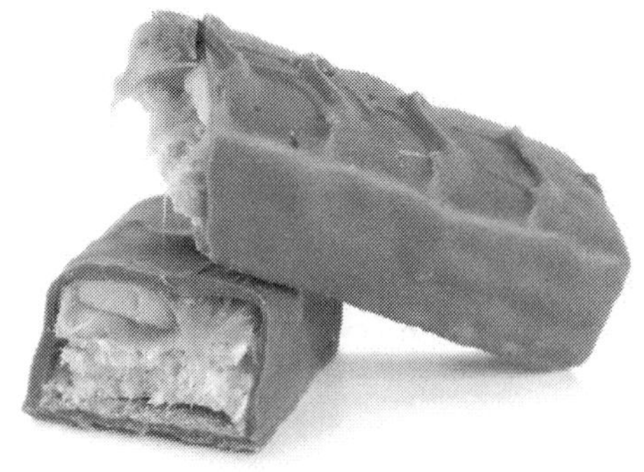

Regular size candy bar

54 grams = 13.5 teaspoons of added sugar

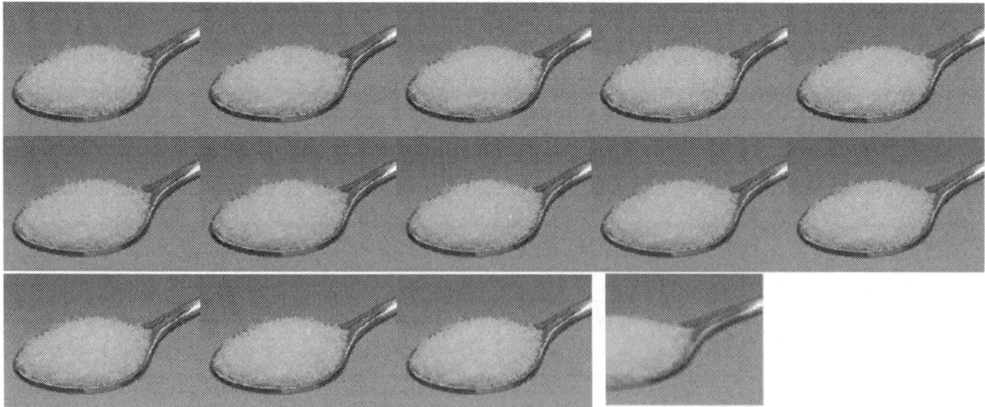

Men:	**50% more than your entire daily sugar allowance**
Women:	**Over 2 times your entire daily sugar allowance**
Children:	**Over 3 times your entire daily sugar allowance**
Teens:	**2 to 3 times your daily sugar allowance**

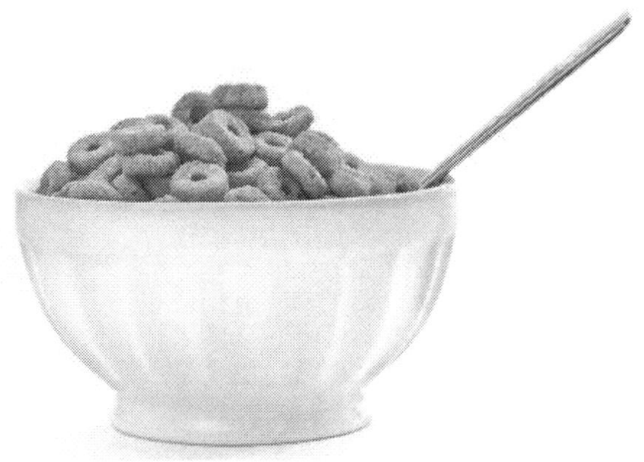

One bowl of sweetened cereal

24 grams = 6 teaspoons of added sugar

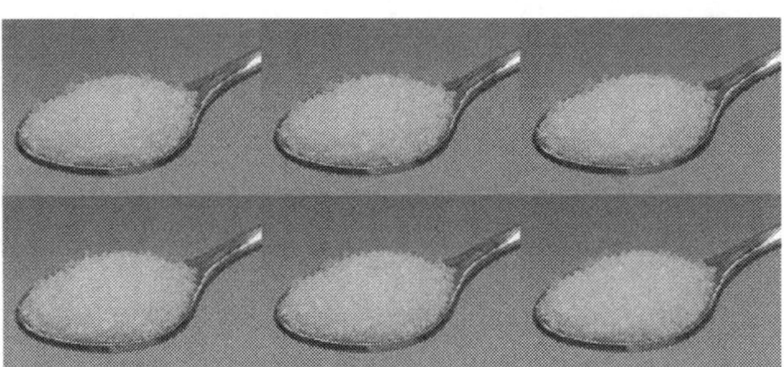

Men: **66% of your entire daily sugar allowance**
Women: **1½ times your entire daily sugar allowance**
Children: **2 times your entire daily sugar allowance**
Teens: **About equal to your daily sugar allowance**

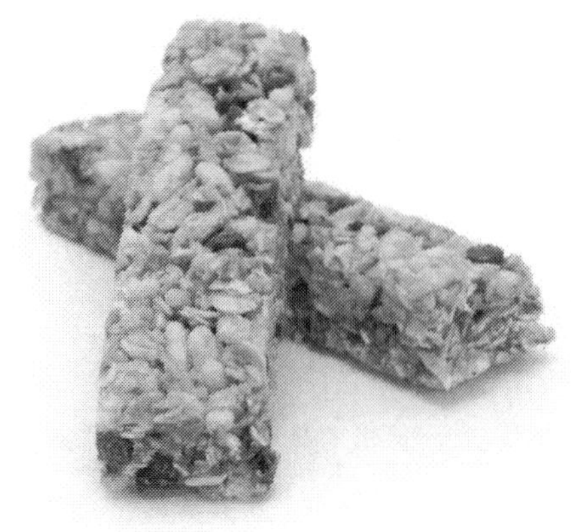

One energy bar

23 grams = 6 teaspoons of added sugar

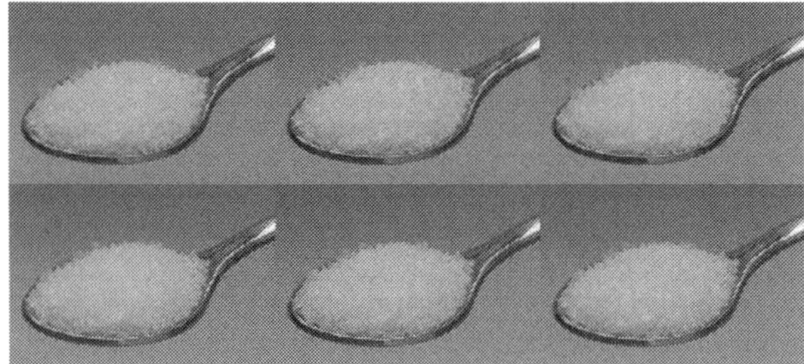

Men:	**66% of your entire daily sugar allowance**
Women:	**Equal to your entire daily sugar allowance**
Children:	**2 times your entire daily sugar allowance**
Teens:	**1 to 1½ times your daily sugar allowance**

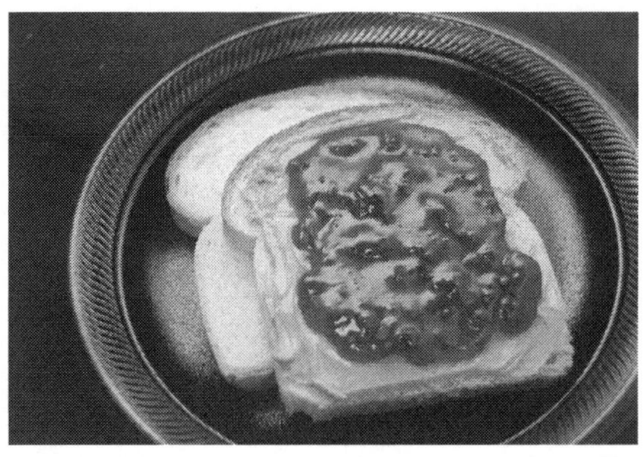

One peanut butter and jelly sandwich

18 grams = 4.5 teaspoons of added sugar

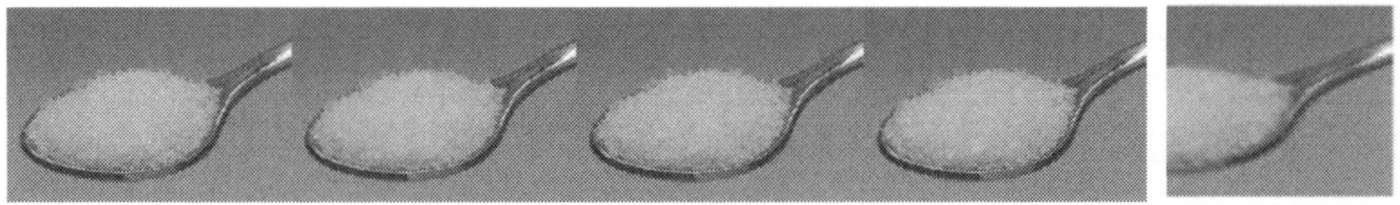

Men:	**50% of your entire daily sugar allowance**
Women:	**75% of your entire daily sugar allowance**
Children:	**1½ times your entire daily sugar allowance**
Teens:	**1 to 1½ times your daily sugar allowance**

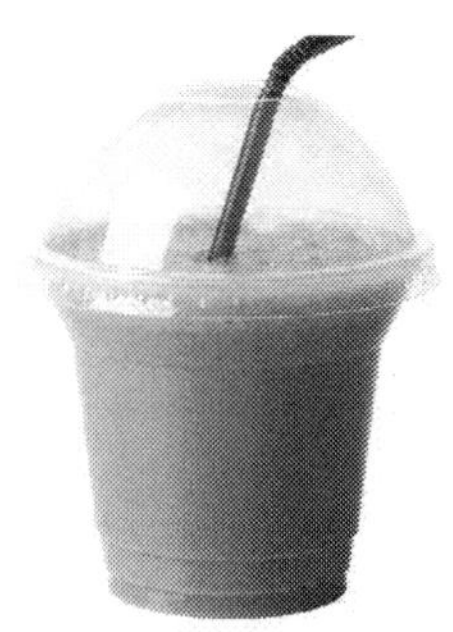

One chocolate shake at a fast food restaurant (21oz)

111 grams = 28 teaspoons of added sugar

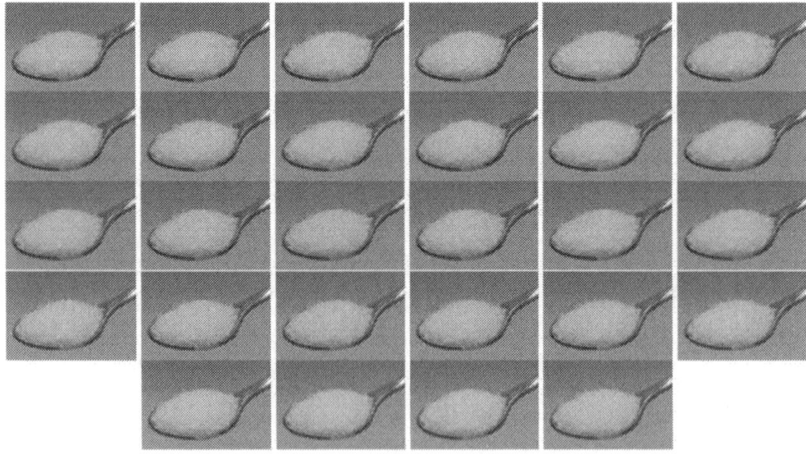

Men:	**3 times your entire daily sugar allowance**
Women:	**Over 4 times your entire daily sugar allowance**
Children:	**Over 9 times your entire daily sugar allowance**
Teens:	**4 to 5 times your daily sugar allowance**

Beware of Unexpected Loads of Sugar In Foods and Drinks

One of the most fascinating facts is how much added sugar there is in foods and beverages that sound like they wouldn't have any sugar. *Summer Tomato* highlights these:

- How about that Thai chicken salad that's popular at many restaurants. That's got 45 grams of added sugar, which is more than double what women should have in ONE entire day.

- Or the vanilla frappuccino grande – 58 grams, almost three days' worth of sugar in one 16 oz drink.

- Blackberry Jamba Juice sound taste good? Of course it does, because it has 49g of added sugar in 16 ounces.

- Some foods that we consider "healthy" like juice, yogurt and dried fruit often have MORE sugar than donuts, ice cream and cookies.

- The popular energy bars are basically candy bars with a fancy name and packaging.

The very worst sugar offenders are beverages of all kinds that have sugar added. Hands down. The *Center for Science in the Public Interest* report "America: Drowning in Sugar" highlights that people who consume a lot of sugar get less calcium, fiber, folate, vitamins, zinc, magnesium, iron and other nutrients.

The Worst of the Worst

100%
Foods that contain about 100% of their calories from added sugar:

- regular sodas
- hard candies
- frozen fruit bars

50% to 99%
Foods that contain 50% to 99% of their calories from added sugar:

- cake icing
- cake mixes
- fudge
- canned fruit in heavy syrup
- pickled beets
- juice drinks
- BBQ sauces
- sherbet/sorbet
- flavored gelatin
- powdered flavored drinks

Note: not all brands contain this much sugar, but many do. Check the labels!

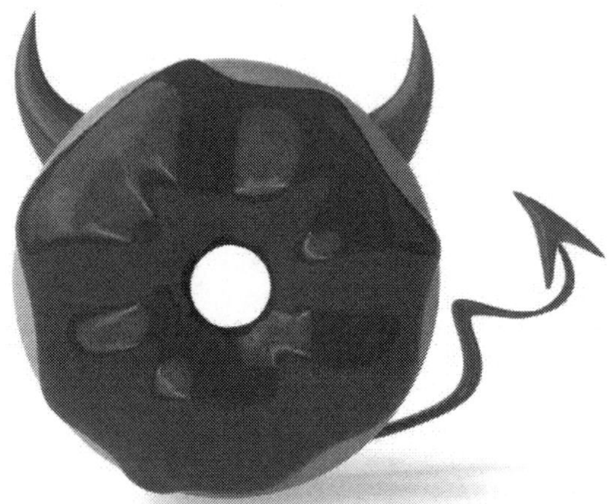

Added sugar *really* is evil: avoid it at all costs

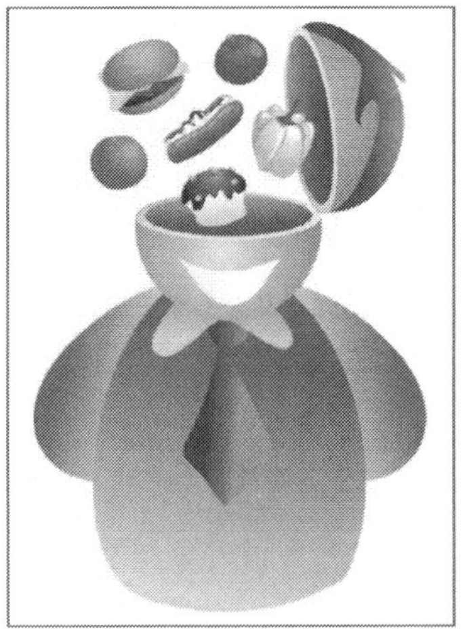

Guidebook #9 *Ingredients Awareness Chart*

Knowing What's in the Foods You Buy is Extremely Important

It's easy to forget what foods contain good or bad ingredients when you're in the supermarket, faced with thousands of choices.

Even when you are choosing between two foods in the same category (i.e. sweet potatoes vs. regular potatoes), there are sometimes big differences in the ingredients they contain.

That's why I put together this "Ingredient Awareness Chart" that presents good and bad ingredients found in 75 popular foods. By no means is this complete, but it should serve as a guide when you're shopping or eating out. I suggest you print it and keep it in your purse or wallet.

How to Use This Chart

Review and Let It Sink In

Take a half hour to go over all the foods in the chart, and make mental images of the foods that are really good and those that are really bad. Green boxes mean good nutrients and red boxes mean bad additives. You can easily see that beans, fish and spinach have a lot of green boxes, and that frozen foods, potato chips and canned soup have a lot of red boxes.

Look for a food that has a lot of green boxes in its row (good for you) or one or more red boxes (not good for you).

Review based on Doctor and Nutrition Specialist Advice

Let's say your doctor tells you that you're deficient in Vitamin D, which is very common. You can use this chart to identify foods rich in Vitamin D, including eggs, fish, milk and oatmeal, to name a few.

Let's say blood tests show you are high in potassium. You can use the chart to stay away from high potassium foods, including bananas, beans, potatoes and peanuts.

Bring to the Supermarket

It's easy to forget which foods are good or bad without having this chart in front of you. Having it handy while shopping will easily reduce the number of foods with bad ingredients you buy and increase the amount of foods with good nutrients you purchase.

Bring to the Restaurant

Similarly, have the chart handy when you eat out. It will help you choose between the good and the bad when you're looking at a menu that undoubtedly is loaded with foods containing ingredients you should not have.

A Word of Caution about This Chart

This chart is a simple guide, and nothing more. To be truly comprehensive, it would be hundreds of pages long, because there are so many differences between foods and brands of foods.

For example, some fishes are extremely healthy and don't contain anything bad for you, while others are borderline and may contain mercury. In consultation with your doctor and nutrition specialist, review this chart to determine which specific foods in each category are desirable and those that should be avoided.

Nutrient and Mineral Definitions and Synonyms

It's a good idea to know a little about each of the good nutrients and minerals that the chart identifies, along with synonyms for each. The more educated you are about these healthy ingredients, the better it is for your food choices.

Antioxidants

- Substances that protect your cells against the effects of "free radicals," which are molecules produced when your body breaks down food, or by exposure to smoke and radiation. Also known as inhibitors and glutathione peroxidase.

Beta Carotene

- A vitamin that aids vision, immune function, bone metabolism, skin and cellular health. Also known as Vitamin A, retinol, retinal and carotenoid.

Calcium

- A mineral that is instrumental in the maintenance of healthy and strong bones, and supports proper functioning of nerves and muscles.

Complex Carbohydrates

- These are chains of three or more single sugar molecules linked together. Longer chains are called starches and store energy. In general, complex carbs are much, much better for you than simple carbs, that include sugar, candy, regular soda, syrups and other processed foods.

Fiber

- Dietary fiber includes all parts of plant foods that your body cannot digest and absorb – found mainly in fruits, vegetables, whole grains and legumes. Also known as roughage and bulk, fiber helps prevent or relieve constipation and helps maintain a healthy weight.

Iron

- Iron is a mineral found in every cell in your body, and is needed to make hemoglobin (found in red blood cells) and myoglobin (found in muscles). Iron also makes up a part of many proteins in the body.

Lycopene

- This nutrient is a powerful antioxidant that can help protect against a wide range of diseases. High levels of lycopene in the blood and fatty tissues are associated with lower risks of cancer, heart disease and macular degeneration. It's classified as a carotenoid and phytonutrient.

Magnesium

- This mineral is needed for more than 300 biochemical reactions in the body. It helps maintain normal muscle and nerve function, keeps heart rhythm steady, supports a healthy immune system, keeps bones strong, helps regulate blood sugar levels, promotes normal blood pressure, and is involved in energy metabolism and protein synthesis.

Omega Fatty Acids

- These are actually polyunsaturated fats, and nutritionists call omega-3 and omega-6 fatty acids "essential" fats for good reason. The human body needs them for many functions, from building healthy cells to maintaining brain and nerve function to lowering the risk of heart disease. Our bodies can't produce them. The only source is food. Omega-3s come primarily from fish (salmon, mackerel, tuna) and walnuts and flaxseed. Omega-6s come from plant oils, nuts and seeds.

Potassium

- This versatile mineral helps your body build proteins, break down and use carbohydrates, build muscle, maintain normal body growth, control the electrical activity of the heart and maintain your acid/base balance.

Protein

- These amino acids are the building blocks of life. Every cell in your body contains protein, is a major part of skin, muscles, organs, glands, and in most body fluids.

Vitamin B1

- Also known as Thiamine or Thiamin, helps the body convert food into fuel, which is used to produce energy. It also supports your nervous system, muscles, carbohydrate metabolism and digestion. Because the body stores very little B1, deficiency can develop if you don't get enough, with potentially serious complications.

Vitamin B2

- B2 or Riboflavin, produces energy for your body, works as an antioxidant by fighting damaging particles called "free radicals," helps convert Vitamin B6 and folate (B9) into forms your body can use, and is also important for body growth and red cell production.

Vitamin B3

- Like other B vitamins, Niacin (B3) helps your body convert food into fuel, used to produce energy. B3 also helps the body make various sex and stress-related hormones in the adrenal glands and other parts of the body, and helps improve circulation.

Vitamin B5

- B5 of pantothenic acid, is needed by your body to synthesize cholesterol, the manufacture of red blood cells and various hormones, maintaining a healthy digestive tract and helps the body use other vitamins. It plays the same role as other B vitamins described above.

Vitamin B6

- Vitamin B6 helps your body make antibodies, necessary to fight many diseases. It also helps maintain normal nerve function, produce hemoglobin (which carries oxygen to the tissues), break down proteins and keep blood sugar in normal ranges.

Vitamin B7

- Biotin (B7), also called Vitamin H, helps your body with metabolism, skin care, tissue maintenance, weight loss, heart health and is a catalyst for various metabolic reactions in our bodies to extract energy.

Vitamin B8

- Vitamin B8 (Inositol) plays a vital role in your body by preventing fatty build-up in the liver and heart, promotes healthy hair growth, aids in nutrient metabolism and in supporting your nerves.

Vitamin B9

- Vitamin B9, also called folate and folic acid, is crucial for proper brain function, and plays a role in mental and emotional health. It aids in the production of DNA and RNA, and is especially important in pregnancy and children. It works closely with B12 to help make red blood cells, and helps iron work properly in your body.

Vitamin B11

- Salicylic acid (B11) functions in DNA and RNA synthesis, necessary for cell division, allows nerve cells to develop properly, helps your cells metabolize protein, carbohydrates and fats, and in the prevention of anemia, tiredness, lack of appetite and other negative changes in your body.

Vitamin B12

- B12, also called cobalamin, is a vitamin that plays a key role in the normal functioning of the brain and nervous system, and the formation of blood. This complicated vitamin also is involved in the metabolism of every cell in your body and affects DNA synthesis and regulation.

Bad Additive Definitions and Synonyms

Similarly, you need to know all about bad food ingredients in order to stay away from them – especially their synonyms. Food manufacturers often use synonyms in order to lead you away from the fact that a specific ingredient is bad for you. For example, most people know that MSG is very bad for you. But how many know that "hydrolyzed plant protein" – doesn't sound too bad, right – always contains MSG?

High Fructose Corn Syrup (HFCS)

- This is one of the most harmful food ingredients you can ingest. HFCS is 24% water and 76% sugars, and is used in soft drinks, processed foods, cereals, baked goods, syrups, ice cream, candy and other foods containing sweeteners. It is very similar to table sugar, but worse.

MSG (Monosodium Glutamate)

- MSG is a flavor enhancer that is added not only to Chinese food but to thousands of foods and used in restaurants. A leading expert in MSG, Dr. Russell Blaylock (author of *Excitotoxins: The Taste That Kills)*, indicates that MSG can contribute to heart disease, obesity, eye damage, headaches, fatigue, disorientation and depression. You need to be aware of food ingredients that contain MSG (courtesy www.healthcentral.com):
    - These always contain MSG:
        - Glutamate
        - Monosodium glutamate
        - Monopotassium glutamate
        - Glutamic acid
        - Gelatin
        - Hydrolyzed vegetable protein
        - Vegetable protein
        - Hydrolyzed protein
        - Plant protein extract
        - Sodium caseinate
        - Calcium caseinate
        - Yeast extract
        - Yeast food
        - Yeast nutrient
        - Textured protein
        - Autolyzed protein
        - Autolyzed yeast
        - Hydrolyzed oat flour
    - These frequently contain MSG:
        - Malt extract
        - Malt flavoring
        - Maltodextrin
        - Bouillon
        - Barley malt
        - Rice and brown rice syrup
        - Gelatin
        - Broth
        - Stock
        - Flavoring (some, not all)
        - Natural flavoring
        - Natural beef flavoring
        - Natural chicken flavoring
        - Seasoning
        - Spices
        - Whey protein
        - Whey protein isolate
        - Whey protein concentrate

    - Protein fortified
    - Pectin
    - Most fermented foods/drinks
  - These **sometimes** contain MSG:
    - Carrageenan
    - Enzymes
    - Soy protein
    - Soy Protein Concentrate
    - Soy Protein Isolate
    - Protein Concentrate
- Note: we all assume that protein is good for you, which it is, but as you can see, the use of the word protein with others often is misleading and hides the fact that MSG is present in many of these additives that contain the word protein.

Sodium (Salt)

- Sodium occurs naturally in most foods, and is necessary for many body functions. What's unnecessary is all of the **added** salt that is found in sauces, processed meats, canned soups and fast food. Too much salt can lead to high blood pressure and a build-up of fluid. I never add salt to any food, and drastically limit the intake of foods high in salt. Other names for sodium include:
  - Sodium alginate
  - Sodium ascorbate
  - Sodium bicarbonate (baking soda)
  - Sodium benzoate
  - Sodium caseinate
  - Sodium chloride
  - Sodium hydroxide
  - Sodium saccharin
  - Sodium stearoyl lactylate
  - Sodium sulfite
  - Disodium phosphate
  - Monosodium glutamate (MDS)
  - Trisodium phosphate
  - Na
  - Sea salt

Saturated Fat

- Fats are organic compounds that are made up of carbon, hydrogen and oxygen, and are a source of energy in foods. Fats belong to a group of substances called lipids, and come in liquid or solid form. Fats are essential for the body and are important for controlling inflammation, blood clotting and brain development. Generally, **unsaturated** fats are considered to be good, and **saturated** fats, not so good. The latter are the biggest dietary cause of high LDL cholesterol ("bad cholesterol"). Fats are a very complex subject – you should discuss it thoroughly with your doctor and nutritionist.

Added Sugar

- As you know from The Mind Diet Guidebook #8, *Sugar Is Evil*, you already know how bad it is for you. Generally, naturally occurring sugar, found in fruits, is not something I worry about. The greater concern is all the sugar added to soda, candy, cake, syrups and juices. Eliminating added sugar is a cornerstone of any successful weight loss strategy.

Trans Fat

- These fats form when vegetable oil hardens during a process called hydrogenation, and can raise LDL ("bad cholesterol") levels. They can also lower HDL levels ("good cholesterol"). Trans fatty acids are found in fried foods, commercial baked goods (donuts, cookies, crackers), processed foods, and margarines.

73 Popular Foods and Drinks and Their Ingredients: Good or Bad For You?

Mind-Diet.com

	GOOD NUTRIENTS/MINERALS																											BAD INGREDIENTS					
	ANTIOXIDANTS	BETA CAROTENE (VITAMIN A)	CALCIUM	COMPLEX CARBOHYDRATES	FIBER	IRON	LYCOPENE	MAGNESIUM	OMEGA FATTY ACIDS (O-3 & O-6)	POTASSIUM	PROTEIN	VITAMIN B1 (THIAMINE)	VITAMIN B2 (RIBOFLAVIN)	VITAMIN B3 (NIACIN)	VITAMIN B5 (PANTOTHENIC ACID)	VITAMIN B6	VITAMIN B7 (BIOTIN)	VITAMIN B8 (INOSITOL)	VITAMIN B9 (FOLATE, FOLIC ACID)	VITAMIN B11 (SALICYLIC ACID)	VITAMIN B12	VITAMIN A	VITAMIN C	VITAMIN D	VITAMIN E	VITAMIN K	ZINC	HIGH FRUCTOSE CORN SYRUP	MSG (MONO SODIUM GLUTAMATE)	SALT/SODIUM	SATURATED FAT	SUGAR (ADDED)	TRANS FAT
Alcohol																																■	
Almonds	■		■	■	■			■					■	■			■		■						■								
Apples	■			■	■												■																
Bacon														■																■	■		
Bananas								■		■							■		■														
Beans	■		■	■	■	■	■	■	■	■	■	■				■		■	■														
Bread					■	■			■					■														■					
Broccoli	■	■	■		■			■							■	■	■		■				■		■	■	■						
Butter		■																													■		
Candy																												■			■	■	■
Carrots		■					■					■					■	■	■			■											
Cashews								■																									
Cereal (boxed)			■			■			■			■		■		■					■			■	■			■		■		■	■
Cheese (hard)		■	■						■		■		■		■						■										■		
Chicken						■					■	■		■			■				■												
Chocolate	■																										■	■			■	■	■
Cookies/Cake/Muffins/Pastries																												■			■	■	■
Corn	■			■	■										■				■						■								
Cottage cheese											■		■								■									■			
Crackers																														■	■		■
Cream cheese			■								■											■								■	■		
Deli meats																					■							■		■	■		
Donuts																												■			■	■	■
Eggs		■				■			■		■	■	■		■		■		■		■			■									
Fish (cold water)			■			■		■	■		■	■	■	■	■	■	■			■	■			■	■								
French fries																														■	■		■
Frozen foods																													■	■	■		■
Grapes																							■										
Greens (leafy)		■	■			■		■							■				■			■	■			■							
Ham						■															■							■		■			
Hot dogs																												■		■	■		
Ice cream																												■			■	■	
Jelly																															■	■	■
Juice																														■		■	
Ketchup																												■		■		■	
Lettuce		■																	■			■	■			■							
Mayonnaise																									■	■				■	■		
Meat						■			■		■		■			■				■	■						■						
Melons										■													■										
Milk		■	■	■					■	■	■		■							■	■			■							■	■	
Oatmeal	■		■		■																			■				■					
Oil									■																■						■		
Onions		■		■								■																					
Oranges			■							■							■	■	■				■										
Pancakes																												■					
Pasta					■				■																			■					

73 Popular Foods and Drinks and Their Ingredients: Good or Bad For You?

Mind-Diet.com

	GOOD NUTRIENTS/MINERALS																											BAD INGREDIENTS					
	ANTIOXIDANTS	BETA CAROTENE (VITAMIN A)	CALCIUM	COMPLEX CARBOHYDRATES	FIBER	IRON	LYCOPENE	MAGNESIUM	OMEGA FATTY ACIDS (O-3 & O-6)	POTASSIUM	PROTEIN	VITAMIN B1 (THIAMINE)	VITAMIN B2 (RIBOFLAVIN)	VITAMIN B3 (NIACIN)	VITAMIN B5 (PANTOTHENIC ACID)	VITAMIN B6	VITAMIN B7 (BIOTIN)	VITAMIN B8 (INOSITOL)	VITAMIN B9 (FOLATE, FOLIC ACID)	VITAMIN B11 (SALICYLIC ACID)	VITAMIN B12	VITAMIN A	VITAMIN C	VITAMIN D	VITAMIN E	VITAMIN K	ZINC	HIGH FRUCTOSE CORN SYRUP	MSG (MONO SODIUM GLUTAMATE)	SALT/SODIUM	SATURATED FAT	SUGAR (ADDED)	TRANS FAT
Pasta sauce																									X					X			
Peas		X		X	X	X		X				X				X																	
Peanuts	X			X						X	X			X		X	X	X	X						X		X		X	X			
Peanut Butter	X									X	X			X			X	X									X					X	
Peppers	X	X					X					X				X		X				X	X		X								
Pickles																												X					
Pineapple	X																						X										
Pizza																												X					X
Popcorn																														X		X	
Pork						X					X	X				X								X									
Potato, White	X			X				X		X		X				X		X	X				X										
Popato, Chips																												X	X	X	X		X
Potato, Sweet	X	X		X		X		X							X		X					X	X		X								
Pretzels																												X	X	X	X		
Raisins										X																							
Rice				X	X	X			X							X																	
Salad dressing																												X	X	X		X	
Shrimp						X					X									X							X						
Soda (not diet)																												X				X	
Soup																												X	X	X	X		X
Spinach	X	X				X		X		X		X	X			X			X			X			X	X	X						
Strawberries	X			X		X											X		X				X										
Tomatoes		X		X			X			X			X	X	X		X	X					X										
Tunafish (canned)						X					X			X		X								X									
Turkey						X					X	X		X			X																
Watermelon						X	X											X					X										
Yogurt (flavored)			X	X				X			X		X		X					X								X			X	X	
Yogurt (plain)			X	X				X		X	X		X		X					X	X			X							X		

These are general guidelines and do NOT apply to ALL foods in each category. You must discuss more specifics with your doctor and nutritionist to get the full value from this chart.

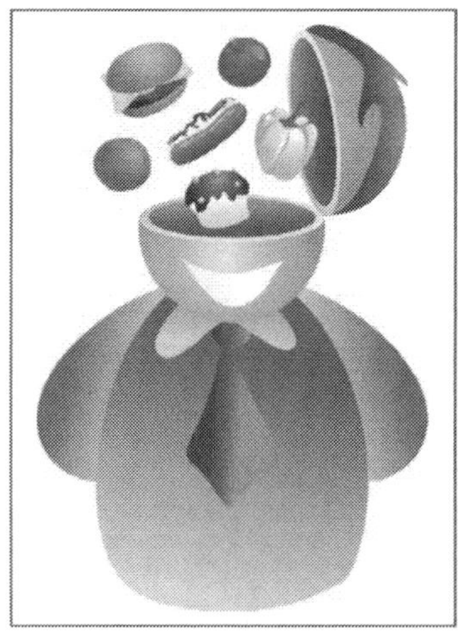

Guidebook #10 *Motivators*

To help you succeed, print or tear out any of these motivators and tape them to your fridge, pantry and other places around your home!

While I've presented a lot of solid arguments to help you reach your Moment of Truth in order to lose a lot of weight safely and keep it off permanently, I've found that clever and/or humorous reminders tend to motivate me as well. Here are more than two dozen of the best motivators I could find!

In a post from several years ago, the CEO of Weight Watchers, David Kirchoff, blogged about motivation. He boiled down weight loss to two components: starting a program and sticking with it. He's absolutely correct. What I've done in *The Mind Diet* is to help you rewire your mind so motivation will come naturally and easy.

By reaching your Moment of Truth, you have a different mindset about weight loss, food choices, the importance of food and more. As Kirchoff states in the post, "Motivation has a nasty habit of not being there when it's most needed." Hopefully your mindset will prevent this.

Use the motivational posters in this section as constant reminders of what you need to do for long-term weight loss.

Eat to Live.

Not the other way around.

Go Slow

Lose just 2/10th of a pound (3.2oz) a day = 72lbs. in one year!

To lengthen your life, shorten your meals.

Nothing tastes as good as being thin feels.

CHOCOLATE CAKE

INGREDIENTS: SUGAR, ENRICHED WHEAT FLOUR (WHEAT FLOUR, NIACIN, FERROUS SULFATE, THIAMIN MONONITRATE, RIBOFLAVIN FOLIC ACID), PARTIALLY HYDROGENATED PALM &/OR PALM KERNEL &/OR COCONUT AND/OR SOYBEAN &/OR COTTONSEED OILS, MILK, EGG WHITES, WATER, COCOA (WITH ALKALI), PASTEURIZED MILK & CREAM, STRAWBERRIES, APRICOT (WITH SULFUR DIOXIDE), CONTAINS 2% OR LESS OF THE FOLLOWING: EMULSIFIERS (PROPYLENE GLYCOL MONO AND DIESTERS OF FATTY ACIDS, MONO & DIGLYCERIDES, SOY LECITHIN, SODIUM STEAROYL LACTYLATE, SORBITAN MONOSTEARATE, POLYGLYCEROL ESTERS OF FATTY ACIDS, POLYSORBATE 60), CORN SUGAR, MODIFIED CORN STARCH, LEAVENING (SODIUM BICARBONATE, SODIUM ALLUMINUM PHOSPHATE, MONOCALCIUM PHOSPHATE, SODIUM PHOSPHATE, DICALCIUM PHOSPHATE), SALT, CARAMEL, COLOR, NONFAT MILK, XANTHAN GUM, CORN STRCH, RICE FLOUR, GUM ARABIC, CELLULOSE GUM, CONFECTIONERS GLAZE, CARRAGE-ENAN, HIGH FRUCTOSE CORN SYRUP, CARBOHYDRATE GUM, NATURAL & ARTIFICIAL FLAVORS, SODIUM CITRATE, DISODIUM PHOSPHATE, BETA CAROTENE (COLOR), MODIFIED FOOD STARCH, CHEESE CULTURE CAROB BEAN GUM, WHEY, CORN SYRUP SOLIDS, SODIUM CASEINATE, CITRIC ACID, DIPOTASSIUM PHOSPHATE, CORN SYRUP, LOCUST BEAN GUM, SODIUM TRISTEARATE, SODIUM ALGINATE, GELLAN GUM, SODIUM BENZOATE & POTASSIUM SORBATE (PRESERVATIVES), ARTIFICIAL COLORS (FD&C RED #3, RED #40, BLUE #1 & #2, YELLOW #5 & #6, BLUE #2 LAKE

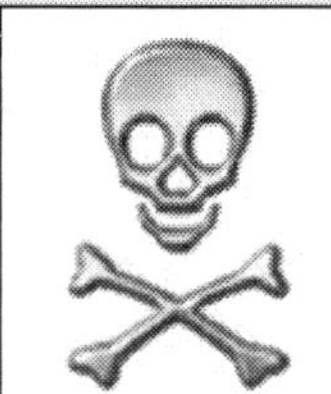

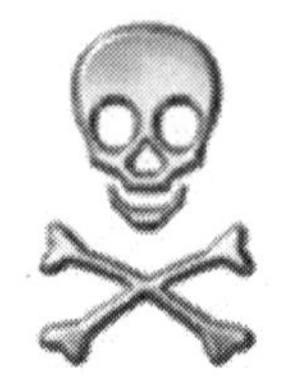

You're Eating This???!!!

Things That Are Addictive

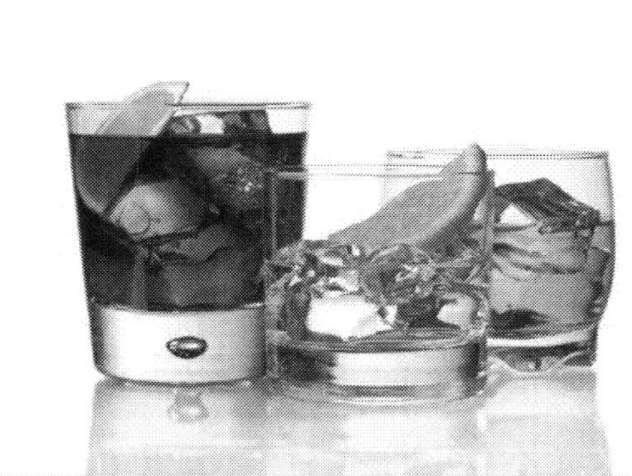

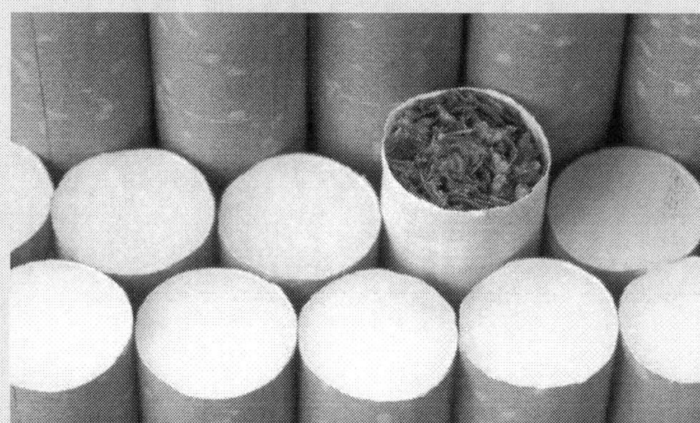

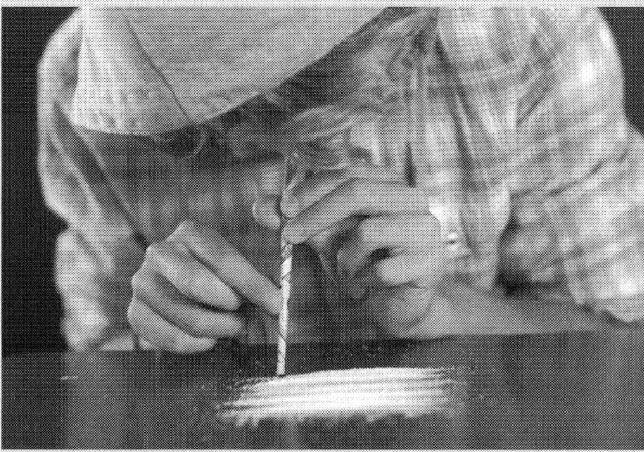

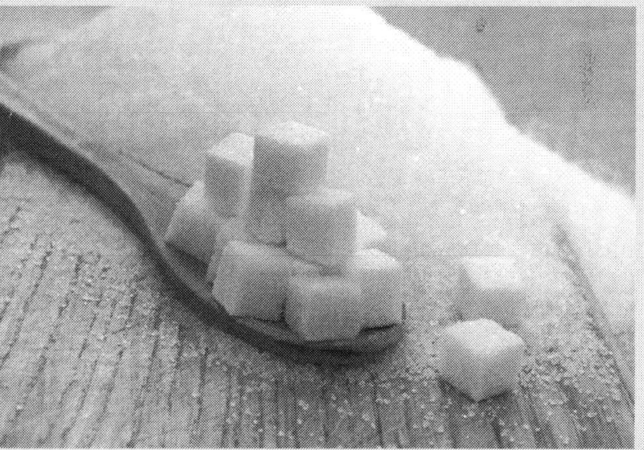

Losing weight is in your mind... ...but it's for your soul

A diet is the penalty we pay for exceeding the feed limit.

If you wish to grow thinner, diminish your dinner.

Take twice as long to eat half as much.

Your stomach should not be a waist basket.

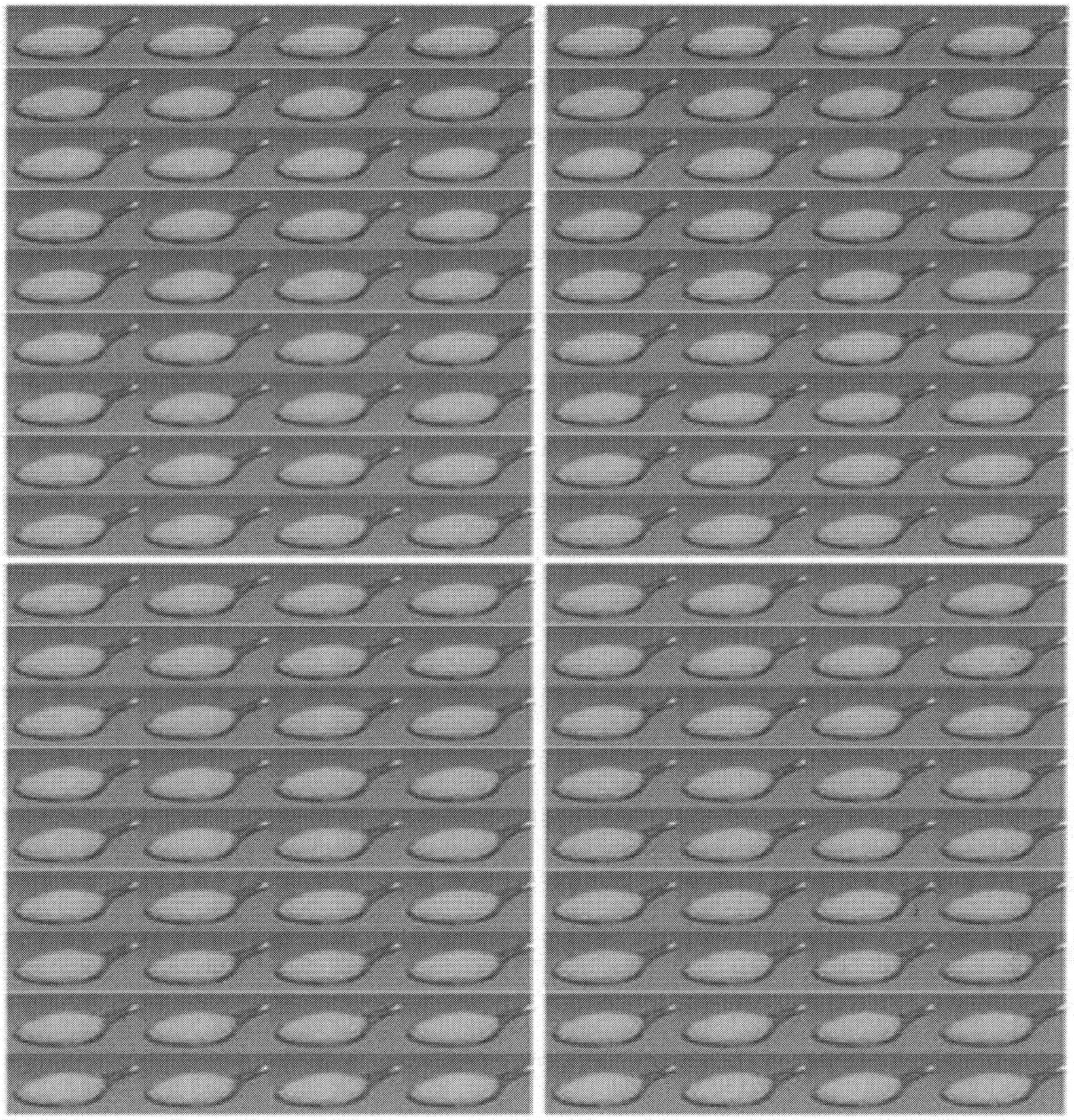

Do you **really** need to eat 660 teaspoons of sugar every month?

No thanks. Not interested in these weight-related conditions:

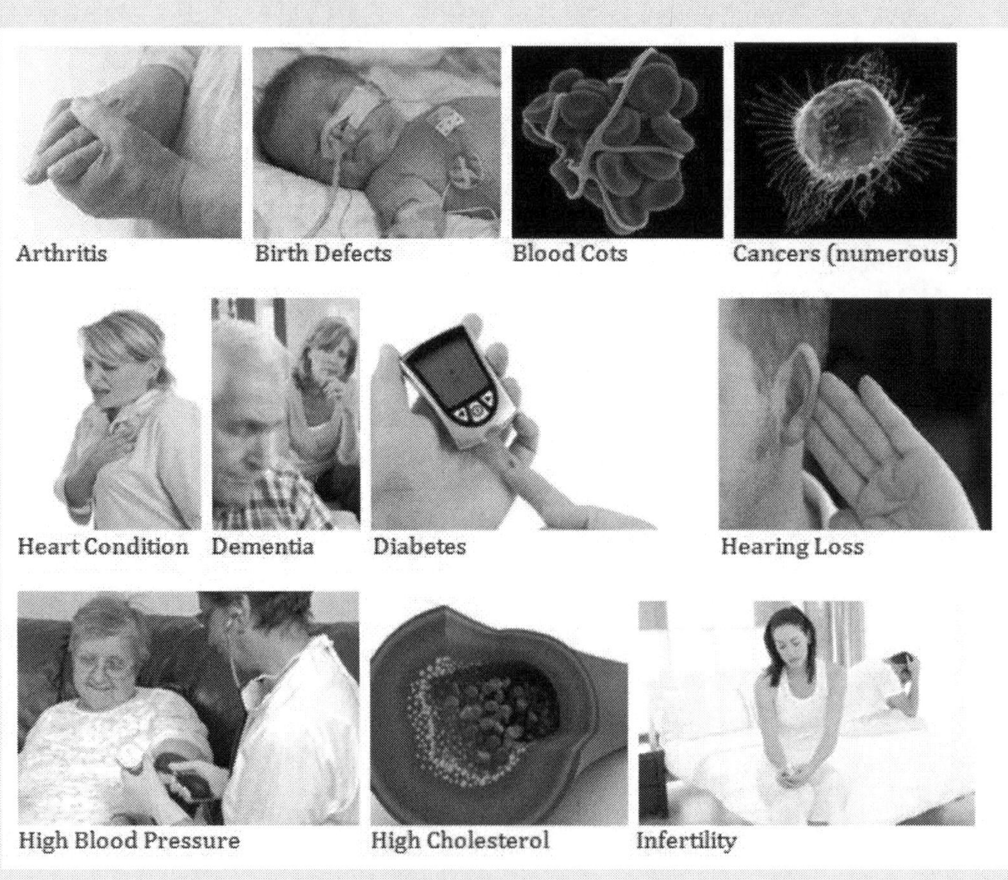

Plus dozens and dozens more. Who needs these?

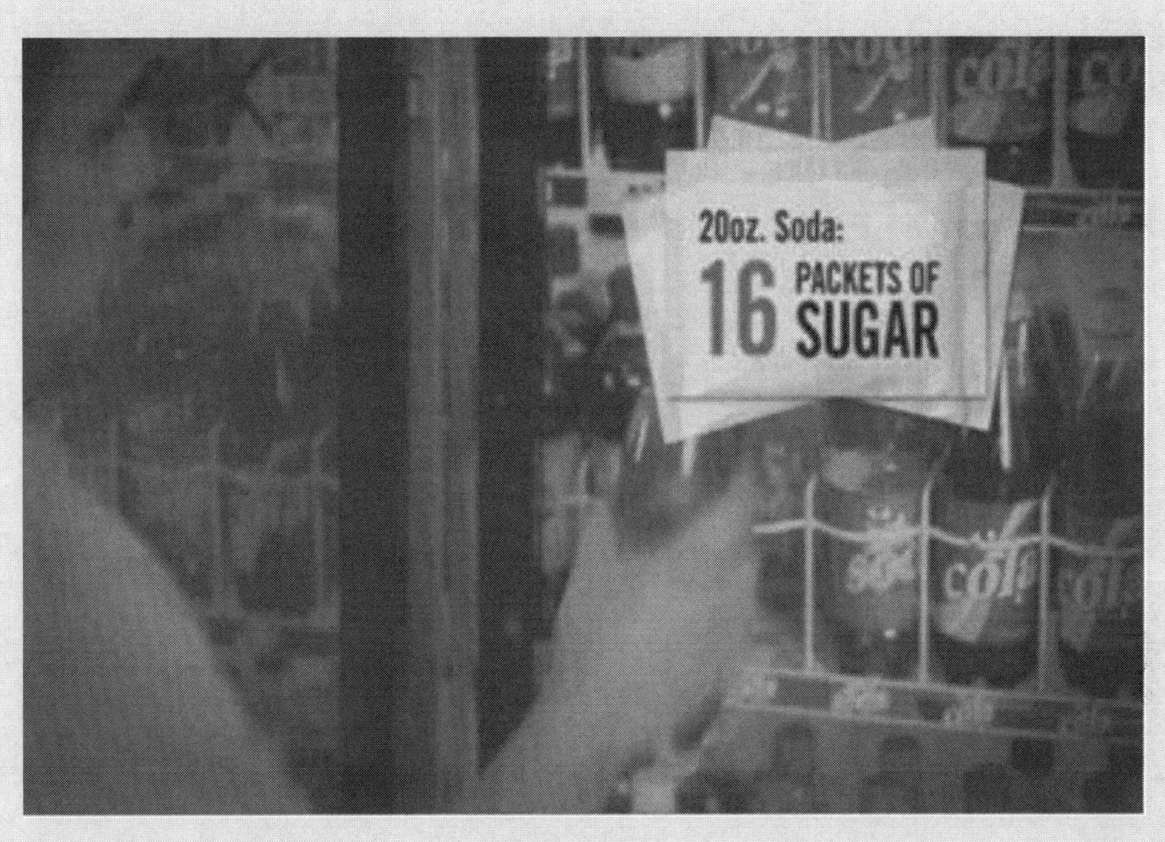
20oz. Soda:
16 PACKETS OF SUGAR

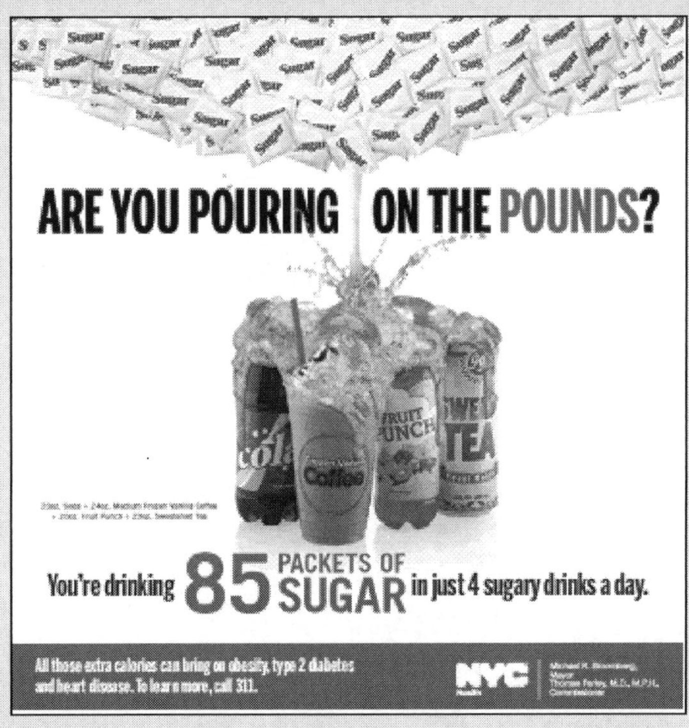
ARE YOU POURING ON THE POUNDS?
You're drinking 85 PACKETS OF SUGAR in just 4 sugary drinks a day.
All those extra calories can bring on obesity, type 2 diabetes and heart disease. To learn more, call 311.
NYC

Ads from the New York City anti-sugar campaign, 2011

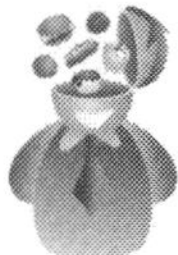

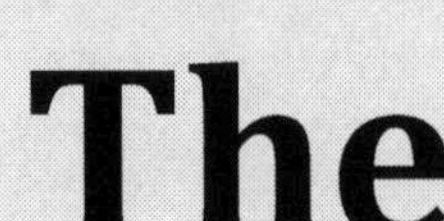

The 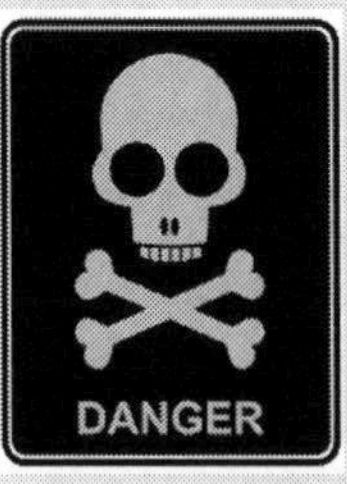 List

Foods and ingredients you absolutely, positively, definitely must avoid.

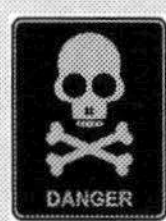 Regular **and** diet soda

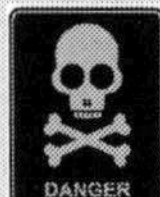 Added sugar

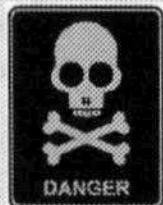 Genetically modified foods

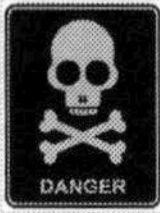 High fructose corn syrup (HFCS) and its cousin, Agave Nectar

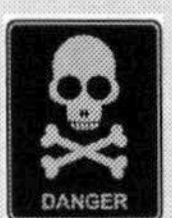 Hydrogenated oils, trans fat

 MSG (Mono Sodium Glutamate)

 Preservatives BHA and BHT

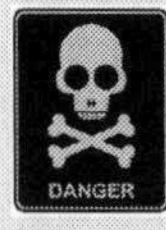 Potassium Bromate

 rBGH, rBST & Brominated Vegetable Oil

1,120 calories

You'd have to climb 1,665 stairs
to burn off 1,120 calories!

Menshealth.com

Have water for dinner tonight!

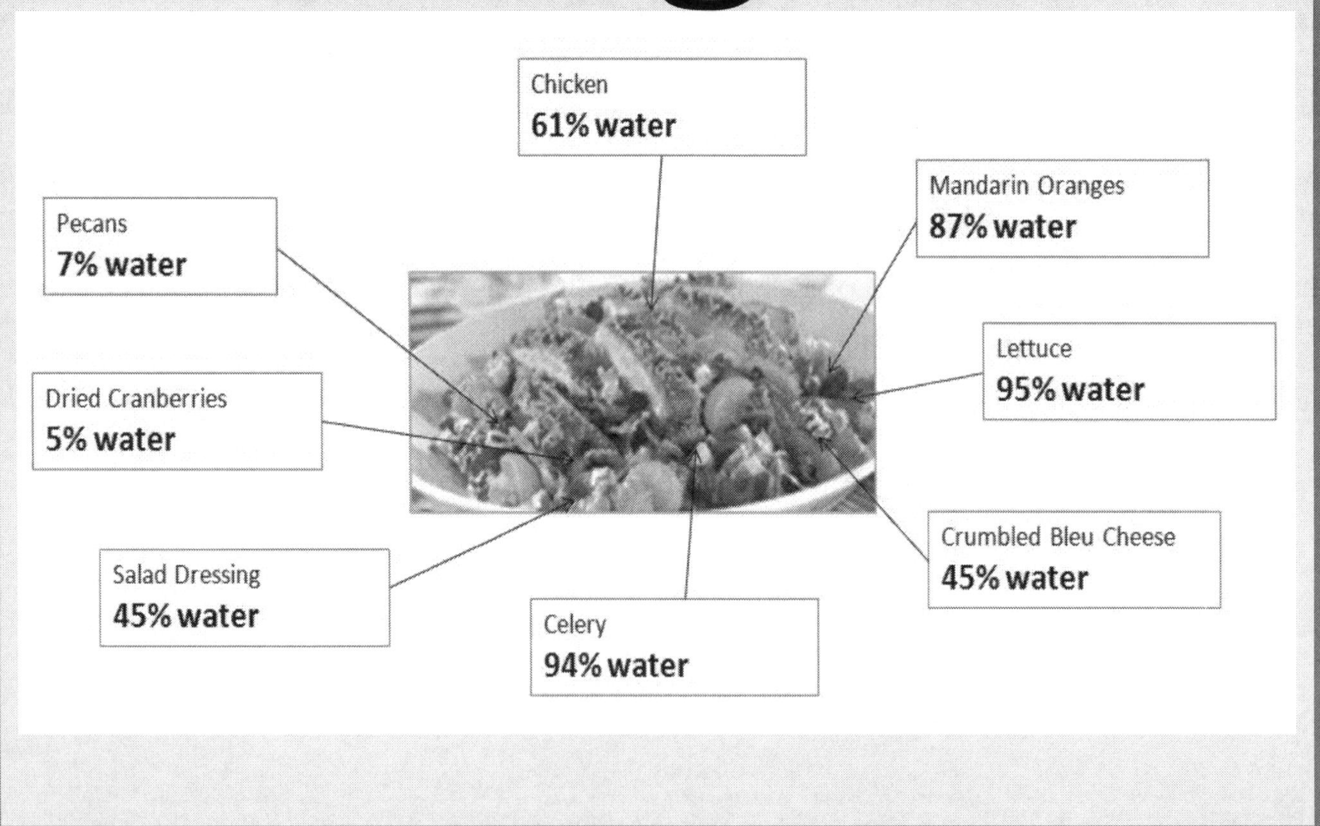

Obesity runs in the family. Only you can stop it.

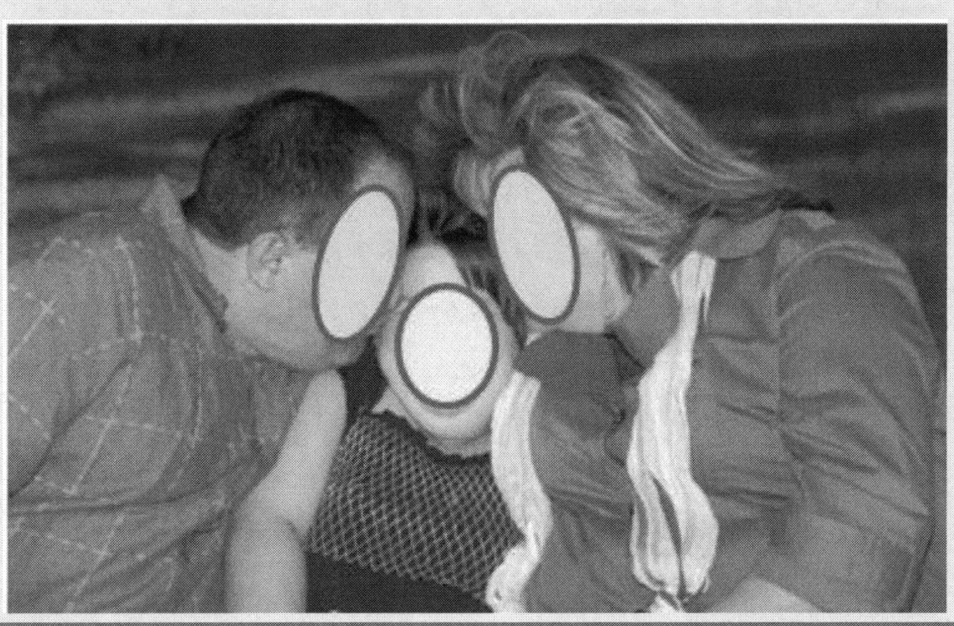

No more "chub rub"

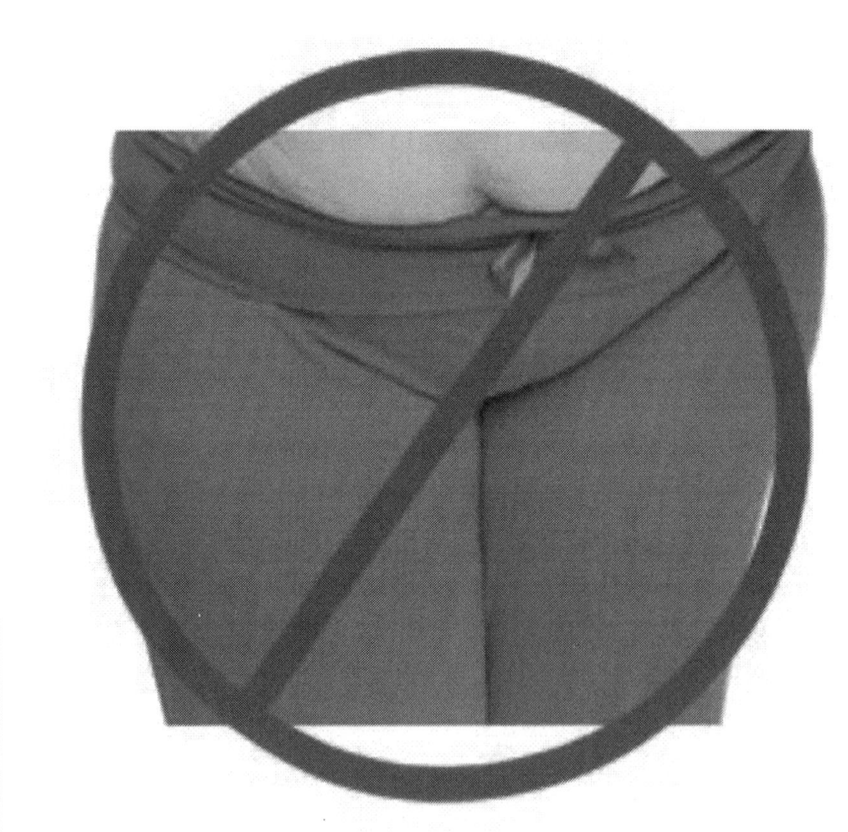

Chub Rub: when thick thighs constantly rub together causing friction, annoyance, and clothes that wear out prematurely.

WHAT'S IN THE Nutrition Label?

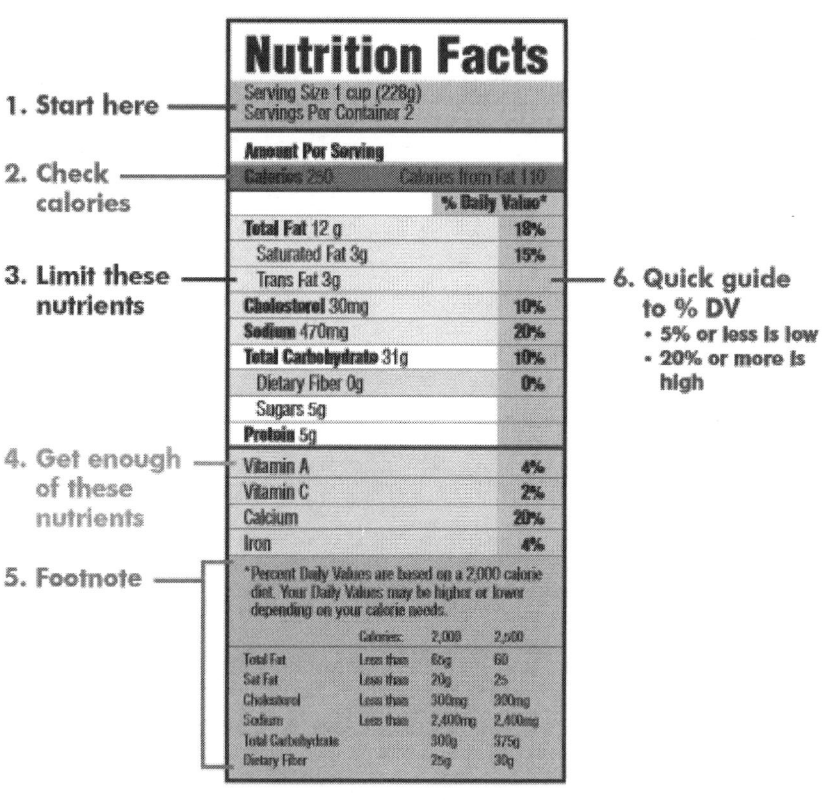

1 All the nutrients listed on the food label pertain to one serving of that food item. Pay attention to the serving size, especially how many servings there are in the food package. Then ask yourself, "How many servings am I consuming?" (1/2, 1 or more)

2 Calories provide a measure of how much energy you get from a serving of that food item. The number of servings you consume determines the number of calories you actually consume.

3 The nutrients identified in yellow should be consumed in limited amounts. Eating too much fat, saturated fat, trans fat, cholesterol or sodium may increase your risk for certain chronic diseases.

4 The nutrients identified in blue should be consumed in enough amounts to improve and maintain health and reduce the risk for some diseases and conditions.

5 The footnote tells that the %DV for the nutrients listed on the food label are based on a 2,000 calorie diet. This statement does not change from product to product; it is always the same.

6 The Percent Daily Value (%DV) helps to determine if a serving of food is high or low in a nutrient. Generally, a 5% DV is considered low and a 20% or more is high.

(Source: U.S. Food and Drug Administration, Center for Food Safety and Applied Nutrition. "How to Understand and Use the Nutrition Facts Label". For detailed information see http://www.cfsan.fda.gov/~dms/foodlab.html)

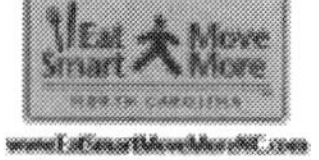

Accessed 5/28/13

What Counts as a Serving?

FOOD	WHAT IT LOOKS LIKE
GRAINS GROUP	
1 slice bread	Size of an audiocassette tape
1 cup ready-to-eat cereal	Size of a fist
1/2 cup cooked cereal, rice or pasta	Size of a cupcake wrapper full
1 pancake	Size of a compact disc
VEGETABLE GROUP	
1 cup raw leafy vegetables	Size of a baseball
1/2 cup other vegetables, cooked or raw	Size of an ice cream scoop or light bulb
3/4 cup vegetable juice	Size of a small Styrofoam cup
1 baked potato	Size of the fist
1/2 cup cooked, dry beans	
FRUIT GROUP	
1 medium fruit	Size of a tennis ball
1/2 cup chopped, cooked or canned fruit	Size of 7 cotton balls
3/4 cup fruit juice	Size of a small Styrofoam cup
1/4 cup raisins	Size of a large egg
DAIRY GROUP	
1 cup milk or yogurt	
1 1/2 ounces of natural cheese (e.g. Cheddar)	Size of a 9-volt battery
2 ounces of processed cheese (e.g. American)	Size of four dice
MEAT & BEANS GROUP	
3 ounces cooked meat, poultry or fish	Size of a deck of cards or palm of hand

Following foods count as 1 ounce of lean meat:
2 tablespoon peanut butter (size of a ping pong ball), 1/2 cup cooked dry beans, 1/2 cup tofu, 2 1/2 ounce soyburger, 1 egg , 1/3 cup nuts

FOOD	WHAT IT LOOKS LIKE
FATS, OILS AND SWEETS GROUP	
1 teaspoon butter, margarine	Size of a fingertip
2 tablespoon salad dressing	Size of a ping pong ball

(Source: Adapted from "Making Sense of Serving Sizes" http://www.mckinley.uiuc.edu/Handouts/maksenseservsizes/maksenseservsizes.html)

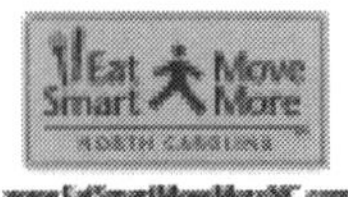

Accessed 5/28/13

“The first wealth is health.”

Ralph Waldo Emerson

"You can't change where you come from. You can change where you are going."

Maya Angelou

“Weight loss is 90% mental and the other half is what you eat.”

Adaptation of Yogi Berra’s famous quote:
“Baseball is 90% mental
and the other half is physical.”

Compare This!

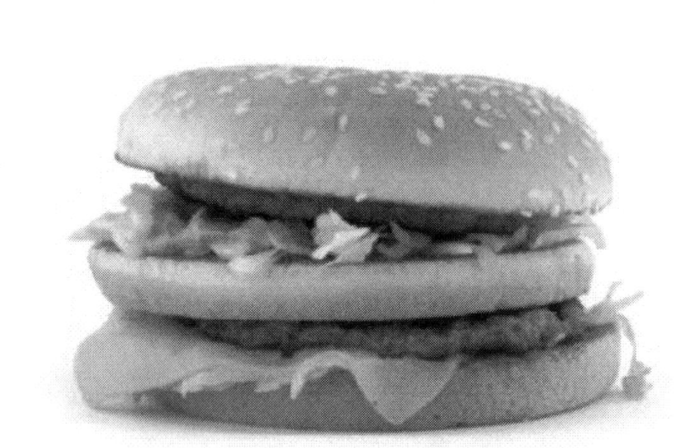

BigMac – 540 unhealthy calories

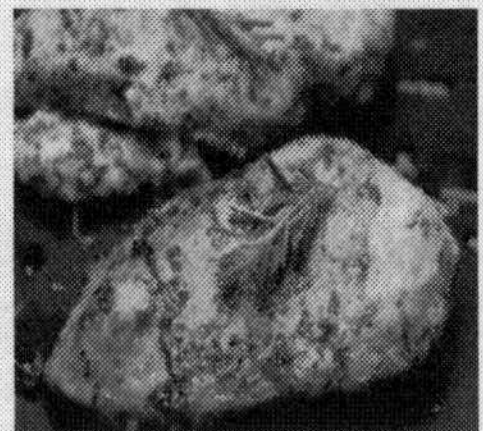

4oz grilled chicken

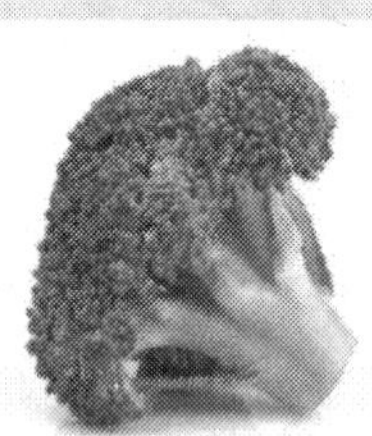

3 cups broccoli

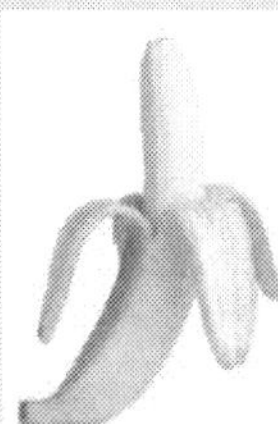

1 med banana

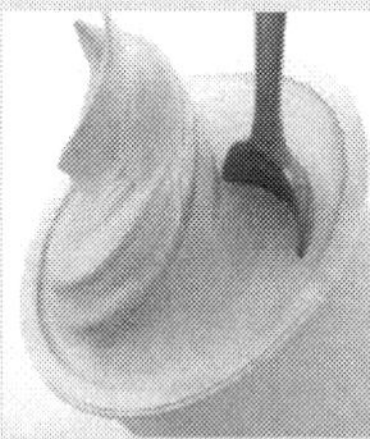

8 oz Greek yogurt

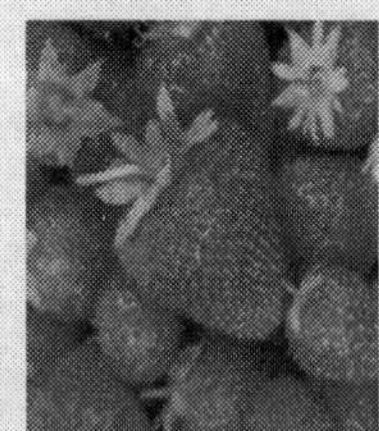

10 med strawberries

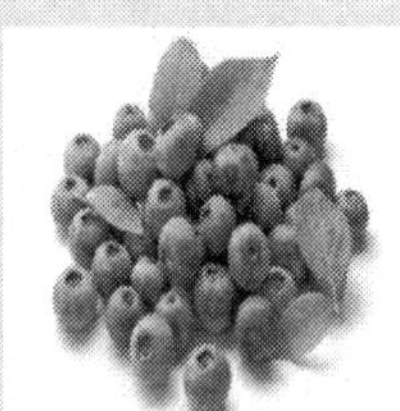

1/2 cup blueberries

ALL of this – 540 healthy calories

Source: BioTrustNews.com

Home Sweet Home

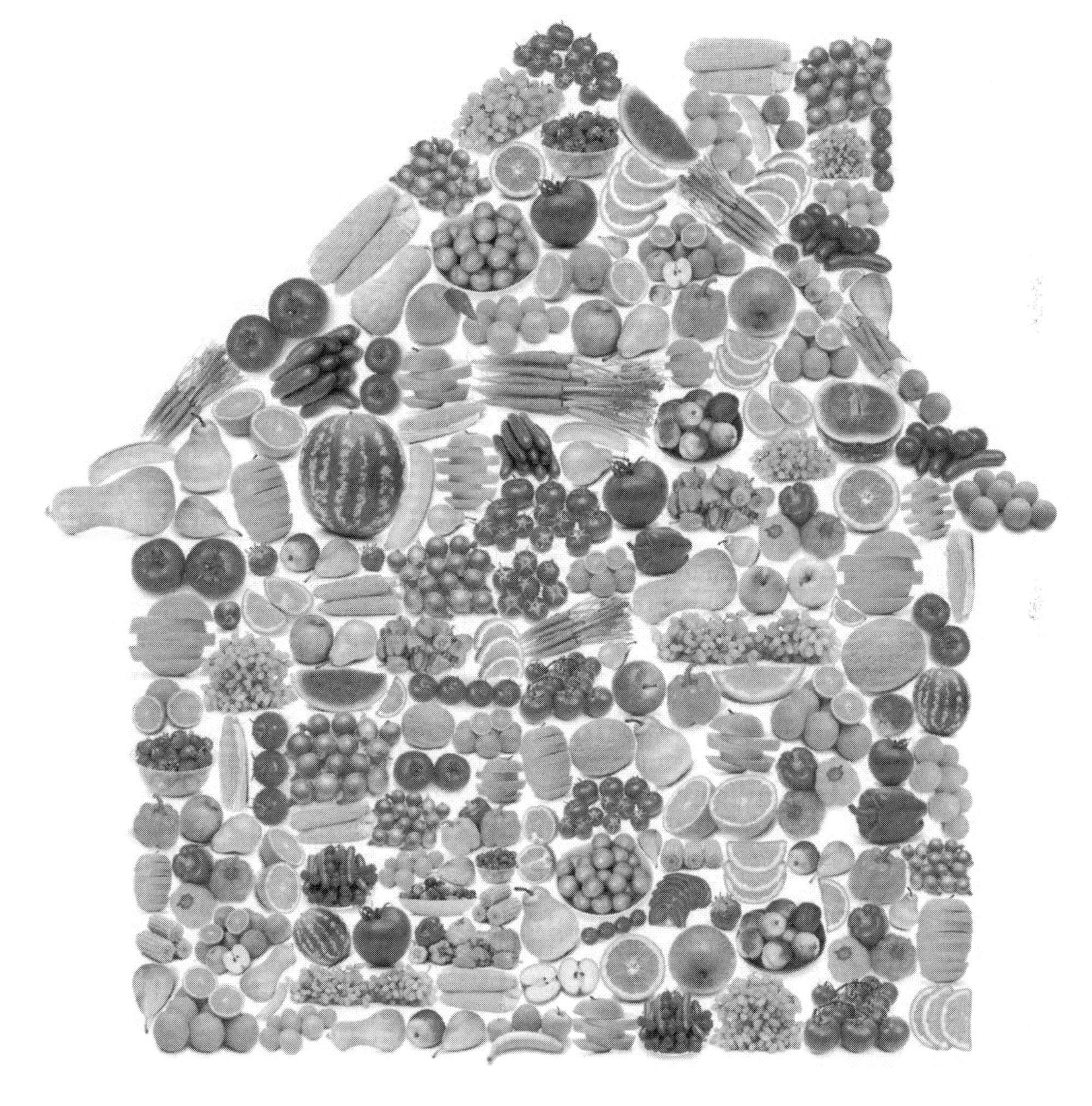

Go Green!

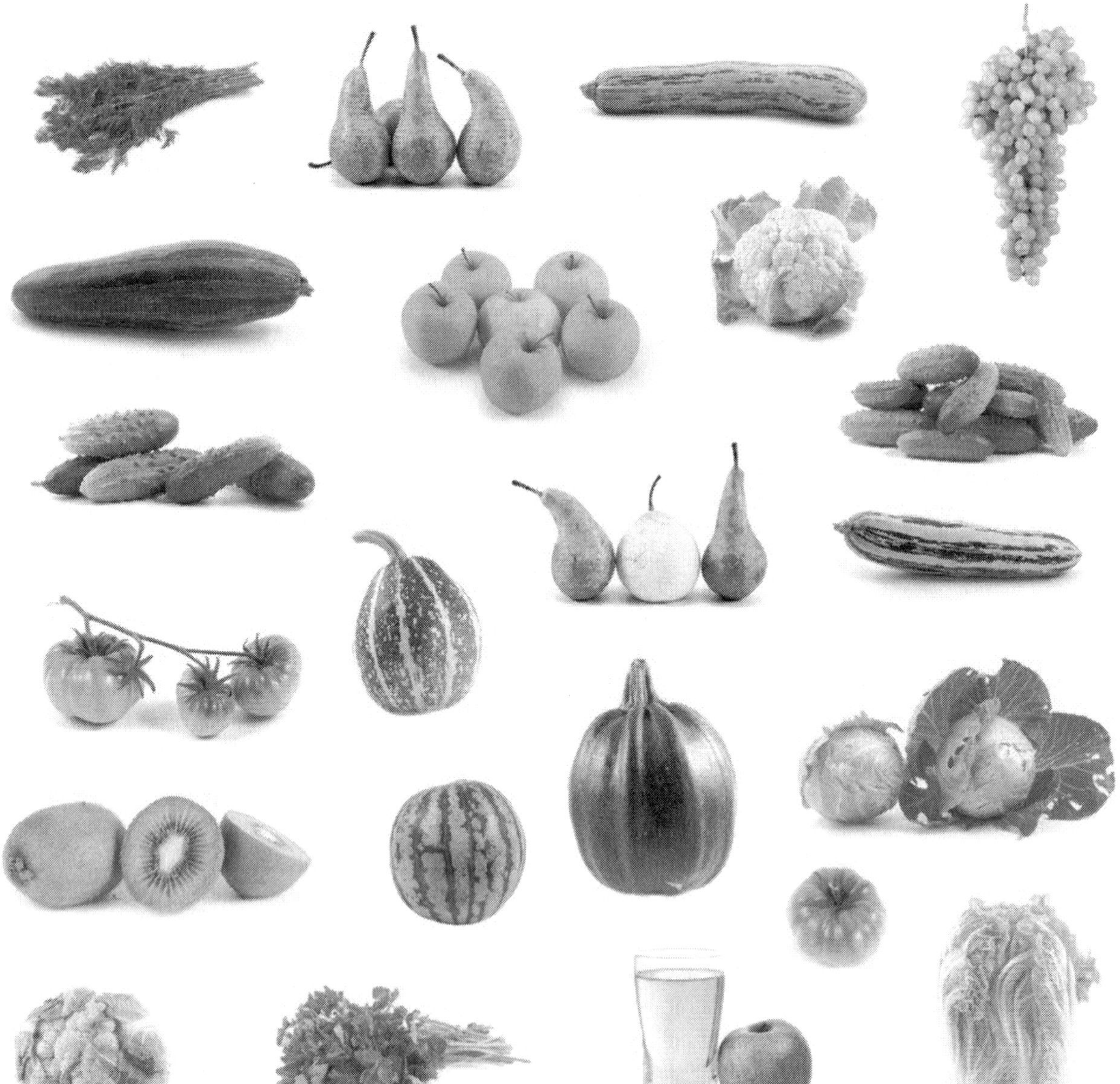

Salad Power

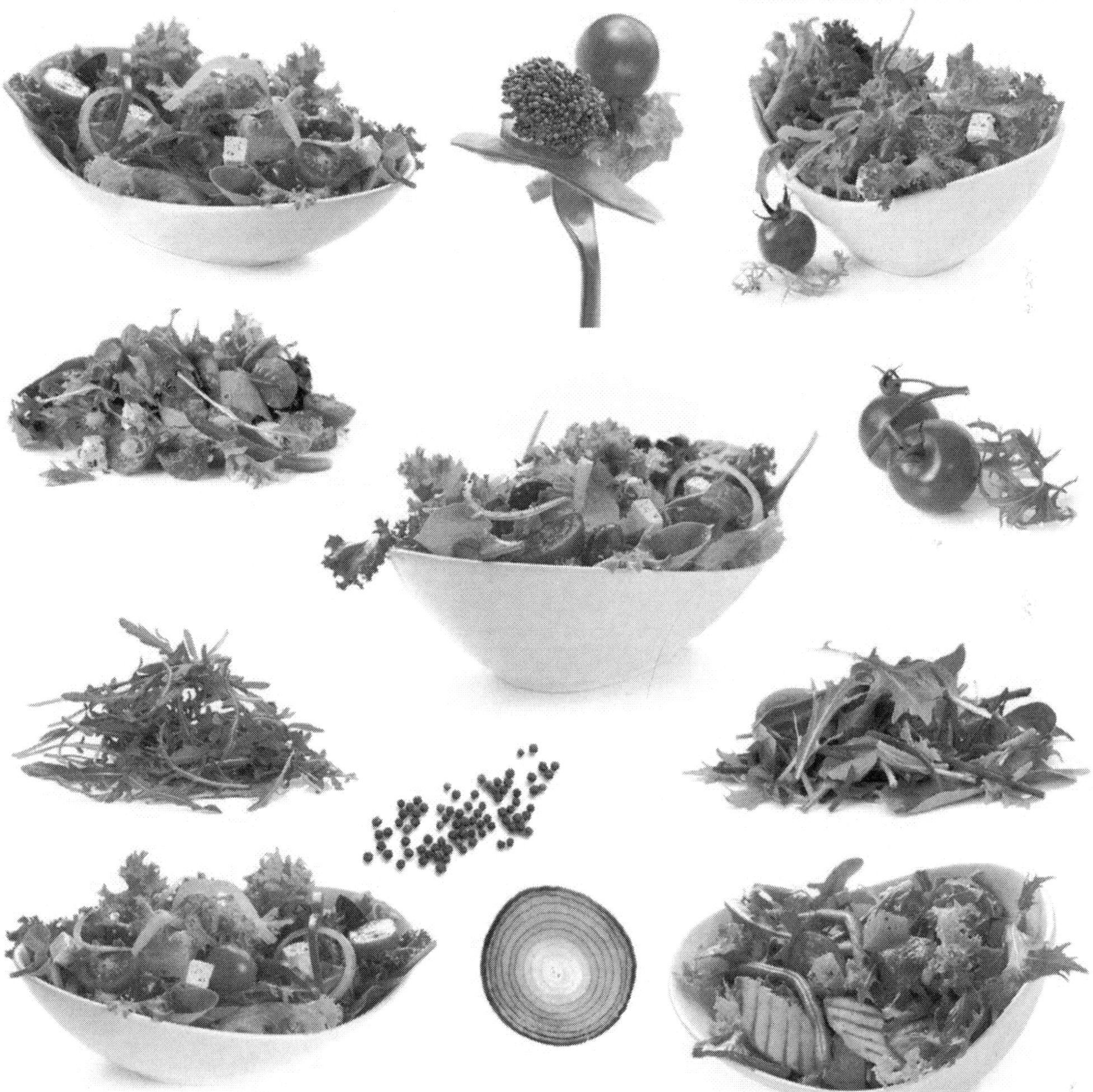

Mmm Mmm Good!

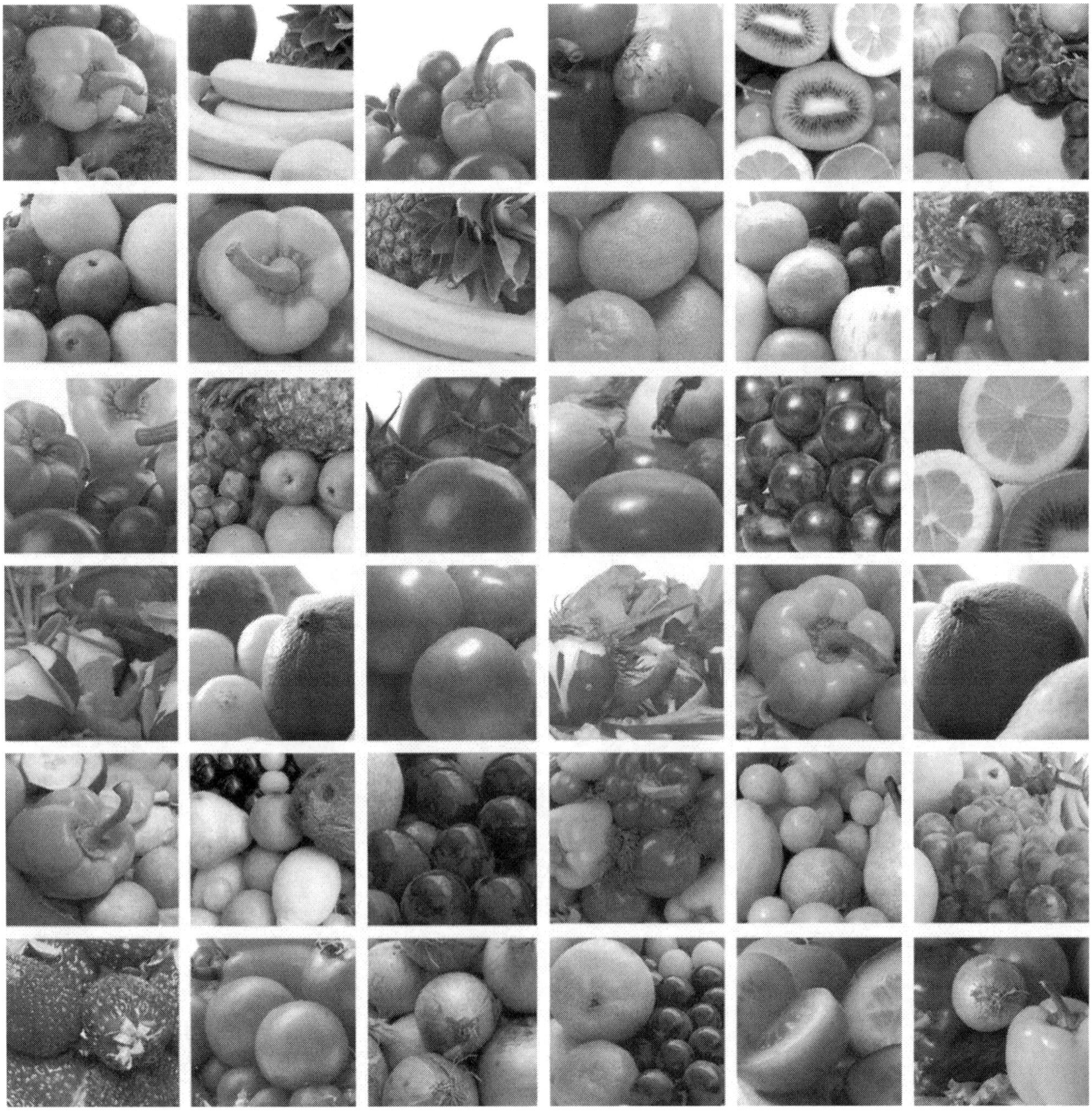

Go Nuts!

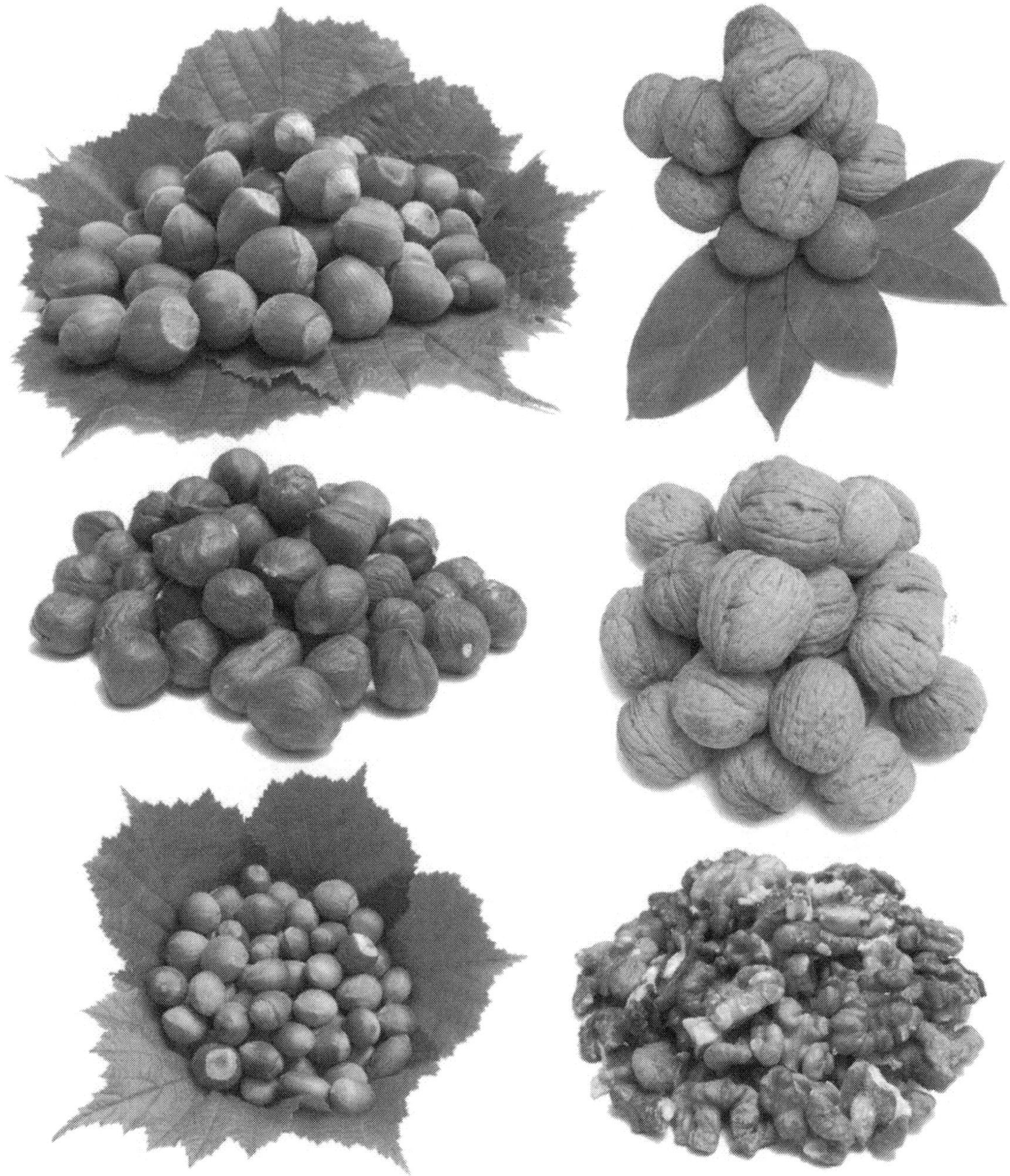

Spice Up Your Health

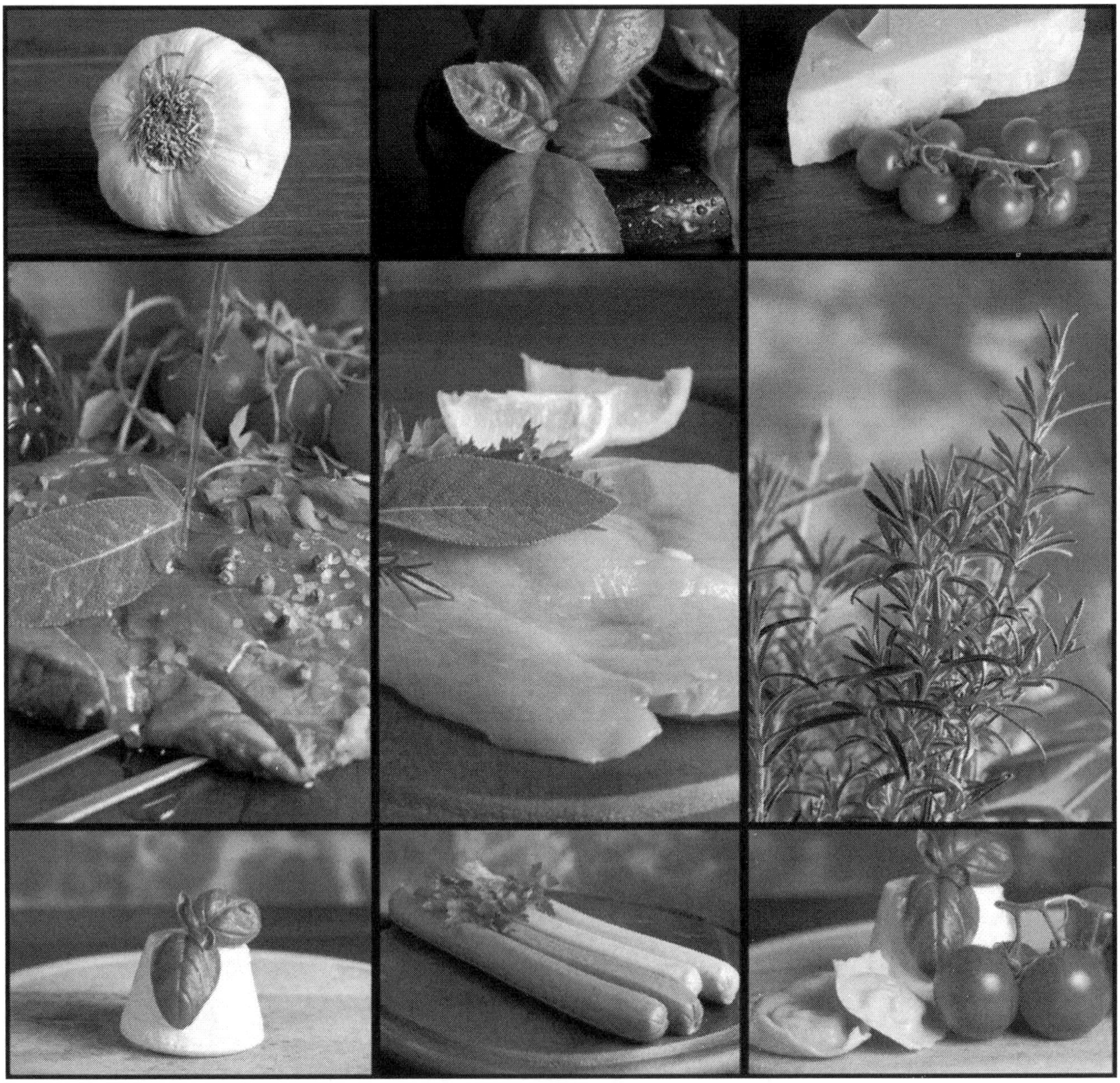

How Sweet It Is!

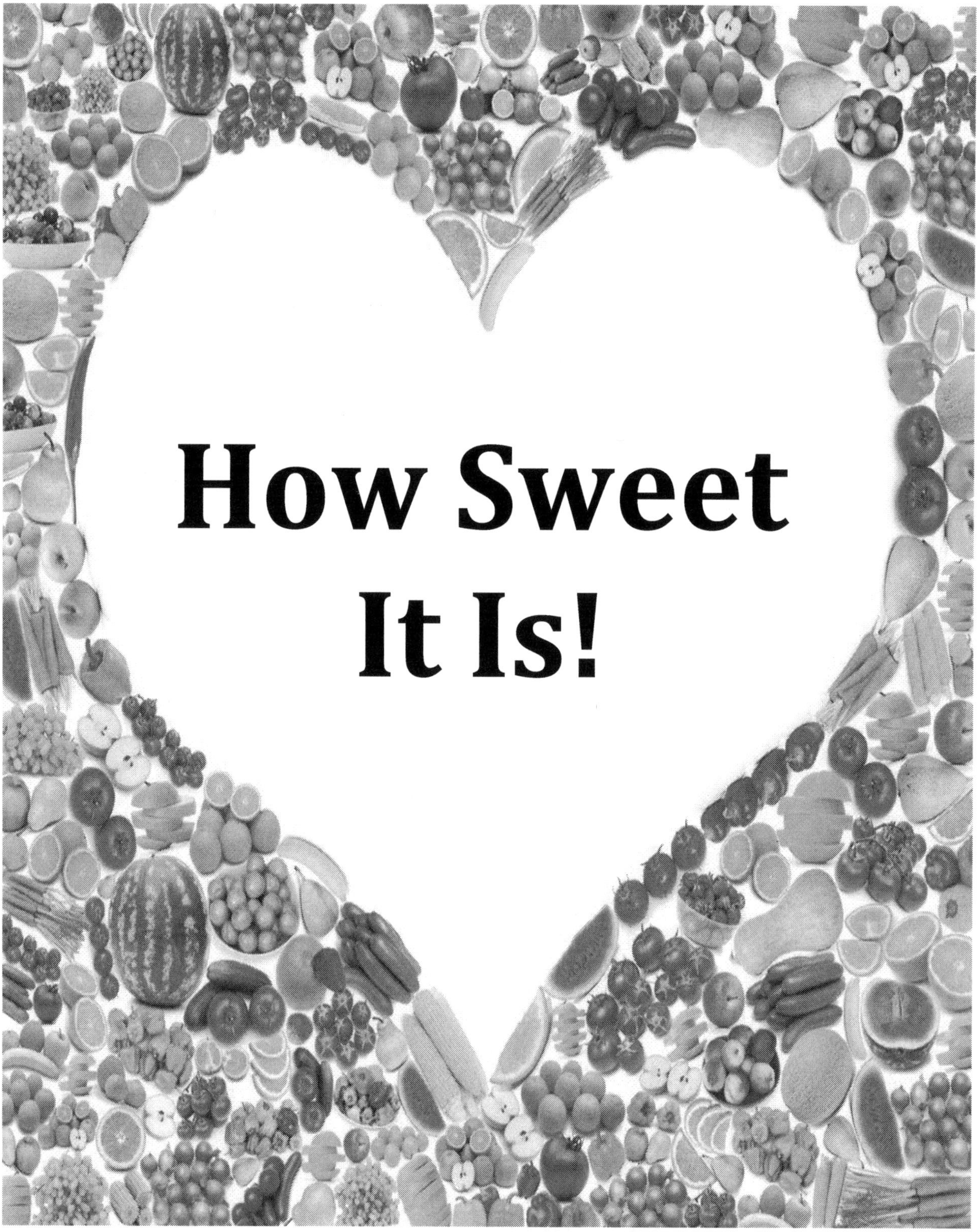

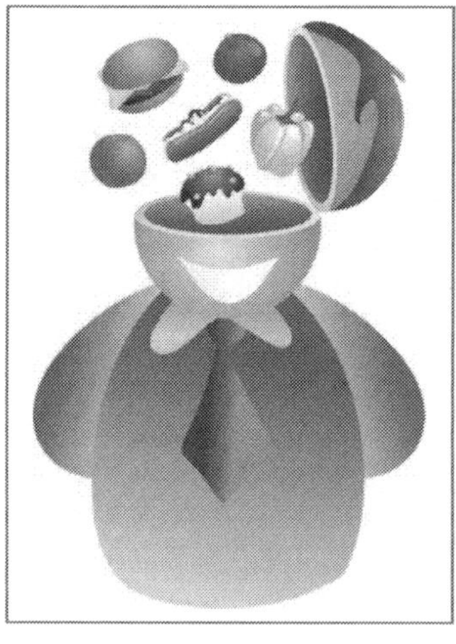

Bonus #1 *My Golden Resources*

Over the course of time, I've come across many great resources, tools, websites and apps. I've summarized what I consider to be the best in this 10th guidebook. I've chosen these websites, books, blogs and products for three main reasons:

- They have consistently produced quality information that is accurate and useful in my personal quest to lose weight.
- They are well-written, easy to understand and provide practical information that I can use.
- They are in line with *The Mind Diet* philosophy of weight loss.

I do not have any financial interest in any of these. While I'm sure that there are plenty of other quality sites, blogs and products, these are the ones I've come across during my weight loss journey. I only have included sites that are free, and they are listed in alphabetical order.

Websites

Diet Review Post
www.dietreviewpost.com

This is quite probably the most comprehensive compendium of reviews of diet programs, everything from fads to mainline companies that are etched in our minds. These impartial reviews are categorized by type of program (i.e. blood type, low carb, low fat) and also includes weight loss centers and camps. As you know from reading *The Mind Diet,* the program you choose to follow must be in conjunction with your doctor and dietician, because it needs to be based on your unique situation. To get the best possible overview of diet programs, look no further than this web site.

EatingWell.com
"Where Good Taste Meets Good Health"
www.EatingWell.com

The focus of this site is on cooking healthy at home. You'll find a wide array of sections including "Cooking for Two," "Kids Cooking," "Quick and Healthy Cooking" and "Budget Cooking." EatingWell.com also features kitchen product reviews, recipe makeovers and "Healthy Cooking 101: Basics and Techniques" for the new or inexperienced cook. Plus, they have dozens of free videos that will help you cook healthy at home.

iVillage
www.ivillage.com

While a massive site addressing a wide range of topics, their health, diet and fitness sections have a wealth of solid information, including videos, community and tools. You can ask their experts questions about weight loss and other topics, and you can sign up for a variety of email newsletters. I've mentioned a few of their slide shows in this book because they are very well done and valuable.

Mercola.com
"Take Control of Your Health"
www.mercola.com

This is one of my favorite sites, and I have learned so much from it. Dr. Mercola provides information that is brutally honest, primarily because he is not beholden to any companies or special interests. The site provides the most up to date natural health information and resources that will most benefit you and, exposes corporate, government and mass media hype that diverts you away from what is truly best for your health and often to a path that leads straight into an early grave. They have a daily email newsletter, and most of the articles feature video interviews with Dr. Mercola, plus footnoted sources that are trustworthy.

MyFitnessPal.com
www.myfitnesspal.com

Believing that the best way to lose weight and keep it off is to simply keep track of the foods you eat. I certainly agree that keeping track is a big part of successful weight loss. This 100% free website and 18 mobile apps and the world's largest nutrition and calorie database make it very easy for you to log your meals quickly and easily. The more you track what you eat, the more likely you are to stay on track and achieve your weight loss goals. They also have a blog and an active community.

NutritionAction.com
"Unbiased Advice to Help You Eat Healthfully and Live Longer"
www.NutritionAction.com

Nutrition Action is loaded with very well-written free offerings in numerous categories. I've been reading their content for years and they've been mentioned elsewhere in this book. You'll find lists of best and worst foods, food specific articles such as "Sugar in Food" and "Salt in Food," plus one of my favorites "Calories in Food: Calories for Dummies." I also subscribed to their newsletter, which is also loaded with valuable information. The information is truly independent and invaluable.

Nutrition Data at Self.com
www.nutritiondata.self.com/
"Know What You Eat"

If you want to dig deeper into understanding what you're eating, this is a great site to do that. You'll find detailed nutrition info for your favorite foods, plus tools that tell you how foods can affect your health. That's the starting point. Self.com is focused on your health, with over a dozen other tools, including one of my favorites, "Are You Actually Hungry?" It's a decision making tool that helps you be really honest with yourself – determining whether you're actually hungry or if you just need a break.

Nutrition Facts
www.NutritionFacts.org

Dr. Michael Greger scours the world's scholarly literature on nutrition and along with a group of dedicated volunteers, distills the most important findings into videos on every health subject under the sun. In addition to over 1,500 videos, there's a "Q&A With the Doctor" section and a blog. A truly wonderful resource, made possible by the dedication of Dr. Greger.

SkinnyChef
"Life Should be Delicious"
www.skinnychef.com

We all love delicious food, but it always seems to put on the pounds. But with the information and recipes at SkinnyChef, you'll be able to enjoy delicious meals, have more energy, maintain a healthier lifestyle, and keep your weight in check. Jennifer Iserloh teaches how to use the right recipes and the right techniques to create amazing food creations that are healthy and don't add weight. Here's proof that delicious doesn't have to mean fattening.

SparkPEOPLE.com
"Sparking Millions of People"
www.sparkpeople.com

This site's mission is to SPARK millions of PEOPLE to reach their goals and lead healthier lives. They offer nutrition, health, and fitness tools, support, and resources that are 100% free, while other sites charge their members for similar services. They have some really cool trackers and a very active community. Sharing experiences, as you know from *The Mind Diet*, is very important. And they have dozens of videos in a number of categories, a radio show and interactive quizzes.

WebMD
"Better Information, Better Health"
www.webmd.com

I find this site to be a treasure trove of solid information and a lot of very useful tools and lists. I especially like their slide shows with titles like "24 Heart-Saving Foods" and "10 Sandwiches to Stop Eating Now" and their "symptom checker." You can communicate with their experts and visit their communities to learn from people that could help you. They have several email newsletters and you can access information on your tablet and smart phone.

Weight Loss Top Blogs Directories

Because blogs are so personal, I chose to direct you to several directories that have researched hundreds of blogs to find the best ones:

- The 100 Most Inspirational Weight Loss Bloggers at DietsToGo.com: http://tinyurl.com/m6rdrje
- Top 100 Weight Loss Blogs to Follow at CouponAudit.com: http://tinyurl.com/mle9zkx
- 20 Inspiring Weight Loss Blogs at Shape.com: http://tinyurl.com/6y92gnu
- 10 Weight Loss Bloggers You Should Follow at msn.com: http://tinyurl.com/boh7zrf

Products

Precise Portions Nutrition Control System
"Making It Easy to Eat Well"
PrecisePortions.com

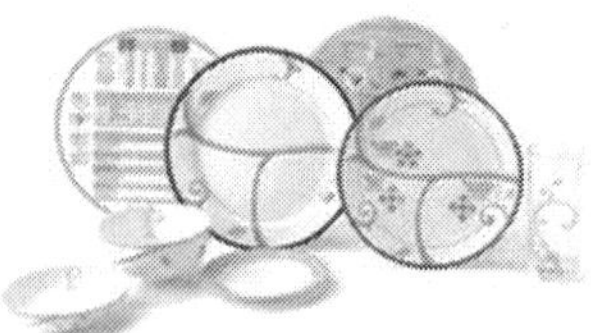

Most people have no idea what a correct portion size is, and consequently overeat at almost every meal. With supersized portions the norm in restaurants, it's no wonder we eat more than we should, whether dining out or eating at home. That's why this product will easily teach yourself (and your kids) what correct portion sizes entail. They also have "Eat and Learn" placements to accompany the dishes and other portion control related products.

NaTUREBOX
"A New Way to Snack"
NatureBox.com

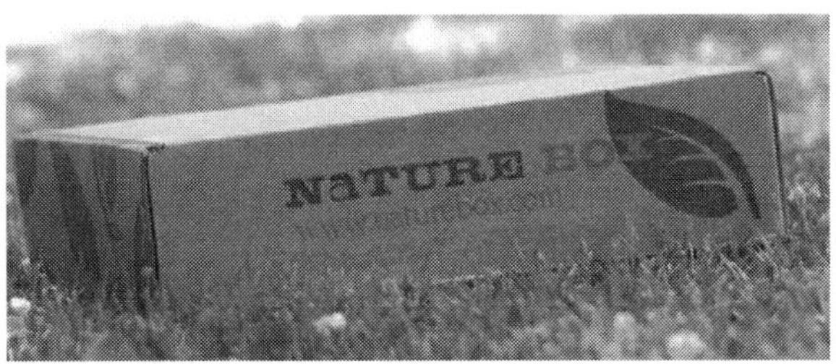

I suspect that people put on as much or more weight snacking than they do eating meals. It's so easy to reach for junk food, unhealthy snacks and candy bars when you need something during the day, whether at home or at work. That's why I think NatureBox is a very smart idea – they ship healthy snacks to you every month, all of which have:

- No high fructose corn syrup (HFCS)
- No partially hydrogenated oils
- No trans fats
- No artificial sweeteners
- No artificial flavors
- No artificial colors

Each box includes 15-20 servings and varies in content by time of year. What a cool idea!

FITBIT
"Will help you tell your weight who's boss"
Fitbit.com

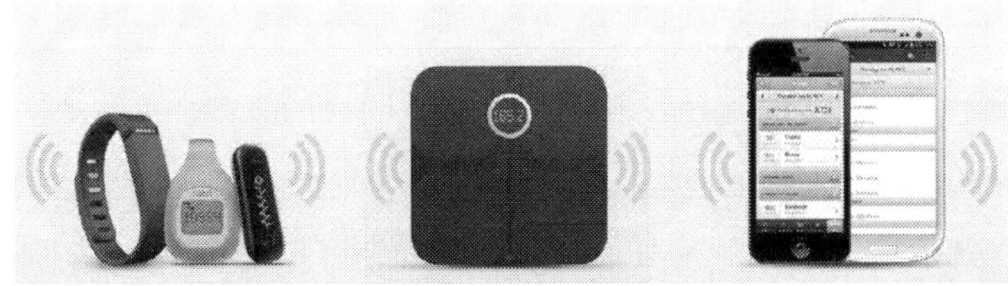

The fitbit family of high tech tools is an integrated set of wireless trackers, a smart scale and mobile tools that motivates you to stay active, live better and reach your goals. All three are synched so that on fitbit.com you see the total picture of how all of your activity –

even going up a flight of steps – is contributing to your overall weight loss program. You'll learn quite a bit, especially how much activity you need to burn calories, and I really like the Wi-Fi scale, which tracks your weight, body fat percentage and BMI, something I've not seen elsewhere.

HEALTHY OUT
"A Healthy Meal Program Made Just For You"
www.healthyout.com

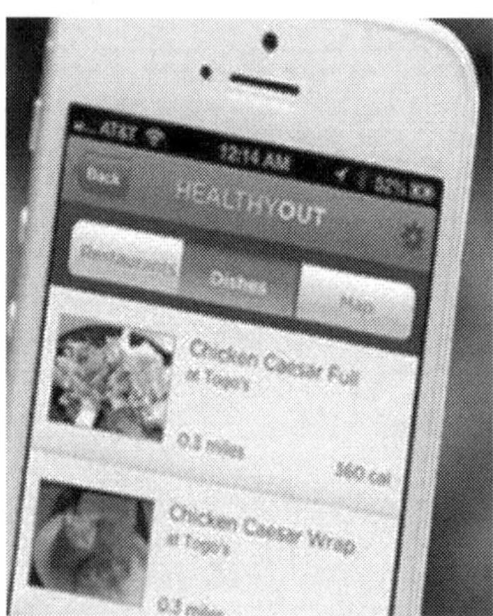

Think of Healthy Out as a restaurant food delivery service (available in NYC) based on your dietary profile. You download their app, fill out the kinds of food you want to eat, and they plan and deliver appropriate foods to your home or office. Based on what your doctor and nutrition specialist and you determine is your optimal diet, Healthy Out can make it happen, making eating right easier for you.

KILLER AT LARGE
Documentary
www.imdb.com/title/tt0903660/

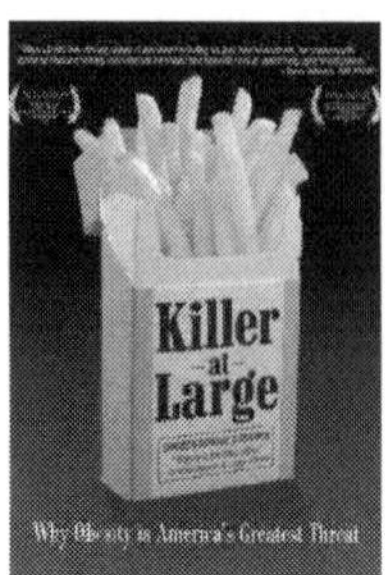

This film by Steven Greenstreet takes an in-depth look at obesity, which it likens to a major threat facing our country. Former Surgeon General Richard Carmona is quoted in the film with a very compelling summary: "Obesity is a terror [threat] within; it's destroying our society from within and unless we do something about it, the magnitude of the dilemma will dwarf 9/11 or any other terrorist event that you can point out."

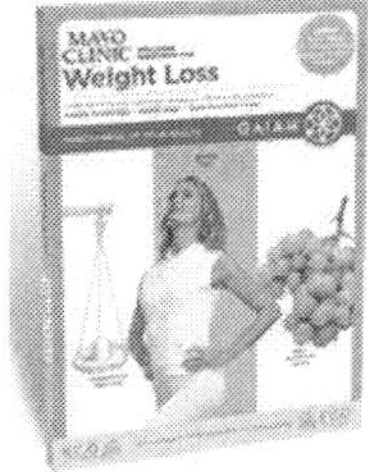

MAYO CLINIC WELLNESS SOLUTIONS FOR WEIGHT LOSS
Video + *My Stress Solution* Book
http://tinyurl.com/kdjmqs8

Mayo Clinic is one of the world's top medical centers. They developed this video with Gaiam, experts in alternative health and wellness that combines traditional medical knowledge with the best of today's alternative therapies. The three sections include understanding your health, eating well to feel better and moderate exercises with stress reducing techniques. Since stress is known to be an underlying factor of obesity, this combination of practical knowledge with stress reduction is a fresh new approach.

Books

The Blood Sugar Solution
Dr. Mark Hyman

Balanced insulin levels are the key to weight loss and health in this cutting-edge book by Dr. Mark Hyman. I've reached pretty much the same conclusion during my weight loss journey. He further identifies seven keys to achieving wellness: nutrition, hormones, inflammation, digestion, detoxification, energy metabolism, and a calm mind. He also goes beyond weight loss with advice on diet, green living, supplements and medication.

Eat Out, Eat Right
Hope Warshaw

Eating out has become more and more commonplace over the decades, and it is a major contributing factor to obesity. We tend to eat more when we dine out, and we often don't know what's in foods prepared at restaurants and other venues. The realistic, informative guidelines in *Eat Out, Eat Right* enable diners to make healthy menu choices from a wide variety of foods and cuisines, including Mexican, Italian, Chinese, Thai, fast food, and many others. This book reflects the latest trends in dining out, with expanded information on "fast casual" restaurants like Applebee's and Chili's; Subway and other sandwich shops; and the myriad of coffee and juice drinks now available. Sample menus, nutritional facts and figures, and diabetic exchanges provide additional information.

Food & Mood
Elizabeth Somer

Nutrition expert Somer explains how what we eat has a direct influence on how we feel, think, sleep, look, and act. She addresses specific food-related issues including health conditions, food cravings, diet struggles, stress, PMS, winter blues, energy levels, depression, memory, and sleep patterns, as well as tackling the issue of supplements and providing the real story on those you need and those you don't. Since food has such a major impact on our lives and in so many ways, this book is recommended because it answers a wide range of questions including: Why do you feel tired after eating a full meal? Why do you have so much trouble concentrating? Why do you crave chocolate? Can diet affect depression? Is there a natural cure for insomnia? Get answers with *Food & Mood.*

Good Calories, Bad Calories
Gary Taubes

Counting calories is one of the staples of diets, as we've been taught that fat is bad for us, carbohydrates better, and that the key to a healthy weight is eating less and exercising more. Yet despite this advice, we have seen unprecedented epidemics of obesity and diabetes. Taubes argues that the problem lies in refined carbohydrates, like white flour, easily digested starches, and sugars, and that the key to good health is the kind of calories we take in, not the number. In this groundbreaking book, this award-winning science writer shows us that almost everything we believe about the nature of a healthy diet is wrong. Reminds me of one section in this book – forget about most of what you know about weight loss because it's wrong. A good read.

Mindless Eating
Brian Wansink

This food psychologist presents a fascinating look into why we eat, focusing on awareness of how much and what we eat, often without our realizing it. He looks at comfort food, plate size and eating patterns based on who we're dining with – friends, family, etc. You'll also learn what "hidden persuaders" are used by restaurants and supermarkets to get us to overeat. His research shows that we are faced with 250 food decisions every day (breakfast or no breakfast, pop-tart or bagel, etc.) and 80% of the decisions we make can't be explained, other than to say they are mindless decisions. The author's web site has the table of contents, additional articles and other resources at http://mindlesseating.org.

Pandora's Lunchbox
Melanie Warner

Because America and the world are hooked on fast food and processed foods sold everywhere, you need to read this book by a journalist who writes about the food industry. You'll be stunned, shocked and amazed by the details she reveals and it should change the way you look at processed food. With all the fast food advertising that sucks us all right in, there's a lot to learn and this book is a great place to supplement what you've read in this book.

Salt Sugar Fat: How the Food Giants Hooked Us
Michael Moss

If you want to read a really fascinating (and sometimes scary) book about why we're addicted to junk food, read this one. Years of researched resulted in this inside look into how top execs at major food companies develop and market products, all, pretty much designed to make us want more and more, translating to obscene profits. Lamented one industry veteran about the amount of salt, sugar and fat in fast and processed foods, "I feel so sorry for the public." Read an adaptation edited by Joel Lovell in the NY Times at http://tinyurl.com/bzvvg6a. Better yet, get the book by this Pulitzer Prize-winning NY Times investigative reporter.

Why You Can't Lose Weight
Dr. Pamela Smith

While I've touched on a variety of reasons why people can't lose weight, Dr. Smith has devoted an entire book to the topic, looking at 18 factors including insufficient exercise, lack of sleep, health disorders such as food allergies and thyroid hormone dysfunction, insulin resistance and depression. For each obstacle to weight loss, Dr. Smith explains how the problem can be recognized, how it contributes to weight gain, and how you can take steps towards a slimmer body.

Smart Phone Apps

Buycott

This clever app lets you scan the barcode of food products and you see the corporate ownership tree of that product. You can then make a decision to buy or not to buy based on other information. For example, you can boycott products from companies that opposed the labeling of genetically modified foods. Conversely, you can buy from companies that are in line with your thinking about social and other issues.

Chemical Cuisine

After reading this book, you know about a lot of food additives, but who can remember them all? With this handy app, you can quickly search additives and learn the truth about those in foods you're considering.

Eat This, Not That! – The Game

You know how important substituting good foods for bad foods is based on reading *The Mind Diet.* Here's a fun way to learn what choices to make when confronted with them. Now you can choose between a chili dog and a cheeseburger, with the full knowledge of which one is better for you.

Food Additives 2

Lets you know what food additives are detrimental to your health, and describes the origin of the substance, general use and functionality, and known or potential side effects.

Fooducate

Use this app when in a food store by scanning the barcodes and the app returns the nutritional content of the food. It highlights ingredients that are bad for you or controversial.

Locavore

Recommends locally produced food based on your location, and tells you which foods are in season or coming into season.

Meal Snap

Ever wonder what's really in the food you eat at a restaurant? Well, now you don't have to wonder with this clever app. With Meal Snap, you take a photo of what's on your plate, and the app estimates the calories and ingredients.

Restaurant Nutrition

With 100 restaurants and some 15,000 food items in its database, this handy app lets you know key facts about the foods you eat at covered restaurants.

Turnyp

This app helps you find local restaurants that serve the food allowed by your diet, such as vegan, gluten-free, high protein, low carb or any other dietary restrictions you need.

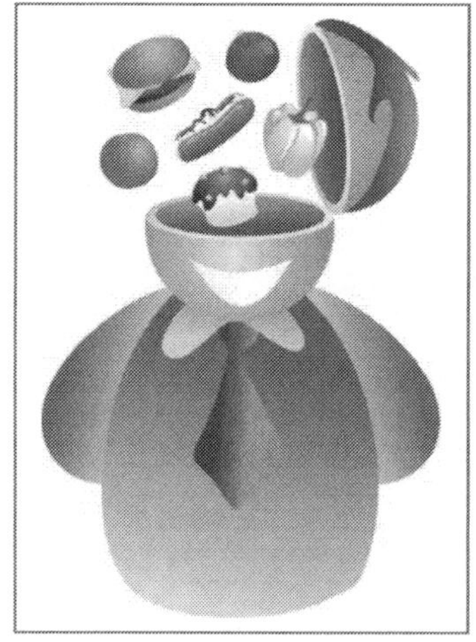

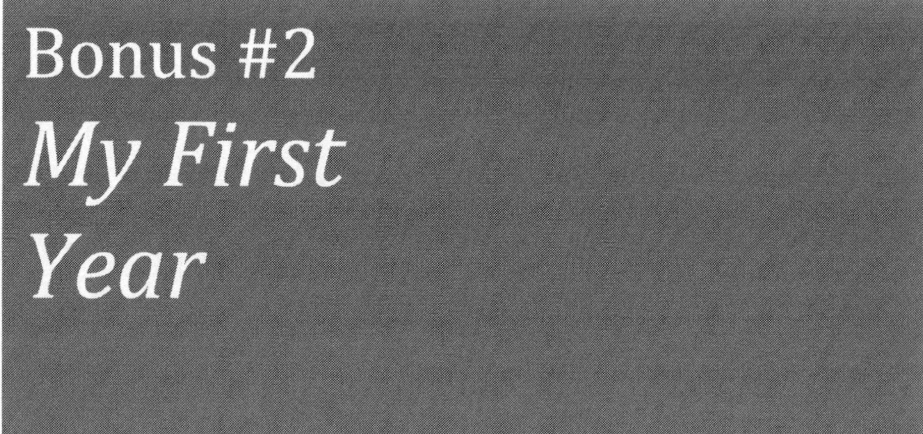

My First Year: Success!

I made notes throughout my first year after reaching my Moment of Truth in July, 2011. The purpose is to give you some insights of how I felt, what I did, and how wonderful a feeling it was to lose a lot of weight safely and keep it off permanently.

DAY #1: FIRST DAY, MY "MOMENT OF TRUTH"

I've spent the last couple of weeks doing a lot of soul-searching, thinking, researching and understanding why I have not been able to lose weight for well over a decade. After seeing all the dreadful diseases that result from being obese, after seeing depressing stats about people who are fat, and after researching why people don't lose weight, I finally had my "a ha" moment. Most people who "try" to lose weight don't have a plan. Like me, they buy the hottest diet book, sign up for the celebrity-endorsed food delivery service and/or join a gym. But ultimately, most fail and it all comes down to not having a well thought-out game plan. Once I understood that, I was able to get to the point where I knew I would be successful, simply because whenever I had a plan at work or other areas of my life, I was successful. Armed with that powerful knowledge, I felt that this time would be different. I **knew** I would not fail, and I had a plan that made a whole lot of sense.

DAY #2: BELIEFS

Once I understood that I needed a plan, I asked "what is that plan?" I looked at business plans I had written and recognized that I needed a **belief system.** It's one thing to reach what I later called my Moment of Truth, but you need to back that up with much more. In the same way I believe that honesty, kindness and laughter are key components of a successful relationship, I created a list of things I needed to believe in for my weight loss journey. Things like sugar is evil, take it slow and share my plan with family and friends.

When I finished my list, I now had firm beliefs to form the basis for my strategies and tactics.

DAY #3: STRATEGIES

Every solid business plan has strategies to help a business grow and succeed. I realized that weight loss was no different. Starting today, and adding to the list every week, I formulated over 120 strategies to help me better think about how to approach situations like buffets, tailgates and dining out. I also realized how well truth, beliefs and strategies feed off each other. I reached the truth, layered in beliefs and created strategies for success.

DAY #4: TACTICS

Armed with truth, beliefs and tactics, I said "what next?" I found over 75,000 diet books on Amazon, read about dozens of programs and food delivery services and on and on and on. I also read numerous times about the importance of getting my doctor and a dietician/nutritionist involved. So I made appointments with both. I learned a lot from both and they both helped me formulate a plan about what to eat, how much and when. My tactics were developed in meetings with my doc and dietician, and I felt very comfortable with them because they were personalized and customized for my body and mind.

DAY #5: IMPLEMENTATION

Today I put my plan in action. I reviewed my beliefs, strategies and the plan I developed with the doctor and dietician. The whole concept of truth, beliefs, strategies and tactics felt so good. I knew it was going to work. Most of all, my mind was very clear and focused, unlike in the past when there was doubts that my diets of the past would even work. What a great feeling to know in advance that what I was doing would succeed. Today I got on the scale for the first time, and started a chart, as weighing myself every single day at the same time was a key component to my plan.

DAY #6: WIPING OUT THE PAST

One of the things I realized I had to do was ignore almost everything people say about dieting and weight loss. Especially clichés like "anything is OK in moderation" and generalizations like "a little candy bar isn't going to hurt you." Sticking to the plan at hand was going to work, and I could not let habits from the past be a part of the present and future. When I weighed myself today for the first time on the new plan, I had lost 3/10th of a pound. In the past, I would have been disappointed, but in my new way of thinking, I was pleased. My plan included some simple math: if I could lose 1/10th to 2/10th of a pound per day (that's just a couple of ounces), I would lose about 3 to 6 pounds a month, which would get me to my goal of losing 40 pounds in about 7 months to a year, give or take. And that it would be a safe and healthy way to lose. I accepted the fact that 99.9999% of people who lose a lot of weight fast gain it back as fast, or even faster. Slow and steady was going to win the race.

DAY #7: ANOTHER SMALL LOSS

Today the scale showed a 1/10th pound loss. Not sure what to expect, I marked it down and now I've lost almost half a pound in two days. Pretty darn good. I've realized that by sticking to my plan, I have not been hungry at all.

DAY #11: MY FIRST MILESTONE

Today I passed the one pound mark. I would come to learn that there are constant milestones the longer you are true to the plan. There will be milestones at every single pound lost, at 5, 10, 15, etc. pounds lost, and at 1 week, 1 month, 2 months, etc. time periods. Having positive reinforcement just by reaching milestones pretty much every week is a pretty cool feeling.

DAY #15: SUGAR vs. FAT

This has emerged as a central issue in people's minds. We have been bombarded with low fat, reducing fat intake and everything fat. I really don't understand this for two reasons: (a) there are many fats that are healthy for you; and (b) most foods that are "low fat" or "no fat" are high in added sugar and/or another common but deadly sweetener, high fructose corn syrup or HFCS. So people that buy into a low-fat diet are in reality getting a high added sugar diet. Just look at labels on low-fat yogurt, for example. Natural sugar, found in fruits, generally is OK, but added sugar, found in a wide range of products, is generally not good for you. Your dietician will help you find the foods that have the right fats and zero or little added sugar.

DAY #19: THIS IS NOT AS HARD AS I THOUGHT IT WOULD BE

Well, I've lost a couple of pounds and am never hungry. I'm eating delicious foods and not food that has no taste. I've seen an increase in my energy and I haven't missed the garbage food I've cut out. Today I'm asking myself, "is this going to be easy in the coming weeks and months?" Well, I don't know, but I believe it will be, simply because I have a plan I believe in, and I can't think of a logical reason why that would change.

DAY #22: THE POWER OF SUBSTITUTION

In my meeting with the dietician, she stressed the importance of substituting healthy and good tasting foods for unhealthy good tasting foods. This has become one of my most important beliefs, as I'm amazed how much junk it cuts out. Take peanut butter, for example. Most brands have added sugar, which I have found is **absolutely unnecessary**. You can easily find peanut (and other nut butters) that have no sugar added, and taste every bit as good as those with sugar added. Once you start seeing how much sugar is in a wide range of juices, cereals and other favorite products, you'll quickly see how easy it is to find substitutes that taste as good and are significantly healthier for you.

DAY #35: ONE MONTH!

30 days have gone by already, and I've not been hungry once while implementing my plan. In fact, I find myself eating less food because I only eat when I'm hungry, and for no other reason. In these first 30 days, I lost a shade over 6 pounds, and as a result, I enjoyed these milestones:

- One for each pound lost
- One for each week on the diet
- One for the first month on the diet

That's a total of 11 reinforcements in 30 days, or about one every 3 days. When you get this type of continual reinforcement on a regular basis, it spurs you on to following the plan and not swerving from it. For the first month, I lose 3.8 pounds. In the past I would have been disappointed about not losing much more, but in this new way of thinking, I'm right on track, according to my plan!

DAY #37: TRICKS OF THE TRADE – THE 14 CHEW RULE

One thing I observe about most people, and I was like this as well, is how darn fast they eat. I watch people at restaurants, and I see the food going in their mouths and down their throats at warp speed. They can't possibly be enjoying the food when they eat that fast. And enjoying the taste of food is the reason we eat, right? Our tastebuds are on our tongues. The longer food stays on your tongue, the more you taste it and enjoy it. So why would you eat fast? I think it's a reflex of some sort, but you can easily do something about it. Whether it's a single pistachio nut, a slice of grilled chicken or a strawberry, aim to chew each piece of food 14 times. Rather than in your mouth and down the hatch in a second or two, chew so each piece lasts 14 seconds. You'll get much more tasteful enjoyment and slowing down your eating will result in less food consumed, and contribute mightily to weight loss.

DAY #44: MY FACE IS GETTING THINNER

While looking in the mirror this morning, I see a definite difference in my face. It's not as puffy as when I was obese, even though I've lost less than 10 pound total. This is another one of those small changes for the better that I've noticed. Combine that with slightly looser pants and similar changes and that means more progress and confidence to continue with the plan!

DAY #49: WHAT'S YOUR SECRET?

As people see that I'm losing weight, I'm starting to be asked "what's your secret?" As if I've found some magic pill. So instead of some half-baked answer, I ask them "are you serious to learn what I'm doing?" Half the people change the conversation, because they're not really interested in losing weight. I tell the other half about my Moment of Truth, about the game plan, and for those that are really interested and sincere, I go into more detail. My observation is that people are so conditioned to instant gratification that they are disappointed when they hear what I'm doing and that it's slow and steady and not a sprint.

DAY #52: WHEN YOU'RE FAT, NO ONE WANTS YOU ON THEIR TEAM

Today I saw a group of kids playing basketball in the local playground. The one kid sitting on the sideline was the fat one. As I looked on with sadness and empathy for him, I thought that no one wants the fat kid (or fat adult) on their team, because they want to win. It's one thing to be a fat adult and not do anything about it, but if your child is obese and you're not taking strong measures to change that, that's just not fair. Your kid deserves to play ball, go to the prom and wear nice clothes – as parents we all need to give them a chance to enjoy life without ridicule. Of course, this is unfair to heavy kids, but it is a fact of life that is very difficult to change without weight loss.

DAY #55: BACKWARDS EATING HABITS

If you're like most people – like I was before I lost my weight – you had a small or no breakfast, a larger or no lunch, and a big dinner. You wound up with the lion's share of food in your stomach before going to bed. Let's think about that for a minute. That's totally backwards. During the day when you're most active, you don't eat much. Then, you have a big dinner when you're least active. Your breakfast should be the largest meal of the day, followed by lunch and dinner should be the smallest. When I made this change, it contributed a lot to my weight loss efforts.

DAY #71: TWO MONTHS IN

Today is my 61st day, and I've lost a total of 9.6 pounds. That's about 2.4 ounces per day, on average. My milestones included:

- Eight weekly milestones
- Nine milestones, one for each pound
- 30- and 60-day milestones
- 20% of my weight loss goal reached

That's 20 milestones in two months! And that doesn't count visible changes in my appearance as well as comments from friends and family, especially those that know what I'm doing. Onward and downward!

DAY #82: FRIDAY NIGHTS --- A NEW ROUTINE

Friends of ours invited us out to a club featuring a live band and dancing. A word about me and dancing: I used to hate it (except for slow ones!). But now our Friday night routine of a big 4-5 course dinner followed by a movie or TV (too much food, too little exercise) has been replaced by a salad and dancing. And guess what – I love it! While I'm not ready for *Dancing With the Stars* just yet, it's a great way to start the weekend, get off my butt and have fun with the one I love. For you it doesn't have to be dancing, but the combination of a light dinner and exercise is a winner. I always lose weight when I weigh myself on Saturday mornings!

DAY #97: MY SECOND "MOMENT OF TRUTH"

I lost my first 10 pounds with just weekend casual walking. Everyone told me that would happen, and that in order to continue losing weight, I'd need to get serious about exercise. On day #97, I reached my second "Moment of Truth." I made up my mind once and for all that I will embark on a consistent exercise program that would not only help me lose more weight, but help my overall health as well. Since I hate working out on machines, I decided to spend a minimum of 30 minutes per day walking briskly, outdoors. Sometimes it would be before working, sometimes as a short lunch hour, and sometimes after work. On weekends, it would be any time. I walk half an hour a day around a big lake, burning 200 to 250 calories, getting lots of fresh air and sunshine, and most of all, enjoying it.

DAY #104: MY FIRST WEEK OF WALKING EVERY DAY

What all the experts say about walking is absolutely true! I've now walked at least 30 minutes every day for a week. And my weight loss has almost doubled during that time period. I'm enjoying being out in the fresh air, even as it begins to get colder here in NJ. I look forward to the spring when I can add shooting some baskets to my daily jaunt. The combination of sun, fresh air, being near water and more gets me more energized and I can tell you that it's a wonderful feeling!

DAY #122: I'M FEELING COOLER ALL OVER

I've noticed that as I lose more and more weight, my body feels cooler and I'm sleeping much better. I guess that a side benefit of losing weight in addition to the obvious health reasons is that my body has less fat and therefore my body temperature seems (maybe it just feels that way) to be lower. In any event, it feels good!

DAY #124: NO MORE HUFFING AND PUFFING

We went to a concert at a grand old theater in New Jersey, and on our way to the cheap sets, discovered there was no elevator. So we had to climb 64 steps (yes, I counted them). A couple of months ago I would have been huffing and puffing, and my leg muscles would have been screaming out in pain. Not this time – we made it up all the steps without a single huff, puff or discomfort. Progress comes in many forms!

DAY #127: MY BMI IS COMING DOWN!

Besides your actual weight, your BMI (Body Mass Index) is a widely used number that is a good predictor of health as it relates to being overweight. Today I checked my BMI at WebMD.com, and it has come down from 36.0 to 32.6 since I started. I have a ways to go to get in the mid 20's which is where I need to be, but along with all the other positives since 7/15/2011, this is more good news.

DAY #147: THANKSGIVING 2011 - MORNING

This is the only holiday where all anyone talks about is the food. It's become a "free pass" for most people to basically stuff your face, and certainly, almost everyone at family gatherings does exactly that. So this morning, as we get ready to leave for our turkey day, my thoughts are unlike every past year. Because of my stunning success (22 pounds lost as of this morning), I'm not going to jeopardize this great progress over food, some of which I like and some of which I don't. I reviewed my "Moment of Thought" process and am now ready to meet this challenge head on. I'll write again when we get back.

DAY #147: THANKSGIVING 2011 – EVENING

Today was a big success. My Turkey Day strategy was to drink a lot of liquid prior to the meal. I had 3 big glasses of water. By the time the food rolled out, I was pretty full. I then sampled very small portions of the foods I liked, and avoided those I didn't. While I did eat more than I usually do, I didn't binge or pig out. I watched other people at this family gathering pile food high on their plates and I felt good inside that I did not. Many of them noticed my weight loss and commented; positive feedback is something we all want and need. It's possible I gained a little bit of weight, but it would be mostly "water weight" which will come off quickly.

DAY #148: THE DAY AFTER THANKSGIVING

8am weigh in: I gained 4/10th of a pound. This is truly amazing. I feel great, and within two days or less, I will have lost that 4/10th. So my first Thanksgiving on my mind diet did not derail me. And it all goes back to the Moment of Truth in which I made a solemn promise to myself never to let any situation cause me to drop off the weight loss bandwagon.

DAY #157: I HAVE "PFD" SYNDROME

We went out of town for a wedding this weekend. The wedding was on Sunday and Saturday night I realized I had forgotten to bring a belt with my suit. When I tried the suit on, I had a bad case of PFD syndrome: Pants Falling Down! Luckily I was able to run out and buy a belt in time for the wedding, so I was able to keep my pants on and dance up a storm without having to constantly "hitch" up my trousers. Looks like I'll need a new suit.

DAY #166: HEAVY WOMAN ON THE AIRPLANE

Boarding a flight last week took a very long time, simply because an extremely overweight woman took forever to walk from the doorway to her seat on the plane. She had to support herself by leaning on every armrest and anything else she could touch. Extremely sad, and maybe it's a medical issue that caused this weight gain. But whatever it is, I felt very sorry for her, but at the same time, it made me question how some people let themselves go that far. On the other hand, we all know that it's never too late to take control of your eating.

DAY #167: NEW YEAR'S EVE DAY

It's been 5 ½ months since my Moment of Truth and the beginning of my complete and total weight loss program. I'm down 23 pounds and looking back, I was rarely hungry, it's been easier than I thought it would be, and what all the experts write in terms of types of food to eat, losing weight slowly and avoid and exercise is true. The #1 reason for my success (among many) is having a salad almost every single night for dinner. I've discussed this in detail before. I'm hoping to get to 30 pounds by 9 months, but if I don't, I'll get there shortly thereafter. And unlike past years, I don't have to make any New Year's resolutions or promises that won't be kept. I'm already doing it – what a great way to go into 2012!

DAY #177: DUCKS ICE DANCING

One of the simple pleasures you get when walking every day is the unexpected. Whether it's around the lake in a park where I walk, or in the middle of a big city where you can take thousands of different routes, there's always something going on that is out of the ordinary. Today the lake was partially frozen, and I saw something I've never seen before. Usually ducks find non-frozen areas where they sit in the water. But this one flock was walking all over the ice, as if in a super slow-motion ice dance. I would have never seen this if I had not started walking several weeks ago!

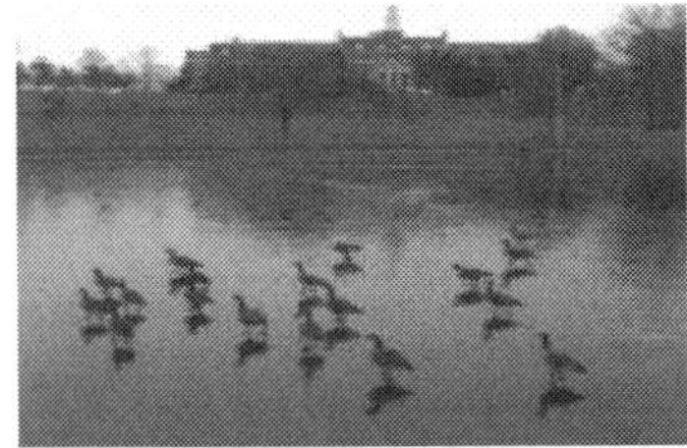

DAY #173: HALFWAY POINT REACHED!

This morning, I weighed myself and the scale said I have lost 25 pounds, half of what I want to lose! I'm actually one week ahead of schedule, as I had aimed for half my weight in six months. Looking back, and I know you're not going to believe this, but I have not felt deprived once, I don't miss all the junk I used to love, and I look forward to my nightly "designer salad" and nothing else. I can only conclude one thing: the power of your mind is so great that it will enable you to achieve something you once thought daunting and impossible.

DAY #181: CHANGE OF PLANS

Today I went to walk, as usual, around the lake in the park. However, it was very cold and even windier, and after one lap (10 minutes), I couldn't keep going. But rather than take a cop-out and quit, I drove to a nearby mall and walked another 40 minutes. It's all a part of a commitment to myself that I won't break, despite the weather.

DAY #192: GOT MY LATEST BLOOD TEST RESULTS

For years, my blood pressure, despite being on BP meds, was hovering at 120-130 over 90. I recently went for a blood test, and for the first time in over a decade, my pressure was 120 over 80, just where it should be. When I lose the rest of my weight, I hope to be off the BP meds, which is a great thing plus it will save me $600 a year to boot!

DAY #196: A REAL SIGN OF SUSTAINED WEIGHT LOSS

My company had a bowling outing last night. When I tried on my usual size shoe, it was too big. I have lost half of a size --- imagine that. And they had great looking pizza for us, but it didn't even tempt me. I went out afterwards and had my usual big salad and was 1/3 of a pound lighter the next morning. Whoo-hoo!

DAY #220: MAJOR MILESTONE!

Today I weighed 199.8 pounds. Having started at 230, today represented three milestones in one: losing a total of 30 pounds, being 60% of the way towards my goal, and most of all, breaking through the "200 pound barrier." So I've lost 30 pounds in a little under 8 months, which is a very good, steady and healthy rate. What am I going to do to celebrate? Go buy some new clothes, because the old ones are getting way too big!

DAY #229: "HI SKINNY"

We got together with some friends I hadn't seen in a while. The first words I heard were "Hi Skinny" and that really made me feel good. Even though I'm not the type of person that needs positive feedback (because I already know that I look much better), it still feels good to hear it.

DAY #276: EMBARASSING GOOD NEWS

Two weeks before my wife's gala last night, I tried on my tuxedo to make sure it fit. A little loose but no problem. Well, I must have reached the "tipping point" because as I'm walking out to the car on the way to the event, my tux pants fell down to the ground. So I'm standing there in my undies in my driveway. Luckily, no one was around. Just imagine if that had happened in the middle of the dance floor! I'll take problems like these any day of the week!

DAY #313: LOADS OF COMPLIMENTS

This weekend was the opening of our pool at the community where we live, and I haven't seen people since last summer. Since I'm now down 32 pounds, people really noticed the difference. No matter how much I tell myself that I don't need compliments, I must admit that they do feel good to hear.

DAY #317: AN OLD SUIT FITS JUST FINE

With a family event coming up in a week, I know that my suit will not fit, and I want to avoid what happened on Day #276. Luckily I had saved some suits from when I was thinner, and when I tried one on, it fit very, very well. Luckily it was a classic design so I all needed to do is get it cleaned. A reader's friend calls this "shopping in her closet!"

DAY #322: ANOTHER IMPORTANT DECISION

While I've been drinking diet soda in place of sweetened sugar for my entire adult life, I reached a decision based on a lot of articles I've read recently. I've decided that artificial sweeteners are just not worth the risk, and I've found substitutes for home and when I'm out. I announced my decision to stop drinking diet soda to my wife and others, and instead I drink flavored seltzer and Stevia flavored sodas. A reader does the same: "I love it! I also drink unsweetened iced tea."

DAY #325: GREAT NUMBERS!

Today I got the results of my six-month checkup and blood test. For the first time in my adult life that I can remember, all of my "vitals" were in the normal range, plus great numbers for blood pressure, cholesterol and sugar. As great as I feel, as light as I am, here's more proof that the "slow and steady" program (now 32.5 pounds in 10.5 months) is working. Nothing better than a clean bill of health!

DAY #365: ONE YEAR!

Exactly a year ago today I reached my Moment of Truth and made up my mind once and for all to lose weight the right way and keep it off forever. Here are my one year stats:

- Weight loss: 34 pounds
- Key blood test numbers: all normal
- How I feel: fantastic!

During this first year (of the rest of my life), I learned so much, especially in reading for *The Mind Diet Guidebooks.* Here are the highlights of my first year:

- It was a lot easier than I thought it would be. I never felt hungry, frustrated, tempted or ready to quit.
- I was correct to do it "the right way" – slow and steady and not a fast weight loss.
- The power of the mind is astounding. Once I truly made up my mind, I pretty much lost interest in all the bad foods I had been eating for most of my adult life.

- The amount of quality information (that I've distilled into these books) is astounding, making it extremely easy to read up on any weight loss related topics that you want to further investigate.

As I enter the second year of this journey, I have no desire to do anything but what I've been doing. I've figured out what foods are good for me and how to prepare them (and how to order in restaurants) so that they taste good. I've learned time and time again how to resist food temptations at parties, tailgates, family dinners, etc.

Bottom line: I'm happier than ever and thankful that I made this momentous decision.

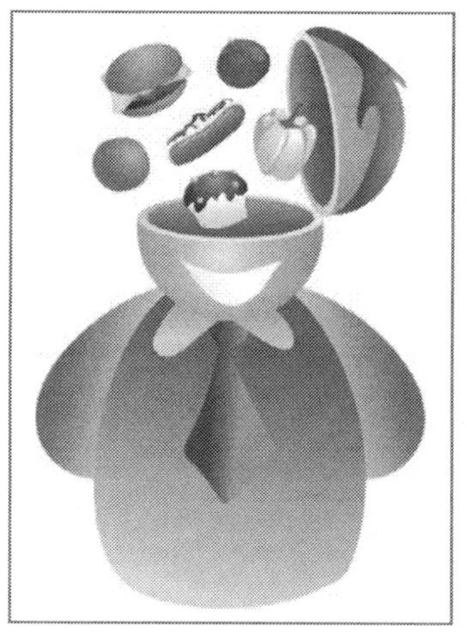

Bonus #3 *Nutrition Facts Labels Explained*

Why It's Important to Understand the Nutrition Facts Labels

You have at your fingertips clear and concise information to help you make good decisions while you shop in supermarkets and other types of stores that sell food and drinks. It is SO easy to learn how to read labels and apply what you know in your food selections. It makes NO sense to avoid learning how to read the nutrition facts labels. Period.

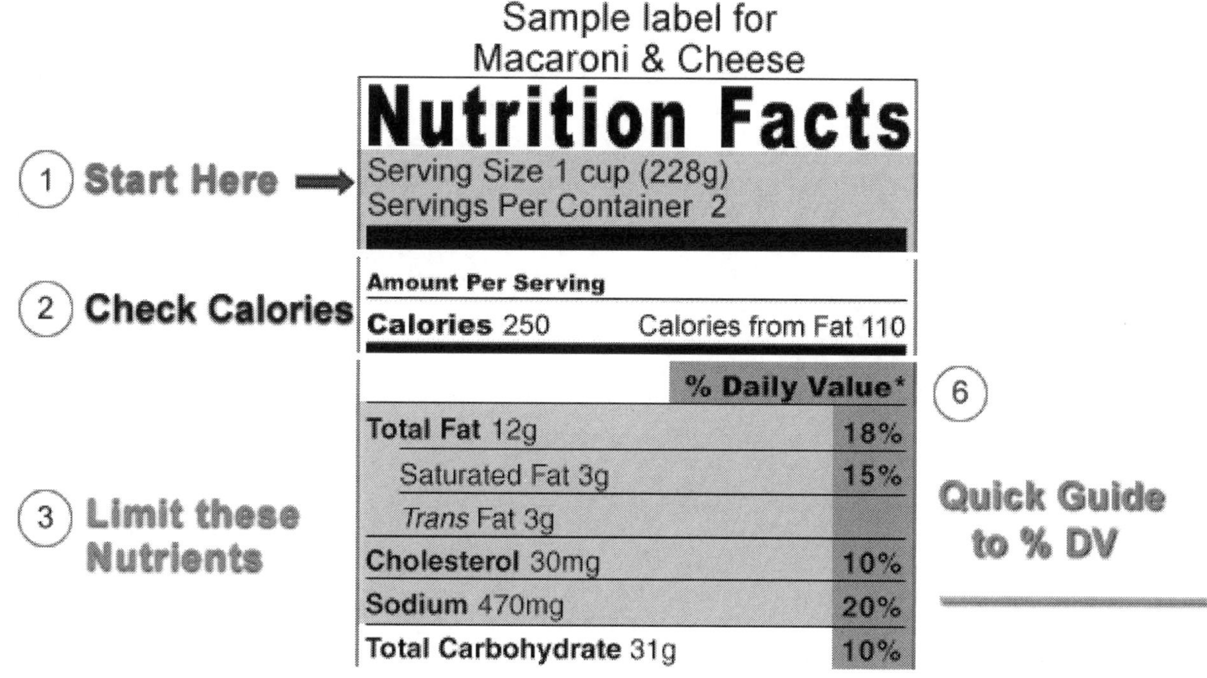
Sample label for
Macaroni & Cheese
Nutrition Facts
1 Start Here
Serving Size 1 cup (228g)
Servings Per Container 2
2 Check Calories
Amount Per Serving
Calories 250 Calories from Fat 110
% Daily Value*
6
Total Fat 12g 18%
Saturated Fat 3g 15%
Trans Fat 3g
Cholesterol 30mg 10%
Sodium 470mg 20%
Total Carbohydrate 31g 10%
3 Limit these Nutrients
Quick Guide to % DV

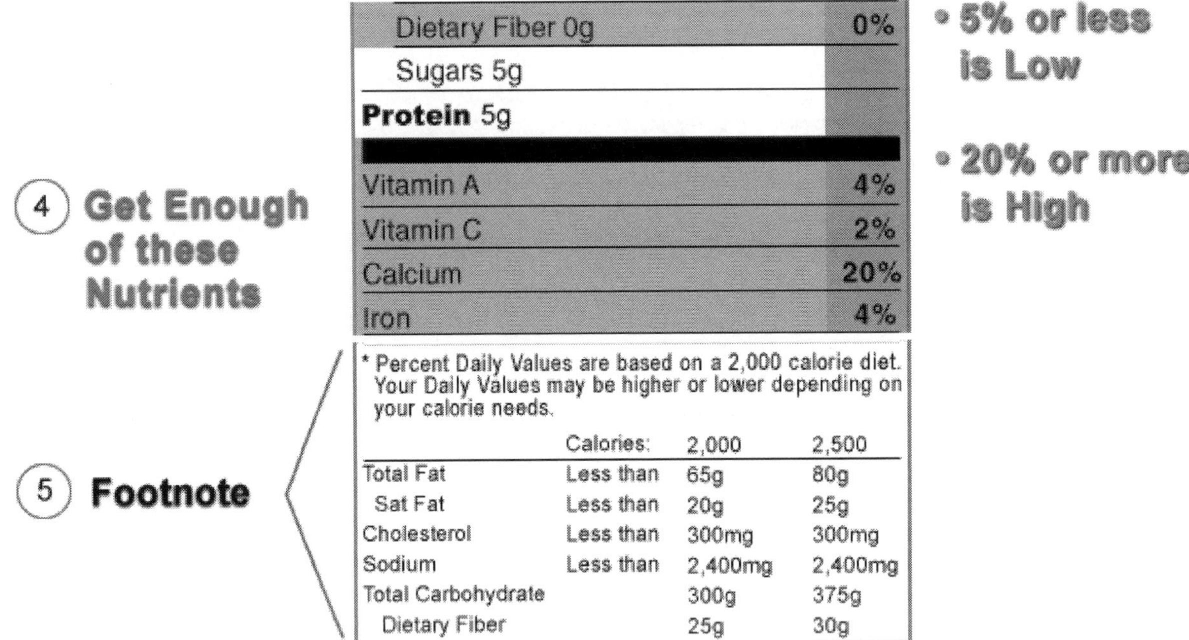

Overview

The information in the main or top section (see #1-4 and #6 on the sample nutrition label above), can vary with each food product; it contains product-specific information (serving size, calories, and nutrient information).

The bottom part (see #5 on the sample label above) contains a footnote with Daily Values (DVs) for 2,000 and 2,500 calorie diets. This footnote provides recommended dietary information for important nutrients, including fats, sodium and fiber. The footnote is found only on larger packages and does not change from product to product. In the following Nutrition Facts Label we have colored certain sections to help you focus on those areas that will be explained in detail. You will not see these colors on the food labels on products you purchase.

① The Serving Size

Serving Size 1 cup (228g)
Servings Per Container 2

The first place to start when you look at the Nutrition Facts label is the serving size and the number of servings in the package. Serving sizes are standardized to make it easier to compare similar foods; they are provided in familiar units, such as cups or pieces, followed by the metric amount, e.g., the number of grams.

The size of the serving on the food package influences the number of calories and all the nutrient amounts listed on the top part of the label. **Pay attention to the serving size, especially how many servings there are in the food package. Then ask yourself, "How many servings am I consuming"?** In the sample label, one serving of macaroni and cheese equals one cup. If you ate the whole package, you would eat **two** cups. That doubles the calories and other nutrient numbers, including the %Daily Values as shown in the sample label.

Example					
	Single Serving	**%DV**		**Double Serving**	**%DV**
Serving Size	1 cup (228g)			2 cups (456g)	
Calories	250			500	
Calories from Fat	110			220	
Total Fat	12g	18%		24g	36%
Trans Fat	1.5g			3g	
Saturated Fat	3g	15%		6g	30%
Cholesterol	30mg	10%		60mg	20%
Sodium	470mg	20%		940mg	40%
Total Carbohydrate	31g	10%		62g	20%
Dietary Fiber	0g	0%		0g	0%
Sugars	5g			10g	
Protein	5g			10g	
Vitamin A		4%			8%
Vitamin C		2%			4%
Calcium		20%			40%
Iron		4%			8%

② Calories (and Calories from Fat)

Calories provide a measure of how much energy you get from a serving of this food. Many Americans consume more calories than they need without meeting recommended intakes for a number of nutrients. The calorie section of the label can help you manage your weight (i.e., gain, lose, or maintain.) **Remember: the number of servings you consume determines the number of calories you actually eat (your portion amount).**

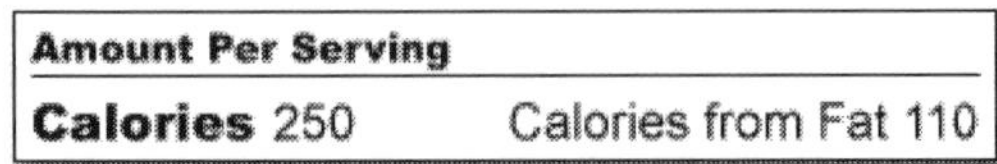

Amount Per Serving	
Calories 250	Calories from Fat 110

In the example, there are 250 calories in one serving of this macaroni and cheese. How many calories from fat are there in ONE serving? Answer: 110 calories, which means almost half the calories in a single serving come from fat. What if you ate the whole package content? You would consume two servings, or 500 calories, and 220 would come from fat.

③④ The Nutrients: How Much?

Look at the top of the nutrient section in the sample label. It shows you some key nutrients that impact on your health and separates them into two main groups:

Limit These Nutrients

Total Fat 12g	**18%**
Saturated Fat 3g	**15%**
Trans Fat 3g	
Cholesterol 30mg	**10%**
Sodium 470mg	**20%**

The nutrients listed first are the ones Americans generally eat in adequate amounts, or even too much. They are identified in yellow as **Limit these Nutrients.** Eating too much fat, saturated fat, *trans* fat, cholesterol, or sodium may increase your risk of certain chronic diseases, like heart disease, some cancers, or high blood pressure.

Important: Health experts recommend that you keep your intake of saturated fat, *trans* fat and cholesterol as low as possible as part of a nutritionally balanced diet.

Get Enough of These

Dietary Fiber 0g	0%

Vitamin A	4%
Vitamin C	2%
Calcium	20%
Iron	4%

Most Americans don't get enough dietary fiber, vitamin A, vitamin C, calcium, and iron in their diets. They are identified in blue as **Get Enough of these Nutrients**. Eating enough of these nutrients can improve your health and help reduce the risk of some diseases and conditions. For example, getting enough calcium may reduce the risk of osteoporosis, a condition that results in brittle bones as one ages (see calcium section below).

Eating a diet high in dietary fiber promotes healthy bowel function. Additionally, a diet rich in fruits, vegetables, and grain products that contain dietary fiber, particularly soluble fiber, and low in saturated fat and cholesterol may reduce the risk of heart disease. **Remember: You can use the Nutrition Facts label not only to help *limit* those nutrients you want to cut back on but also to *increase* those nutrients you need to consume in greater amounts.**

⑤ Understanding the Footnote on the Bottom of the Nutrition Facts Label

* Percent Daily Values are based on a 2,000 calorie diet. Your Daily Values may be higher or lower depending on your calorie needs.

	Calories:	2,000	2,500
Total Fat	Less than	65g	80g
Sat Fat	Less than	20g	25g
Cholesterol	Less than	300mg	300mg
Sodium	Less than	2,400mg	2,400mg
Total Carbohydrate		300g	375g
Dietary Fiber		25g	30g

Note the * used after the heading "%Daily Value" on the Nutrition Facts label. It refers to the Footnote in the lower part of the nutrition label, which tells you "**%DVs are based on a 2,000 calorie diet**". This statement must be on all food labels. But the remaining information in the full footnote may not be on the package if the size of the label is too small. When the full footnote does appear, it will always be the same. It doesn't change from product to product, because it shows recommended dietary advice for all Americans--it is not about a specific food product.

Look at the amounts circled in red in the footnote--these are the Daily Values (DV) for each nutrient listed and are based on public health experts' advice. DVs are recommended levels of intakes. DVs in the footnote are based on a 2,000 or 2,500 calorie diet. Note how the DVs for some nutrients change, while others (for cholesterol and sodium) remain the same for both calorie amounts.

How the Daily Values Relate to the %DVs

Look at the example below for another way to see how the Daily Values (DVs) relate to the %DVs and dietary guidance. For each nutrient listed there is a DV, a %DV, and dietary advice or a goal. If you follow this dietary advice, you will stay within public health experts' recommended upper or lower limits for the nutrients listed, based on a 2,000 calorie daily diet.

Examples of DVs versus %DVs

Based on a 2,000 Calorie Diet

Nutrient	**DV**	**%DV**	**Goal**
Total Fat	65g	= 100%DV	Less than
Sat Fat	20g	= 100%DV	Less than
Cholesterol	300mg	= 100%DV	Less than
Sodium	2400mg	= 100%DV	Less than
Total Carbohydrate	300g	= 100%DV	At least
Dietary Fiber	25g	= 100%DV	At least

Upper Limit - Eat "Less than"...

The nutrients that have "upper daily limits" are listed first on the footnote of larger labels and on the example above. Upper limits means it is recommended that you stay below - eat "less than" - the Daily Value nutrient amounts listed per day. For example, the DV for Saturated fat (in the yellow section) is 20g. This amount is 100% DV for this nutrient. What is the goal or dietary advice? To eat "less than" 20 g or 100%DV for the day.

Lower Limit - Eat "At least"...

Now look at the section in blue where dietary fiber is listed. The DV for dietary fiber is 25g, which is 100% DV. This means it is recommended that you eat "at least" this amount of dietary fiber per day.

The DV for Total Carbohydrate (section in white) is 300g or 100%DV. This amount is recommended for a balanced daily diet that is based on 2,000 calories, but can vary, depending on your daily intake of fat and protein.

18%
15%
10%
20%
10%
0%

⑥ The Percent Daily Value (%DV)

% Daily Value*

4%
2%
20%
4%

The % Daily Values (%DVs) are based on the Daily Value recommendations for key nutrients but only for a 2,000 calorie daily diet--not 2,500 calories. You, like most people, may not know how many calories you consume in a day. But you can still use the %DV as a frame of reference whether or not you consume more or less than 2,000 calories.

The %DV helps you determine if a serving of food is high or low in a nutrient. Note: a few nutrients, like *trans* fat, do not have a %DV--they will be discussed later.

Do you need to know how to calculate percentages to use the %DV? No, the label (the %DV) does the math for you. It helps you interpret the numbers (grams and milligrams) by putting them all on the same scale for the day (0-100%DV). The %DV column doesn't add up vertically to 100%. Instead each nutrient is based on 100% of the daily requirements for that nutrient (for a 2,000 calorie diet). This way you can tell high from low and know which nutrients contribute a lot, or a little, to your **daily** recommended allowance (upper or lower).

Quick Guide to %DV

	% Daily Value*
Total Fat 12g	18%
Saturated Fat 3g	15%
Trans Fat 3g	
Cholesterol 30mg	10%
Sodium 470mg	20%
Total Carbohydrate 31g	10%
Dietary Fiber 0g	0%
Sugars 5g	
Protein 5g	
Vitamin A	4%
Vitamin C	2%
Calcium	20%
Iron	4%

This guide tells you that **5%DV or less is low** for all nutrients, those you want to limit (e.g., fat, saturated fat, cholesterol, and sodium), or for those that you want to consume in greater amounts (fiber, calcium, etc). As the **Quick Guide** shows, **20%DV or more is high** for all nutrients.

Example: Look at the amount of Total Fat in one serving listed on the sample nutrition label. Is 18%DV contributing a lot or a little to your fat limit of 100% DV? Check the **Quick Guide to %DV**. 18%DV, which is below 20%DV, is not yet high, but what if you ate the whole package (two servings)? You would double that amount, eating 36% of your daily allowance for Total Fat. Coming from just one food, that amount leaves you with 64% of your fat allowance (100%-36%=64%) for *all* of the other foods you eat that day, snacks and drinks included.

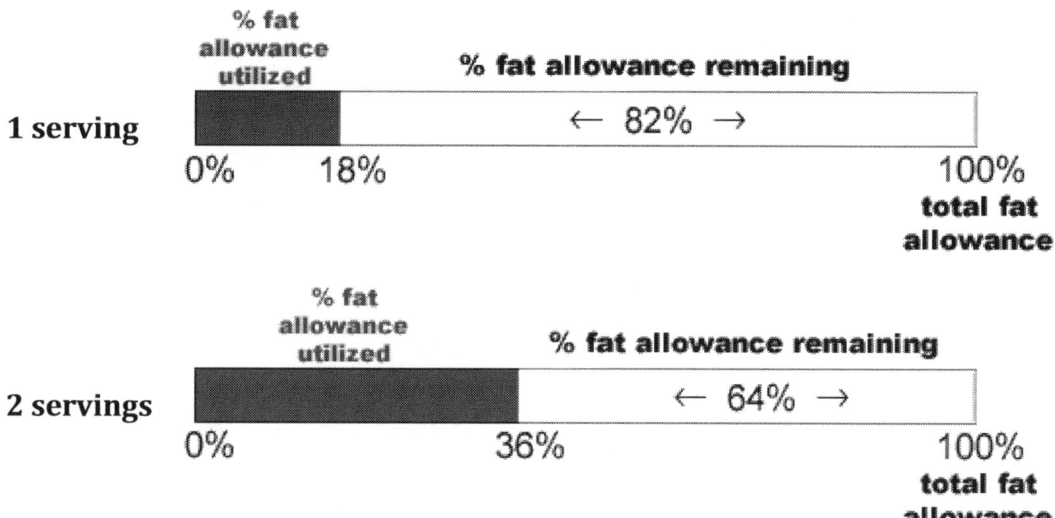

Using the %DV

Comparisons: The %DV also makes it easy for you to make comparisons. You can compare one product or brand to a similar product. Just make sure the serving sizes are similar, especially the weight (e.g. gram, milligram, ounces) of each product. It's easy to see which foods are higher or lower in nutrients because the serving sizes are generally consistent for similar types of foods, (see the comparison example at the end) except in a few cases like cereals.

Nutrient Content Claims: Use the %DV to help you quickly distinguish one claim from another, such as "reduced fat" vs. "light" or "nonfat." Just compare the %DVs for Total Fat in each food product to see which one is higher or lower in that nutrient--**there is no need to memorize definitions.** This works when comparing all nutrient content claims, e.g., less, light, low, free, more, high, etc.

Dietary Trade-Offs: You can **use the %DV to help you make dietary trade-offs** with other foods throughout the day. You don't have to give up a favorite food to eat a healthy diet. When a food you like is high in fat, balance it with foods that are low in fat at other times of the day. Also, pay attention to how much you eat so that the **total** amount of fat for the day stays below 100%DV.

Nutrients With a %DV but No Weight Listed Spotlight on Calcium:

Nutrition Facts

Serving Size 1 cup (236ml)
Servings Per Container 1

Amount Per Serving	
Calories 80	Calories from Fat 0
	% Daily Value*
Total Fat 0g	**0%**
Saturated Fat 0g	**0%**
Trans Fat 0g	
Cholesterol Less than 5mg	**0%**
Sodium 120mg	**5%**
Total Carbohydrate 11g	**4%**
Dietary Fiber 0g	**0%**
Sugars 11g	
Protein 9g	**17%**

Vitamin A 10% • Vitamin C 4%
Calcium 30% • Iron 0% • Vitamin D 25%

*Percent Daily Values are based on a 2,000 calorie diet. Your daily values may be higher or lower depending on your calorie needs.

Calcium: Look at the %DV for calcium on food packages so you know how much one serving contributes to the *total amount you need* per day. Remember, a food with 20%DV or more contributes a lot of calcium to your daily total, while one with 5%DV or less contributes a little.

Experts advise adult consumers to consume adequate amounts of calcium, that is, 1,200mg or 100%DV in a daily 2,000 calorie diet. This advice is often given in milligrams (mg), but the Nutrition Facts label **only** lists a %DV for calcium.

For certain populations, they advise that adolescents, especially girls, consume 1,300mg (130%DV) and post-menopausal women consume 1,200mg (120%DV) of calcium daily. The DV for calcium on food labels is 1,000mg.

Don't be fooled -- always check the label for calcium because you can't make assumptions about the amount of calcium in specific food categories. Example: the amount of calcium in milk, whether skim or whole, is generally the same per serving, whereas the amount of calcium in the same size yogurt container (8oz) can vary from 20-45 %DV.

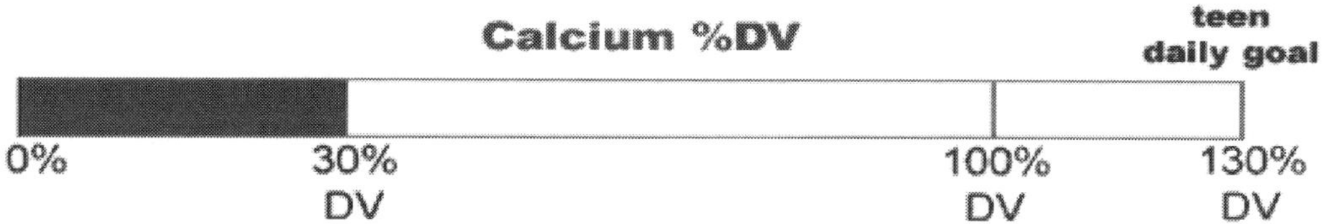

Equivalencies
30% DV = 300mg calcium = one cup of milk
100% DV = 1,000mg calcium
130% DV = 1,300mg calcium

Nutrients Without a %DV:

Trans Fats, Protein, and Sugars:

Note that *Trans* fat, Sugars and, Protein do not list a %DV on the Nutrition Facts label.

Plain Yogurt **Fruit Yogurt**

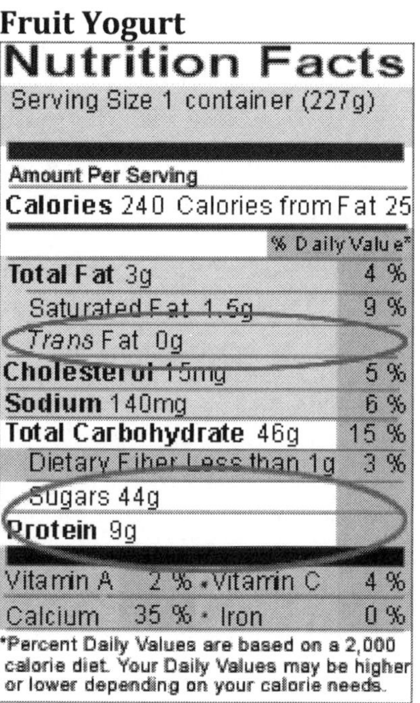

Plain Yogurt

Nutrition Facts	
Serving Size 1 container (226g)	
Amount Per Serving	
Calories 110 Calories from Fat 0	
	% Daily Value*
Total Fat 0g	0 %
Saturated Fat 0g	0 %
Trans Fat 0g	
Cholesterol Less than 5mg	1 %
Sodium 160mg	7 %
Total Carbohydrate 15g	5 %
Dietary Fiber 0g	0 %
Sugars 10g	
Protein 13g	
Vitamin A 0 % • Vitamin C	4 %
Calcium 45 % • Iron	0 %

*Percent Daily Values are based on a 2,000 calorie diet. Your Daily Values may be higher or lower depending on your calorie needs.

Fruit Yogurt

Nutrition Facts	
Serving Size 1 container (227g)	
Amount Per Serving	
Calories 240 Calories from Fat 25	
	% Daily Value*
Total Fat 3g	4 %
Saturated Fat 1.5g	9 %
Trans Fat 0g	
Cholesterol 15mg	5 %
Sodium 140mg	6 %
Total Carbohydrate 46g	15 %
Dietary Fiber Less than 1g	3 %
Sugars 44g	
Protein 9g	
Vitamin A 2 % • Vitamin C	4 %
Calcium 35 % • Iron	0 %

*Percent Daily Values are based on a 2,000 calorie diet. Your Daily Values may be higher or lower depending on your calorie needs.

Trans Fat: Experts could not provide a reference value for *trans* fat nor any other information that FDA believes is sufficient to establish a Daily Value or %DV. Scientific reports link *trans* fat (and saturated fat) with raising blood LDL ("bad") cholesterol levels, both of which increase your risk of coronary heart disease, a leading cause of death in the US.

Important: Health experts recommend that you keep your intake of saturated fat, *trans* fat and cholesterol as low as possible as part of a nutritionally balanced diet.

Protein: A %DV is required to be listed if a claim is made for protein, such as "high in protein". Otherwise, unless the food is meant for use by infants and children under 4 years old, none is needed. Current scientific evidence indicates that protein intake is not a public health concern for adults and children over 4 years of age.

Sugars: No daily reference value has been established for sugars because no recommendations have been made for the total amount to eat in a day. Keep in mind, the sugars listed on the Nutrition Facts label include naturally occurring sugars (like those in fruit and milk) as well as those added to a food or drink. Check the ingredient list for specifics on added sugars.

Take a look at the Nutrition Facts label for the two yogurt examples. The plain yogurt on the left has 10g of sugars, while the fruit yogurt on the right has 44g of sugars in one serving.

Now look below at the ingredient lists for the two yogurts. Ingredients are listed in descending order of weight (from most to least). Note that no added sugars or sweeteners are in the list of ingredients for the plain yogurt, yet 10g of sugars were listed on the Nutrition Facts label. This is because there are no added sugars in plain yogurt, only naturally occurring sugars (lactose in the milk).

Plain Yogurt - contains no added sugars
INGREDIENTS: CULTURED PASTEURIZED GRADE A NONFAT MILK, WHEY PROTEIN CONCENTRATE, PECTIN, CARRAGEENAN.

Fruit Yogurt - contains added sugars
INGREDIENTS: CULTURED GRADE A REDUCED FAT MILK, APPLES, HIGH FRUCTOSE CORN SYRUP, CINNAMON, NUTMEG, NATURAL FLAVORS, AND PECTIN. CONTAINS ACTIVE YOGURT AND L. ACIDOPHILUS CULTURES.

If you are concerned about your intake of sugars, make sure that added sugars are not listed as one of the first few ingredients. Other names for added sugars include: corn syrup, high-fructose corn syrup, fruit juice concentrate, maltose, dextrose, sucrose, honey, and maple syrup.

To limit nutrients that have no %DV, like *trans* fat and sugars, compare the labels of similar products and choose the food with the lowest amount.

Comparison Example

Below are two kinds of milk- one is "Reduced Fat," the other is "Nonfat" milk. Each serving size is one cup. Which has more calories and more saturated fat? Which one has more calcium?

REDUCED FAT MILK
2% Milkfat

Nutrition Facts

Serving Size 1 cup (236ml)
Servings Per Container 1

Amount Per Serving	
Calories 120	Calories from Fat 45
	% Daily Value*
Total Fat 5g	8%
Saturated Fat 3g	15%
Trans Fat 0g	
Cholesterol 20mg	7%
Sodium 120mg	5%
Total Carbohydrate 11g	4%
Dietary Fiber 0g	0%
Sugars 11g	
Protein 9g	17%

Vitamin A 10% • Vitamin C 4%
Calcium 30% • Iron 0% • Vitamin D 25%

*Percent Daily Values are based on a 2,000 calorie diet. Your daily values may be higher or lower depending on your calorie needs.

NONFAT MILK

Nutrition Facts

Serving Size 1 cup (236ml)
Servings Per Container 1

Amount Per Serving	
Calories 80	Calories from Fat 0
	% Daily Value*
Total Fat 0g	0%
Saturated Fat 0g	0%
Trans Fat 0g	
Cholesterol Less than 5mg	0%
Sodium 120mg	5%
Total Carbohydrate 11g	4%
Dietary Fiber 0g	0%
Sugars 11g	
Protein 9g	17%

Vitamin A 10% • Vitamin C 4%
Calcium 30% • Iron 0% • Vitamin D 25%

*Percent Daily Values are based on a 2,000 calorie diet. Your daily values may be higher or lower depending on your calorie needs.

As you can see, they both have the same amount of calcium, but the nonfat milk has no saturated fat, and has 40 calories less per serving than the reduced fat milk.

Source: http://tinyurl.com/3yz34zy

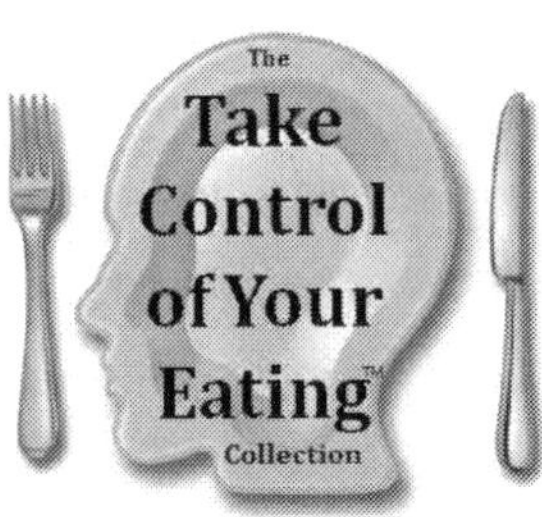

Learn More at www.Mind-Diet.com

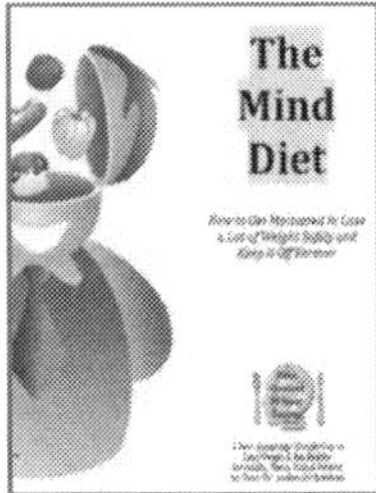

THE MIND DIET – how to lose a lot of weight safely and keep it off permanently. Written for teens and adults of all ages. 250+ graphics/photos, inspirations from Gloria Gaynor ("I Will Survive") and golfer Gary Player. Contributions from medical obesity expert Dr. Ethan Lazarus. Brand new approach to weight loss that helps people get in the right state of mind – a key strategy necessary for success. 26 beliefs, 122 strategies, Ingredients Awareness Chart, much more.

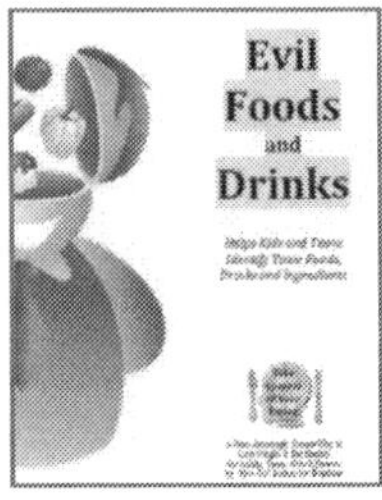

EVIL FOODS & DRINKS – helps kids and teens identify toxic foods, drinks and ingredients that are addictive and causing them to live in a never-ending cycle of weight gain and unhealthy eating. Includes a shocking sugar quiz and covers sugar, HFCS, saturated fat, trans fat, processed food and more. Large type, simple and clear messages make "getting it" easy for kids age 7 and up. Dramatically shows sugar content for 12 common foods and drinks.

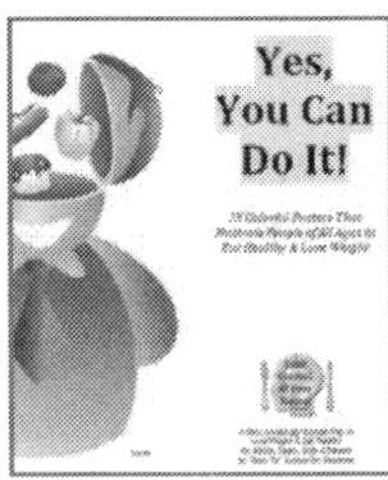

YES, YOU CAN DO IT! – 25 colorful motivational posters helps people of all ages stay motivated and on track to lose weight and keep it off. Printed on heavy paper and packaged loose. Includes a special "If He Can Do It, So Can You!" poster about a very obese British boy who got stuck in a slide in the playground, which motivated him to lose 75% of his body weight – a remarkable story.

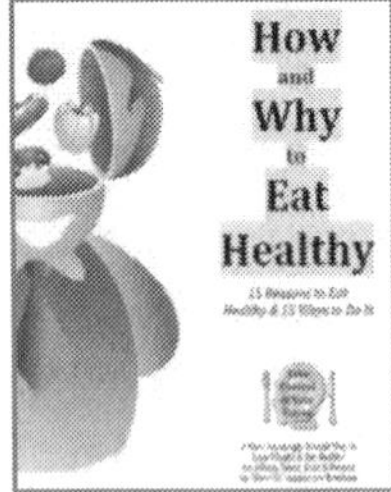

HOW AND WHY TO EAT HEALTHY – clear and simple messages for kids and teens and gives them 15 bite-size reasons why they should achieve a healthy weight, plus 15 ways to do it. Drives home the importance of making the right food choices and is great discussion material, both in classrooms and with parents. Includes a simple food substitution chart to make it easy for kids to replace harmful foods and drinks with healthy ones.

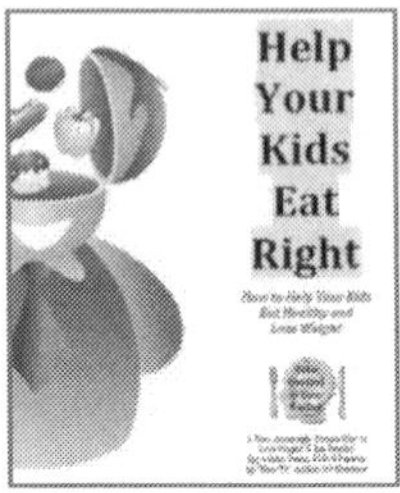

HELP YOUR KIDS EAT RIGHT – a guide for parents of kids and teens to give them tools to lose weight and make good food/drink choices. A modern guide for parents, it covers the 5 P's of successful healthy eating, 25 strategies, 8 posters, 11 great meals and snacks recipes kids love and a portion size chart. Helps parents become involved with a simple book loaded with proven strategies.

Photo/Graphic Credits

Section	Description	Artist/Source
Cover	Food in Head Icon	Dawn Hudson/Shutterstock.com
Cover	Plate Icon	Digitalista/BigStockPhoto.com
Intro	Gloria Gaynor	Troy Word
Intro	Gary Player	Black Knight International Archives
Intro	2 Year Old Toddler	News.com.au
Truth	Google Str View	Popfi.com
Truth	Mission Statement	Pixels Away
Truth	Boy in Slide	SWNS.com
Truth	Silver Lining	Vepar5
Truth	Shocked Woman	Konstantinov
Truth	Thinker	R. Ramirezlee/BigStockPhoto.com
Truth	Arthritis	Aliced/BigStockPhoto.com
Truth	Birth Defects	SloveGrove/BigStockPhoto.com
Truth	Blood Clots	Eraxion/BigStockPhoto.com
Truth	Cancer	Pseudo Longino/BigStockPhoto.com
Truth	Heart Condition	Digitalista/BigStockPhoto.com
Truth	Dementia	Monkey Biz/BigStockPhoto.com
Truth	Diabetes	Zothen/BigStockPhoto.com
Truth	Hearing Loss	Flynt/BigStockPhoto.com
Truth	Blood Pressure	VW Photo/BigStockPhoto.com
Truth	Cholesterol	Alexmit/BigStockPhoto.com
Truth	Infertility	Wavebreak/BigStockPhoto.com
Truth	Liver Disease	Eraxion/BigStockPhoto.com
Truth	Back Pain	Pressmaster/BigStockPhoto.com
Truth	Nerve Damage	Sergey Nivens/BigStockPhoto.com
Truth	Bone Problems	Erdosain/BigStockPhoto.com
Truth	Skin Problems	TovaWWW/BigStockPhoto.com
Truth	Sleep Apnea	BVDC/BigStockPhoto.com
Truth	Gallbladder Surgery	BVDC/BigStockPhoto.com
Truth	Vision Problems	Ostill/BigStockPhoto.com
Truth	Pain	DJMA/BigStockPhoto.com
Truth	Osteoarthritis	Bus023/BigStockPhoto.com
Truth	Muscle Problems	Maridav/BigStockPhoto.com
Truth	Tingling in Hands	AliceD/BigStockPhoto.com
Truth	Pancreas Disease	Eraxion/BigStockPhoto.com
Truth	Wound Infections	Olegd/BigStockPhoto.com
Truth	Carpal Tunnel	WebRx/BigStockPhoto.com
Truth	Depression	Gina Sanders/BigStockPhoto.com
Truth	Sleepiness	Zog/BigStockPhoto.com
Truth	Respiratory	Radist/BigStockPhoto.com
Truth	Metabolic	Ishihara Shojiro/BigStockPhoto.com
Truth	Neck Pain	Wavebreak/BigStockPhoto.com
Truth	Vein Problems	HKannn/BigStockPhoto.com
Truth	Heel Spurs	Wavebreak/BigStockPhoto.com
Truth	Atrial Fibrillation	Max Borovkov/BigStockPhoto.com
Truth	Chronic Odor	Hugh Stonelan/BigStockPhoto.com
Truth	Heart Disease	Digitalista/BigStockPhoto.com
Truth	Gastric Reflux	HKannn/BigStockPhoto.com
Truth	Immune System	Spectral Design/BigStockPhoto.com
Truth	Joint Problems	Juriah/BigStockPhoto.com
Truth	Swelling	Marcovarro/BigStockPhoto.com
Truth	Memory Loss	DJ Photo/BigStockPhoto.com
Truth	Pregnancy	Wavebreak/BigStockPhoto.com
Truth	Kidney/Dialysis	Pics Five/BigStockPhoto.com
Truth	Stroke	Digitalista/BigStockPhoto.com
Truth	Surgical	Monkey Biz/BigStockPhoto.com
Truth	Urinary/Bowel	Sinisa Botas/BigStockPhoto.com
Truth	Shop in Market	Gina Sanders/BigStockPhoto.com
Truth	Couple Eating	Monkey Business/BigStockPhoto.com
Truth	At The Movies	NYUL/BigStockPhoto.com
Truth	Couple Dining	East West/BigStockphoto.com
Truth	Man in Office	Dolgachov/BigStockPhoto.com
Truth	Eating Styles	Freeflyer/BigStockPhoto.com
Truth	Discrimination	Ivelin Radkov/BigStockPhoto.com
Truth	Stop & Think	Kikkerdirk/BigStockPhoto.com
Truth	Tomorrow	Vepar5/BigStockPhoto.com
Truth	Time for Healthy	Don Skarpo/BigStockPhoto.com
Truth	Moment of Truth	iQoncept/BigStockPhoto.com
Beliefs	Obesity Factors	Hartman Group
Beliefs	Muscle Maker Chart	Muscle Maker
Beliefs	Trade Up Comps	NuVal
Beliefs	New ABNorman	MakingHealthEasier.com
Beliefs	Choose/Weigh Less	ChooseHealthLA.com
Beliefs	Brain Scans	Oak Ridge National Laboratory
Beliefs	Smash Your Food	Big Food Exhibit/Yale Peabody
Beliefs	Donut Nut Facts	Google
Beliefs	Food Ingredients	Choice.com.au
Beliefs	Sources of Sugar	US Dep't of Agriculture
Beliefs	Raising Hands	Khorzhevska/BigStockPhoto.com
Beliefs	Satiety of Food	Massive Health
Beliefs	Fats	Blog.friendseat.com
Beliefs	Soda/Sugar Comp	fit.WebMD.com
Beliefs	Non GMO Logo	NonGMOProject.org
Beliefs	Childhood Obesity	TheLunchTray.com
Beliefs	Snooze/Lose	SixStepstoSleep.com
Beliefs	#1: Power of Mind	Digitalista/BigStockPhoto.com
Beliefs	#2: Diets Failing	Michael Jung/BigStockPhoto.com
Beliefs	#3: Words	Kheng Guan Toh/BigStockPhoto.com
Beliefs	#4: Why Eat	Joey Gil/BigstockPhoto.com
Beliefs	#5: Numbers	Suen Hoppe/BigStockPhoto.com
Beliefs	#6: Substitution	Gus Photo/BigStockPhoto.com
Beliefs	#7: Slow/Small	Burly/BigStockPhoto.com
Beliefs	#8: Knowledge	IJDema/BigStockPhoto.com
Beliefs	#9: Honesty	Vepar5/BigStockPhoto.com
Beliefs	#9: Sharing	Velin Radkov/BigStockPhoto.com
Beliefs	#10: Proc Foods	L. Iordache/BigStockPhoto.com
Beliefs	#11: Sugar	McFields/BigStockPhoto.com
Beliefs	#12: Exercise	W. Goldswain/BigStockPhoto.com
Beliefs	#13: Insulin/Carbs	Dmitry Lobanov/BigStockPhoto.com
Beliefs	#14: Water	Dolgachov/BigStockPhoto.com
Beliefs	#15: Cheating	Dashek/BigStockPhoto.com
Beliefs	#16: Visualizing	Sergey Nivens/BigStockPhoto.com
Beliefs	#17: Myths	Pixels Away/BigStockphoto.com
Beliefs	#18: Fat	Pixels Away/BigStockPhoto.com
Beliefs	#19: Soda	Scanrail/BigStockPhoto.com
Beliefs	#20: Timing	iQoncept/BigStockPhoto.com
Beliefs	#21: Milestones	Nasir1164/BigStockPhoto.com
Beliefs	#22: GMO	Eltoto69/BigStockPhoto.com
Beliefs	#23: Children	Michael Jung/BigStockPhoto.com
Beliefs	#24: Sleep	Deklo Fenak/BigStockPhoto.com
Beliefs	#25: Calories	iQoncept/BigStockPhoto.com
Beliefs	#26: Forget	ElvinStar/BigStockPhoto.com

Strats	Cooking Oils	BalancedBites on Wikipedia
Strats	King Cartoon	YaYaYoYo/BigStockPhoto.com
Strats	Prince Cartoon	Memo Angeles/BigStockPhoto.com
Strats	Pauper Cartoon	Davi Sales/BigStockPhoto.com
Tactics	Blood Test	John Kwan/BigStockPhoto.com
Tactics	Nutrition Elements	Flynt/BigStockPhoto.com
Reasons	Touching Toes	Forgiss/BigStockPhoto.com
Reasons	Love Handles	Kzenon/BigStockPhoto.com
Reasons	Beer Belly	Forewer/BigStockPhoto.com
Reasons	Steaming Ears	Kelpfish/BigStockPhoto.com
Reasons	Lonely Woman	Gina Sanders/BigStockPhoto.com
Reasons	Woman Jumping	Ari Wasabi/BigStockPhoto.com
Reasons	Double Chin	Nosnibor137/BigStockPhoto.com
Reasons	Tennis Player	Agency BY/BigStockPhoto.com
Reasons	Couple on Beach	Alta Fulla/BigStockPhoto.com
Reasons	Fat Fingers	Bee-Nana/BigStockPhoto.com
Reasons	Woman on Plane	Pressmaster/BigStockPhoto.com
Reasons	Fat Foot	Marco Varro/BigStockPhoto.com
Reasons	Pudgy Face	Cherry Merry/Shutterstock.com
Reasons	Size XXL Tag	Radubalint/BigStockPhoto.com
Reasons	Couple Jogging	Candy Bar/BigStockPhoto.com
Reasons	Fat Legs	Voronin76/BigStockPhoto.com
Reasons	Woman in Jeans	SBorisov/BigStockPhoto.com
Reasons	Couple Dancing	Kurhan/BigStockPhoto.com
Reasons	Holding Head	Wavebreak/BigStockPhoto.com
Reasons	Crossing Legs	Viorel Sima/BigStockPhoto.com
Reasons	Buttoning Pants	Zurljeta/BigStockPhoto.com
Reasons	Thumbs Up	Andres/BigStockPhoto.com
Reasons	Woman's Legs	VKJR/BigStockPhoto.com
Reasons	Rubbing Lower Back	PDB1/BigStockPhoto.com
Reasons	Doctor Scolding	Style Photos/BigStockPhoto.com
Reasons	Father Scolding	V. Lebedev/BigStockPhoto.com
Reasons	Beached Whale	Devon/BigStockPhoto.com
Reasons	Rubbing Knee	Juriah/BigStockPhoto.com
Reasons	Taunting	Auremar/BigStockPhoto.com
Reasons	Tying Shoelaces	Llike/BigStockPhoto.com
Reasons	Thigh Pain	Maridav/BigStockPhoto.com
Reasons	Lifting Weights	Kee Wee Boy/BigStockPhoto.com
Reasons	Cellulite	Kurhan/BigStockPhoto.com
Reasons	Sagging Belly	Gelpi/BigStockPhoto.com
Reasons	Smiling Woman	Gus Photo/BigStockPhoto.com
Reasons	Woman Yoga	Maridav/BigStockPhoto.com
Reasons	Fat Behind	Hannamariah/BigStockPhoto.com
Reasons	Class Reunion	Alex Millos/BigStockPhoto.com
Reasons	Rejection	Dolgachov/BigStockPhoto.com
Reasons	Climbing Ladder	Ifoto com/BigStockPhoto.com
Reasons	Fat Cartoon	YaYaYoYo/BigStockPhoto.com
Reasons	Clothes in Closet	Crystal Photo/BigStockPhoto.com
Reasons	Man and Woman	Conrado/BigStockPhoto.com
Reasons	Depressed Man	Hikcrn/BigStockPhoto.com
Reasons	Family Bicycling	Darren Baker/BigStockPhoto.com
Reasons	Dementia	Lisa FX/BigStockPhoto.com
Reasons	Liver on Man	Decade 3D/BigStockPhoto.com
Reasons	Skiier	Shock/BigStockPhoto.com
Reasons	Nerves	Sergey Nivens/BigStockPhoto.com
Reasons	Sleep Apnea Mask	BVDC/BigStockPhoto.com
Reasons	Man Preg Woman	A. Chiriac/Shutterstock.com
Reasons	Man Pigging Out	Sumners/BigStockPhoto.com
Reasons	Buttoning Pants	Zurljeta/BigStockPhoto.com
Reasons	Oversize Jeans	Wavebreak/BigStockPhoto.com
Reasons	Looking in Mirror	Elnur/BigStockPhoto.com
Reasons	Sports Balls	Jut/BigStockPhoto.com

Reasons	Female Singer	Stokkete/BigStockPhoto.com
Reasons	BP Monitor	Lisa fx/BigStockPhoto.com
Reasons	Sickly Woman	Warren Goldswain/BigStockPhoto.com
Reasons	Rubbing Elbow	Phakimata/BigStockPhoto.com
Reasons	Large Chest	Kletr/Shutterstock.com
Reasons	Heavy Fashion	Ostill/BigStockPhoto.com
Reasons	Sharing Clothes	Hasloo Group/Shutterstock.com
Reasons	Woman in Tight Shirt	Otna Ydur/BigStockPhoto.com
Reasons	Woman in Dress	Yeko Photo/BigStockPhoto.com
Reasons	Man Sweating	Dandaman/BigStockPhoto.com
Reasons	Happy Woman	Ariwasabi/BigStockPhoto.com
Reasons	Man Carry Woman	Pictrough/BigStockPhoe.com
Reasons	Happy Woman	Dirima/BigStockPhoto.com
Reasons	Relaxed Fit Jeans	Taigi/Shutterstock.com
Reasons	Woman on Scale	Michael Jung/BigStockPhoto.com
Reasons	Chores List	R. Mackay/BigStockPhoto.com
Reasons	Dad and Son	Monkey Business/BigStockPhoto.com
Reasons	BMI Collage	Karen Roach/BigStockPhoto.com
Reasons	Girl Taunted	Monkey Business/BigStockPhoto.com
Reasons	Woman Jumping	Andres/BigStockPhoto.com
Reasons	Woman in Bikini	Wavebreak/BigStockPhoto.com
Reasons	Pills Collage	Coprid/BigStockPhoto.com
Reasons	Tape Around Money	LHW/BigStockPhoto.com
Reasons	Food Happy Plate	L. Iordache/BigStockPhoto.com
Reasons	In Control Scale	Alex Millos/BigStockPhoto.com
Reasons	Person/Water/Sun	Sangoiri/BigStockPhoto.com
Reasons	Woman	Andres/BigStockPhoto.com
Reasons	Eating Strawberry	Sol.Ru/BigStockPhoto.com
Reasons	Friends	Dolgachov/BigStockPhoto.com
Reasons	Mom Holding Baby	Monkey Biz/BigStockPhoto.com
Reasons	Fit Into Clothes	Andres/BigStockPhoto.com
Reasons	Sleeping	Wavebreak/BigStockPhoto.com
Reasons	Grocery Receipt	Flippo/BigStockPhoto.com
Reasons	Back Pain	StylePhotos/BigStockPhoto.com
Reasons	Oversized Jeans	Gajus/BigStockPhoto.com
Reasons	Trendy Clothing	M. Goldbehear/BigStockPhoto.com
Reasons	Cancer Ribbon Tree	Trish/BigStockPhoto.com
Reasons	Glucose Meter	Zothen/BigStockPhoto.com
Reasons	Money and Pills	Yastremska/BigStockPhoto.com
Reasons	Woman Hold Heart	G. Sanders/BigStockPhoto.com
Reasons	Couple Make Love	G. Sanders/BigStockPhoto.com
Reasons	Holding Hands	Szefei/BigStockPhoto.com
Reasons	Couple Arms Spread	S. Ana/BigStockPhoto.com
Reasons	4 Person Family	Monkey Biz/BigStockPhoto.com
Reasons	6 Person Family	Andy Dean/BigStockPhoto.com
Reasons	6 Person Family	Monkey Biz/BigStockPhoto.com
Sugar	Sugar in Spoon	C. Tan Teck Hean/Shutterstock.com
Sugar	Soda Cans	Scanrall/BigStockPhoto.com
Sugar	Energy Drinks	Scanrall/BigStockPhoto.com
Sugar	Ice Cream	SVRY/BigStockPhoto.com
Sugar	Chocolate Cake	Kesuo1/BigStockPhoto.com
Sugar	Chocolate Milk	Elena The Wise/BigStockPhoto.com
Sugar	Fruit Pie	Bhofack22/BigStockPhoto.com
Sugar	Blueberry Muffin	Oysy/BigStockPhoto.com
Sugar	Candy Bar	Givaga/BigStockPhoto.com
Sugar	Cereal	Kmitu/BigStockPhoto.com
Sugar	Energy Bar	Devon/BigStockPhoto.com
Sugar	PB&J Sandwich	Dragon Child/BigStockPhoto.com
Sugar	Chocolate Shake	Chris Elwell/BigStockPhoto.com
Sugar	Devil Donut	Julien Tromeur/Shutterstock.com
Sugar	Bad Guys	YaYaYoYo/BigStockPhoto.com
Marriage	Blackboard	Almoond/BigStockPhoto.com

Sugar	Beware	Real Callahan/BigStockPhoto.com
Motivators	Beer	Kesuoi/BigStockPhoto.com
Motivators	Cigarettes	M. Mainka/BigStockPhotl.com
Motivators	Snorting Drugs	Natulrich/BigStockPhoto.com
Motivators	Sugar	Shock/BigStockPhoto.com
Motivators	Sugar Packets	NYC Anti-Soda Ad Campaign
Motivators	Pouring on Pounds?	NYC Anti-Soda Ad Campaign
Motivators	Skull & Crossbones	Jazzia/BigStockPhoto.com
Motivators	Popcorn	G. Tuledo/BigStockPhoto.com
Motivators	Salad Ingredients	TGI Fridays
Motivators	Fat Family	Nosnibor/BigStockPhoto.com
Motivators	Chub Rub	Shutterstock.com
Motivators	Nutrition Label	EatSmartMoveMoreNC.com
Motivators	Serving Size	EatSmartMoveMoreNC.com
Motivators	Cheeseburger	Puercoespan/BigStockPhoto.com
Motivators	Grilled Chicken	GBH007/BigStockPhoto.com
Motivators	Broccoli	Nito/BigStockPhoto.com
Motivators	Banana	Mazzzur/BigStockPhoto.com
Motivators	Yogurt	Sideways/BigStockPhoto.com
Motivators	Strawberries	Mr. Smith/BigStockPhoto.com
Motivators	Blueberries	Maksheb/BigStockPhoto.com
Motivators	Home Sweet Home	Elnur/BigStockPhoto.com
Motivators	Go Green	iFong/BigStockPhoto.com
Motivators	Salad Power	R. Mackenzie/BigStockPhoto.com
Motivators	Mmmm Mmmm Good	Schmeljov/BigStockPhoto.com
Motivators	Go Nuts	Margo555/BigStockPhoto.com
Motivators	Spice	O6Photo/BigStockPhoto.com
Motivators	How Sweet It Is	Elnur/BigStockPhoto.com
Nut Label	Nutrition Labels	FDA.gov